NurseAdviser

Taking Your
Medications
Safely

Springhouse Corporation
Springhouse, PA

Staff

Senior Publisher
Matthew Cahill

Art Director
John Hubbard

Senior Editor
H. Nancy Holmes

Editors
Virginia Alpaugh, Jane V. Cray, Anthony Prete, Elizabeth Blizard Whitman

Copy Editors
Cynthia C. Breuninger (manager), Lynette High, Kathy Marino, Doris Weinstock

Designers
Stephanie Peters (associate art director), Matie Patterson (assistant art director)

Illustrators
John Gist, Robert Jackson

Cover
SuperStock

Typography
Diane Paluba (manager), Elizabeth Bergman, Joyce Rossi Biletz, Phyllis Marron, Valerie Rosenberger

Manufacturing
Deborah Meiris (director), Pat Dorshaw (manager), T.A. Landis

Production Coordination
Margaret A. Rastiello

Editorial Assistants
Beverly Lane, Mary Madden

TYMS-020396

A member of the Reed Elsevier plc group

Library of Congress Cataloging-in-Publication Data
Taking your medications safely.
   p. cm.
Includes index.
1. Drugs — Popular works. 2. Drugs — Side effects. 3. Drug interactions. I. Springhouse Corporation.
RM301.15. T35   1996
615".1 — dc20   956698
ISBN 0-87434-824-2   CIP

Contents

ADMINISTRATION TECHNIQUES

CHECKING PULSE AND BLOOD PRESSURE

MEDICATIONS

Nurses are perhaps the most common source of information about medications. In a hospital, nurses are the ones who actually give the medications that doctors prescribe — and talk to patients about them. They're specially trained for this task. And because they give medications to millions of people each year, they've heard just about every question a person may have.

Now, the world's largest publisher for nurses has put together the advice, directions, and tips of its expert NurseAdviser team for you. In your hands, you have the first book that anticipates your questions and gives you accurate, easy-to-understand answers from trusted health professionals — a book that looks out for you.

That's important. After all, directions and warnings about medications generate many questions — whether you're a person who takes one medication a day or several. *Do I take this pill 1 hour before meals, or was that the other pill? Which side effects are dangerous? Can I have my usual cocktail? What about the dose I forgot to take?*

Avoid danger

When it comes to medications, not having the answers can be dangerous. If you stop taking your antibiotic the minute you start feeling better, you invite your infection to rebound. If you don't take the right dose of your antihypertensive drug on schedule, your high blood pressure could lead to a stroke. If you pass off stomach pains as mere indigestion, you risk not recognizing this dangerous ulcer symptom caused by some pain medications.

An equally serious — and all too common — problem stems from taking two drugs that react badly with each other. Taking Advil for a headache while you're taking a blood thinner such as Coumadin can cause internal bleeding. If you're an insulin-dependent diabetic, you'd better avoid Deltasone, which neutralizes insulin. If you take large doses of aspirin for arthritis and add Benadryl to fight a cold, beware; Benadryl hides an aspirin overdose. Experts say that drug reactions like these account for hundreds of thousands of avoidable hospitalizations (even deaths) annually.

Become informed

Clearly, by becoming informed about the medications you take, you act as your own best friend. Sticking to your medication schedule and overall treatment plan can help you recover faster, reduce drug side effects, and even avoid side effects entirely. It can help keep you out of the doctor's office and out of the hospital. And that can help reduce your health care costs.

Taking Your Medications Safely covers just about all of the common and important prescription and over-the-counter drugs and tells how you can best take them to prevent problems. For each of the drugs, you'll learn answers to the following questions:

— Why is this drug used? What forms are available?

— What's the recommended way to take the drug?

— What should you do if you miss a dose?

— What side effects may occur? And what can you do?

— Which dangerous symptoms need your doctor's immediate attention?

— When must you eliminate alcohol? Other drugs?

— What do you especially need to know if you're pregnant, breast-feeding, an athlete, or an older adult?

Besides this core information, you'll find illustrated, step-by-step directions for taking tablets and capsules, using inhalers, applying ointments, and putting drops in your eyes, ears, or nose. You'll even learn the correct way to do pulse and blood pressure checks, a safety measure for certain drugs.

Get answers to your questions

Have you ever left your doctor's office, then thought of a question that didn't come to mind before? Or tried to remember an important point about a new medication?

Question no more. *Taking Your Medications Safely* helps you steer clear of the dangers of drug therapy and get the most benefit from your medication. It's the one drug guide you'll turn to time and again.

Mark E. Rosenthal, MD
Director of Cardiac Electrophysiology
Abington (Pa.) Memorial Hospital
Clinical Assistant Professor of Medicine
University of Pennsylvania School of Medicine
Philadelphia

Administration Techniques

To get the most benefit from the medication your doctor has prescribed, it's important that you take it properly. This section of *Taking Your Medications Safely* shows you — step by step — how to best follow your doctor's instructions. It helps you use the right techniques for taking any type of drug.

The section begins with reminders about filling your prescription and taking and storing your medication as well as advice for staying on schedule. It proceeds to illustrated guidelines for taking, using, or giving every form of medication your doctor may prescribe: from simple tablets, capsules, and liquid medications to ointments, suppositories, bath products, aerosols, and injections.

Also included are special tips on how to adapt your techniques to give medications successfully to a child.

Taking your medication correctly

To benefit from the medication your doctor has prescribed, you must take it and store it correctly. Here's how.

Filling your prescription
• Have your prescription filled at the pharmacy you ordinarily use. That way, the pharmacist can keep a complete record of all your medications. Make sure the record includes a notation on which medications you're allergic to.
• Refill your prescription before you run out of medication. Don't wait until the last minute.

Taking your medication
• Double-check the label under a bright light to make sure you're taking the right medication. If you don't understand the directions, call your pharmacist or doctor.
• If you forget to take a dose or several doses, don't try to "catch up" by taking two or more doses together. Instead, consult your pharmacist or doctor.
• Don't stop taking your medication unless your doctor tells you to. And don't save it for another time.

Storing your medication
• Keep your medication in its original container or in a properly labeled prescription bottle. If you're taking more than one medication, don't store them together in a pillbox. For convenience, however, you may count them out into daily, weekly, or even monthly containers. (See the entry "Taking medications on schedule.")
• Store your medication in a cool, dry place or as directed by your pharmacist. Avoid the bathroom medicine cabinet where heat and humidity may cause it to lose its effectiveness.
• If you have young children in the house, make sure your medication containers have childproof caps. Keep the containers out of children's reach.

Avoiding problems
• Use index cards or a chart to record the following information about each medication you take: its name, its purpose, its appearance, how to take it, when to take it, how much to take, and any special precautions or side effects connected with it.

• If you have any questions about any symptoms you experience while taking your medication, call your doctor.

• If you're pregnant or breast-feeding, talk to your doctor before taking any medication or home remedy. Some medications can harm the baby.

• Never take a medication that doesn't look right or that has passed its expiration date. It may not work. Worse, it may harm you.

• Don't take nonprescription medications along with your prescription medications until you have first checked the combination with your pharmacist. Sometimes a nonprescription product can change the way your prescribed medication works.

• Alcoholic beverages and some foods can also change the way some medications work. Read the label on your prescription. It may tell you what to avoid.

• Don't share your medication with family or friends. It could hurt them.

Taking medications on schedule

Taking the right amount of medication at the right time is a crucial part of your treatment. But many people have trouble getting this important task down to a routine. The following tips may help.

Premeasure your medication Your pharmacy sells several kinds of plastic "medication planners." One type separates your tablets or capsules into individual doses and is helpful if you take your medication more than once a day. Compartments with flip-top lids indicate the time of day — for example, breakfast, lunch, supper, and bedtime, as shown below.

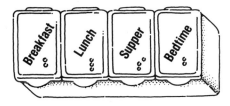

Another type of planner compartmentalizes and stores your medications for an entire week. The illustrations that follow show two versions of this type.

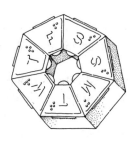
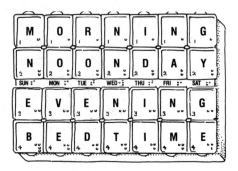

A third type is designed to hold your entire prescription, bottle and all. Computerized numbers on top of the lid show the last time (hour and day) you opened the medication bottle, as shown below.

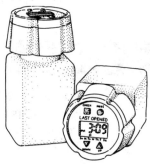

If you prefer, you can make your own medication planner. Here's how: Place a single medication dose in a small envelope, and write on the envelope what time you need to take that dose. Do this for each dose you need to take during the day.

Then put all the small envelopes into a larger one and label the larger one with the day of the week. Do this for each day of the week. Arrange the envelopes chronologically in an empty shoe box.

Make a medication clock

To remind you to take your medication at the right time, make a simple device called a medication clock. Using our sample clocks (opposite) as guidelines, make two large clock faces. (If you have access to a Xerox machine that enlarges, you can simply enlarge one of the samples to the size of a kitchen clock and then make a copy of it so you'll have two.)

Write A.M. in the center of one clockface and P.M. in the center of the other. Then write the names of your medications in the spaces for the hours when you're supposed to take them. Use one color ink for the A.M. clock and a different color ink for the P.M. clock so you can tell them apart easily. Check the clock often during the day so you don't miss any doses.

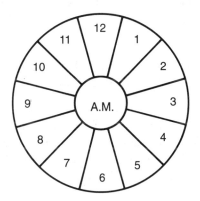 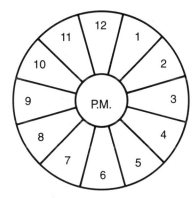

Check the calendar   Another way to keep track of your medications is on a calendar. Dedicate a new calendar—one with plenty of space for daily notes—just for this purpose. In each daily space, write down the names of your medications and the times you're supposed to take them. You can fill in your schedule for a few days at a time or for the whole month. Draw a line through your notation after you take each medication. This method lets you see at a glance what you've taken.

Set an alarm or   If you're still having trouble, set your wristwatch or
ask a friend   alarm clock to ring at medication time. Or ask a relative, friend, or coworker to remind you to take your medication until you know your schedule.

Taking tablets, capsules, and liquid medications

Whether your medication comes in a solid form (tablets, capsules) or in a liquid form (syrup, elixir, emulsion, suspension), make sure you take it correctly. Here are some guidelines.

Taking tablets and capsules
First, wash your hands. Then gather everything you need, such as the medication, a glass of water or juice and, if you plan to crush a tablet, a mortar and pestle or a commercial pill crusher. If you need to divide a scored tablet, get a knife. Now follow these steps:

1 Look at the medication container to make sure you have the right medication and the right dose.

2 Pour the prescribed number of tablets or capsules into the bottle cap. If you accidentally pour out too many, tap the extra tablets or capsules back into the container without touching them (to avoid contamination). Now pour the medication from the cap into your hand.

3 Place the tablets or capsules as far back on your tongue as you can. You may do this with one tablet or capsule at a time or with all of them at once.

4 Tip your head slightly *forward*, take a drink of water or juice, and swallow.

Special tips
• Take coated tablets and capsules with plenty of water or juice.
• If you have trouble swallowing a tablet or capsule, moisten your mouth with some water or juice first. If that doesn't do the trick, you can crush an uncoated tablet, open a soft capsule, or split a tablet.
• *Never* crush tablets or open capsules that have a special coating. Doing so may alter the medication's effectiveness by changing the way your body absorbs it. If you're in doubt, ask your doctor or pharmacist whether it's safe for you to crush or open your medication.
• Protect tablets and capsules from light, humidity, and air. If your medication changes color or has an unusual odor, discard it. Also discard all outdated medications.

Taking liquid medication First, wash your hands. Then get the medication bottle and a medicine cup or measuring spoon. Look at the container to make sure you have the right medication and are about to take the prescribed dose. If the medication is in a suspension, shake it vigorously before proceeding with the following steps:

1 Uncap the bottle and place the cap upside down on a clean surface.

2 Locate the marking for the prescribed dose on your medicine cup. Keeping your thumbnail on the mark, hold the cup at eye level and pour in the correct amount of medication. If you're using a measuring spoon, pour the correct dose into the spoon. Place the bottle safely on a flat surface; then swallow the medication.

3 Wipe the bottle's lip with a damp paper towel, taking care not to touch the inside of the bottle. Replace the bottle cap.

4 Rinse the medicine cup or spoon and store your medication properly.

Special tips • When pouring liquid medication, keep the label next to your palm. This way, if any liquid spills or drips, it won't deface the label.
• If you pour out too much liquid, discard the excess. Don't return it to the bottle.
• If a liquid medication has an unpleasant taste, ask your doctor or pharmacist about diluting it with water or juice. You can also try sucking on ice first to numb your taste buds or, if the dose is large enough, pouring the medication over ice and then drinking it through a straw. You may want to chill an oily liquid before taking it.
• To relieve any bitter taste left in your mouth after swallowing the medication, suck on a piece of sugarless hard candy or chew gum. Gargling or rinsing your mouth with water or mouthwash may also help.

Taking precautions • Keep all medications out of the reach of children.
• Don't hesitate to ask your doctor or pharmacist about medications and directions you don't understand.
• Never share your medication with anyone else.

Giving children medication by mouth

Giving medication to a child doesn't have to be a problem — for you or the child — if you go about it with patience and care.

Take a positive approach

• Use a matter-of-fact but friendly manner to put the child at ease. Act as though you expect cooperation, and give praise when the child cooperates.

• Offer older children choices, if possible, to give them a sense of control. For example, let them decide which beverage to take with (or after) their medication. (Exclude from their options anything the doctor has advised you against; some medications cannot be taken with certain beverages or foods.)

• Taste a liquid medication (just a drop) before giving it to a child. This gives you an idea of how the medication will taste and helps you decide whether to improve the medication's taste by mixing it with a small amount of syrup or food, if appropriate. (Of course, don't taste a medication if you think you may be sensitive to it.)

• Explain to older children how the treatment relates to the illness. They may be more cooperative if they realize that the medication will help them get better.

• Double-check the basics: Are you giving the right medication and dose to the right child at the right time?

• Place a tablet or capsule near the back of the child's tongue, and give plenty of water or flavored drink to help ease swallowing. Then make sure the child swallows it.

• Encourage the child to tip his or her head forward when swallowing a tablet or capsule. Throwing the head back increases the risk of inhaling the medication and choking.

• Give an infant medication as though you were feeding it to him or her—for example, through a bottle's nipple to take advantage of the natural sucking reflex. Don't mix the medication with formula, though, unless the doctor has advised it because if the formula isn't finished, the infant won't get a full dose of medication.

• Observe a child closely to see if the medication has the intended effect or is causing side effects.

Be honest and careful

- Never try to trick children into taking medication; they may resist and distrust you the next time.
- Don't tell children that medication is candy. If they like the taste, they may try to take more than the prescribed dose; if they don't, they may distrust you the next time you tell them something.
- Don't promise that the medication will taste good if you've never tasted it or if you know it won't.
- Never threaten, insult, or embarrass a child if he or she doesn't cooperate. These actions can lead to further resistance.
- Keep medication out of children's reach to avoid accidents.
- Don't force children to swallow the medication or try to hold their nose or mouth shut to promote swallowing. This may cause choking.
- Don't try to give medication to a crying child; he or she could choke on it.

Using an oral metered-dose inhaler

Inhaling your medication through a metered-dose inhaler (also called a nebulizer) will help you breathe more easily. Use the nebulizer exactly as demonstrated here, and follow your doctor's instructions for when to use it and how much medication to take.

Getting ready

1 Remove the mouthpiece and cap from the bottle. Then remove the cap from the mouthpiece.

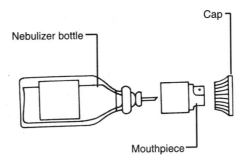

Cap

Nebulizer bottle

Mouthpiece

2 Turn the mouthpiece sideways. On one side of the flattened tip is a small hole. Fit the metal stem of the bottle into the hole to assemble the nebulizer.

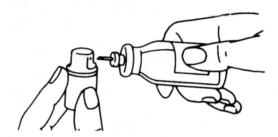

Using the inhaler **1** Exhale fully through pursed lips. Hold the inhaler upside down, as shown below. Close your lips and teeth loosely around the mouthpiece.

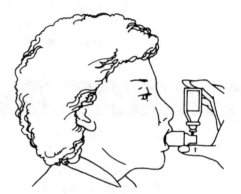

2 Tilt your head back slightly. Take a slow, deep breath. As you do this, firmly push the bottle against the mouthpiece — one time only — to release one dose of medication. Continue inhaling until your lungs feel full.

To make sure you're taking the correct amount of medication, be careful to take only one inhalation at a time.

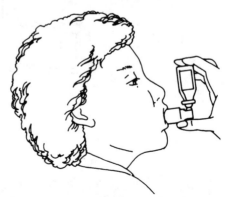

3 Remove the mouthpiece from your mouth, and hold your breath for several seconds.

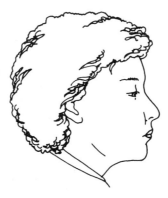

4 Purse your lips and exhale slowly. If your doctor wants you to take more than one dose, wait a few minutes and then repeat steps 1 through 3. Now rinse your mouth, gargle, and drink a few sips of fluid.

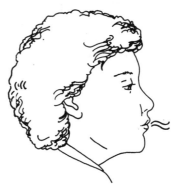

Taking precautions

• Remember to discard the inhalation solution if it turns brown or contains solid particles. Store your medication in its original container and put it in the refrigerator, if that's what the label directs.

• Remember to clean the inhaler once a day by taking it apart and rinsing the mouthpiece and cap under warm running water for 1 minute (or immersing them in alcohol). Shake off the excess fluid, let the parts dry, and then reassemble them. This prevents clogging and sanitizes the mouthpiece.

• *Never overuse your oral inhaler.* Follow your doctor's instructions exactly.

Using an oral inhaler with a holding chamber

Your doctor has prescribed an oral inhaler to help open your breathing passages. In this treatment, you'll inhale a medication called a *bronchodilator* through a small device that you put in your mouth. A holding chamber attached to the inhaler helps the medication reach deeply into your lungs.

Common inhalation devices include the InspirEase System and the Aerochamber System.

InspirEase System This system has a holding chamber that collapses when you breathe in and inflates when you breathe out. To operate this inhaler, follow these steps:

1 Insert the inhaler into the mouthpiece and shake the inhaler. Then place the mouthpiece into the opening of the holding chamber, and twist the mouthpiece to lock it in place.

2 Extend the holding chamber, breathe out, and place the mouthpiece in your mouth.

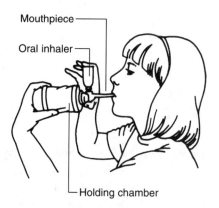

Mouthpiece

Oral inhaler

Holding chamber

3 Firmly press down once on the inhaler. Then breathe in slowly and deeply so that the bag collapses completely. If you breathe incorrectly, the bag will whistle. Hold your breath for 5 to 10 seconds; then breathe out slowly into the bag. Repeat breathing in and out.

4 Wait 5 minutes. Then shake the inhaler again and repeat the dose, following steps 2 and 3.

Aerochamber System

This system uses a small cylinder called a *valved chamber* to trap medication. It may also include a mask that helps deliver the medication more easily. Follow these steps for use:

1 Remove the cap from the inhaler and from the mouthpiece of the Aerochamber. Then insert the mouthpiece into the wider rubber-sealed end of the Aerochamber. Inspect for foreign objects, and check that all parts are secure.

2 Shake the device three or four times.

3 Breathe out normally, and close your lips over the mouthpiece.

If your device has a mask, place the mask firmly over your nose and mouth.

With either device, aim for a good seal. Leaks will reduce effectiveness.

4 Spray *only one puff* from the inhaler into the Aerochamber. Take in one full breath slowly and deeply. If you hear a whistling sound, you're breathing too fast. Now hold your breath for 5 to 10 seconds.

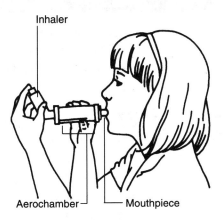

Inhaler

Aerochamber — Mouthpiece

If your device has a mask, hold it firmly in place, as shown at the top of the next page, and breathe in at least six times.

Caution: Spraying more than one puff into the Aerochamber will give you the wrong dose of medication.

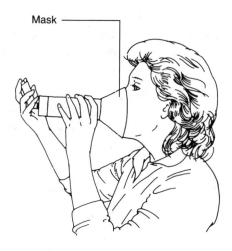

Mask

5 Repeat the steps as directed by your doctor.

6 Remove the inhaler. Follow the manufacturer's directions for cleaning and storing the mouthpiece. Rinse any remaining medication from your face.

Using an AeroVent inhaler

An AeroVent inhaler holds medication supplied by a metered-dose inhaler and delivers the medication through a ventilator breathing circuit. Following are some guidelines for using the device.

Connecting the AeroVent to the circuit

1 Remove the AeroVent from its box. The device will join the ventilator circuit between the ventilator tubing and the Y-connector that leads to you.

2 Now collapse the AeroVent holding chamber gently by compressing the device as you would an accordion. Push and rotate the springlike chamber slightly until the ends come together. Then press the bracketlike clasp down until it clicks into place.

3 Connect one end of the holding chamber to the Y-connector and the other end to the ventilator tubing.
Caution: Don't use too much force. If you do, you could damage the device or make it difficult to remove.

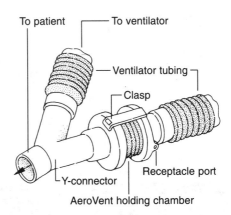

To patient — To ventilator
Ventilator tubing
Clasp
Receptacle port
Y-connector
AeroVent holding chamber

Make sure that the receptacle port (which will hold the inhaler) faces upward and away from you.

Opening the circuit

1 Before giving medication through the AeroVent, you'll need to expand the device. To begin, unlatch the external clasp and swing it open (180 degrees).

2 Grasp the connected ends of the holding chamber. Then lightly rotate and stretch the device to the open position. Be careful not to damage the AeroVent by bending or rocking it.

3 Reposition the receptacle, if needed, because it may be displaced when the chamber expands. To give medication correctly, you must make sure that the nozzle of the inhaler canister points directly down and that the receptacle port points up to receive the inhaler.

Taking the medication

1 Shake the inhaler canister and insert its nozzle into the AeroVent receptacle port. Don't press on the inhaler yet.

2 When a ventilator exhalation ends, activate the inhaler by pressing on the canister's base as many times as the doctor has instructed you to. Don't press with too much force; you could jam the nozzle and damage the equipment.

After several uses, you may notice cloudiness in the chamber. Don't be alarmed. This results from collected moisture and medication particles.

Taking precautions

• Once you've taken the medication, remove the inhaler canister and collapse the AeroVent by gently pushing the ends together. Use a slight rotating motion until you compress the device securely. Now relatch the external clasp.

• Observe safety precautions at all times. For example, replace a damaged AeroVent at once, and attach a new AeroVent when you change the tubing.

Giving yourself eyedrops

Your doctor has prescribed eyedrops for you. Here's how to put them in your eye.

Getting ready

1 Begin by washing your hands thoroughly.

2 Hold the medication bottle up to the light and examine it. If the medication is discolored or contains sediment, don't use it. Take it back to the pharmacy and have it checked.

If the medication looks okay, warm it to room temperature by holding the bottle between your hands for 2 minutes.

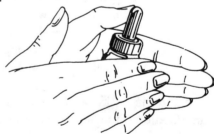

3 Moisten a cosmetic puff or a tissue with water, and clean any secretions from around your eyes. Use a fresh puff or tissue for each eye. Be sure to wipe outward in one motion, starting from the area nearest your nose.

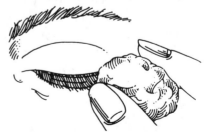

4 Stand or sit before a mirror or lie on your back, whichever is most comfortable for you. Squeeze the bulb of the eyedropper and slowly release it to fill the dropper with medication.

Using the eyedrops   **1** Tilt your head back slightly and toward the eye you're treating. Pull down your lower eyelid to expose the conjunctival sac.

2 Position the dropper over the conjunctival sac, and steady your hand by resting two fingers against your cheek or nose.

3 Look up at the ceiling, and then squeeze the prescribed number of drops into the sac. Take care not to touch the dropper to your eye, eyelashes, or fingers. Wipe away excess medication with a clean tissue.

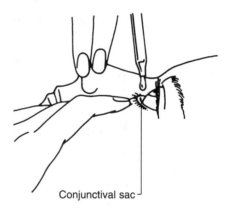

Conjunctival sac

4 Release the lower lid and gently close your eye. Try not to blink for at least 30 seconds. Apply gentle pressure to the corner of your eye nearest your nose for 1 minute. This will prevent the medication from being absorbed through your tear ducts.

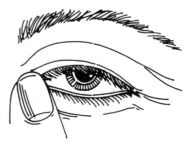

5 Repeat the procedure in the other eye if the doctor has instructed you to do so.

6 Recap the bottle and store it away from light and heat.

Taking precautions
• If you're using more than one kind of drop, wait 5 minutes before giving yourself the next one.
• *Call your doctor immediately if you have any unusual side effects,* such as blisters on your eyelids, red and peeling skin, or extremely swollen, itchy, or burning eyelids.
• Never put medication in your eyes unless the label reads "For Ophthalmic Use" or "For Use in Eyes."

Putting ointment in your eye

Your doctor has prescribed eye ointment for you. Here's how to apply it.

Getting ready
1 Wash your hands thoroughly; then hold the ointment tube in your hand for several minutes to warm up the medication.

2 Moisten a cosmetic puff or a tissue with water, and clean any secretions from around your eye. Wipe outward in one motion, starting at the corner of the eye near the nose. Remember to avoid touching the uninfected eye.

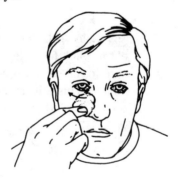

Using the ointment
1 Gently pull down your lower eyelid to expose the conjunctival sac, and look up toward the ceiling. Squeeze a small amount of ointment (about ¼ to ½ inch

[½ to 1 centimeter]) into the conjunctival sac. Steady your hand by resting two fingers against your cheek or nose, as shown below. Hold the tube close to its tip to avoid accidentally poking the tip into your eye.

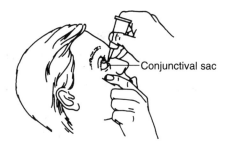

Conjunctival sac

2 Without touching the tube's tip with your eyelashes, close your eye to pinch off the ointment. With your eyes still closed, roll your eyeball in all directions. After a minute or two, open your eyes again.

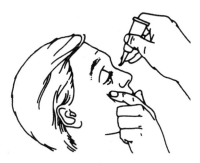

3 Recap the medication tube. If you're using more than one ointment, wait about 10 minutes before you use the next one. It's normal for your vision to be blurred temporarily after you use the ointment.

Giving yourself eardrops

Your doctor has prescribed eardrops. Use them exactly as the label directs you to. Here are some guidelines.

Getting ready　　**1** Wash your hands thoroughly and then check your medication. If it's discolored or contains sediment, notify your doctor and have your prescription refilled. If your eardrops are okay, proceed.

2 For comfort, warm the eardrops by holding the bottle in your hands for 2 minutes. Then shake the bottle, if that's what the directions say, and open it.

3 Fill the dropper by squeezing the bulb; then place the open bottle and dropper within easy reach.

Using the eardrops **1** Lie on your side with your "bad ear" up.

2 To straighten your ear canal, gently pull the top of your ear up and back, as shown.

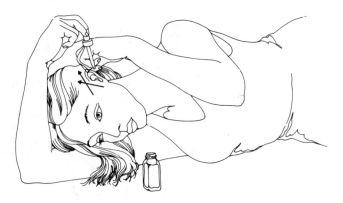

3 Position the dropper above your ear, taking care not to touch it to your ear. Squeeze the dropper's bulb to release 1 drop.

4 Wait until you feel the drop in your ear. Then, if directed, release another drop. Repeat these steps until you have given yourself the prescribed number of drops. To keep the drops from running out of your ear, remain on your side for about 10 minutes.

5 If you wish, you can plug your ear with a piece of cotton moistened with eardrops. Unless your doctor directs you to, don't use dry cotton. It will absorb your medication.

6 Treat your other ear, if necessary, following the same procedure.

7 Recap the eardrop bottle, and store it away from light and extreme heat.

Giving eardrops to a child

To treat your child's ear problem, use the prescribed eardrops exactly as directed on the label.

Getting ready   **1** First, wash your hands thoroughly. Then examine the medication. Does it look discolored or contain sediment? If it does, notify the doctor and have the prescription refilled. If it looks normal, you can proceed.

2 For your child's comfort, warm the medication by holding the bottle in your hands for about 2 minutes.

3 Shake the bottle (if directed), open it, and fill the dropper by squeezing the bulb. Place the open bottle and dropper within easy reach.

Giving the eardrops   **1** Have your child lie on his or her side with the "bad ear" up. Now gently pull the earlobe down and back to straighten the ear canal.

2 Position the filled dropper above—but not touching—the opening of the canal. Gently squeeze the dropper's bulb once to release one drop.

Watch the drop slide into the ear canal or have your child tell you when he or she feels the drop enter the ear.

Then gently squeeze the bulb again to release the rest of the drops prescribed.

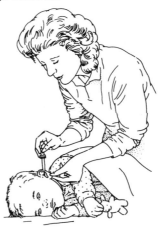

3 Continue holding your child's ear as the eardrops disappear down the canal. Now massage the area in front of the ear. Ask your child to tell you when he or she no longer feels the drops moving around; then release the ear.

4 Tell your child to remain on his or her side and to avoid touching the ear for about 10 minutes. If your child is active, place an eardrop-moistened cotton plug in the ear to help keep the medication in the ear canal. Don't use dry cotton because it may absorb the medication.

If both ears require medication, repeat the procedure in the child's other ear.

5 Finally, return the dropper to the medication bottle (or recap the dropper bottle). Store the bottle away from light and extreme heat.

Using a metered-dose nasal pump

A metered-dose nasal pump delivers an exact amount of medication. Here's how to use it.

Getting ready   **1** Remove the protective cap and prime the pump as directed by the manufacturer. (Usually, pressing down about four times primes the pump. If it's refrigerated, the pump will stay primed for about 1 week. After that, you'll need to prime it again.)

2 To get the right dose, tilt the pump bottle so that the strawlike tube inside draws medication from the deepest part, as shown below.

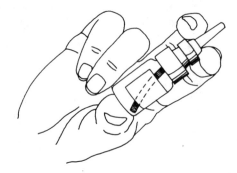

Using the pump   **1** Insert the pump's applicator tip about half an inch into your nostril. Point the tip straight up your nose and toward the inner corner of your eye. (Don't angle the pump or the medication may run into your throat.)

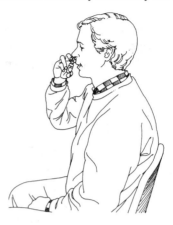

2 Without inhaling, squeeze the pump once, quickly and firmly. Try to use just enough force to coat the inside of your nostril, but not so much that you inject the medication into your sinuses. (That will cause a headache.) Spray again if the package directions instruct you to, or repeat the procedure in the other nostril if your doctor directs you to do so.

3 Keep your head still for several minutes so the medication has time to work. And don't blow your nose for a while.

4 Store the medication in the refrigerator.

Giving yourself nose drops

Here is what you need to know about using nose drops.

Getting ready   **1** Look at the container to make sure you have the right medication and that you know how much to take.

2 Warm the medication container by holding it in your hands for about 2 minutes.

3 With the dropper still in the bottle, squeeze the bulb to load the dropper chamber with medication.

The method you use to instill the drops will vary, depending on the problem you're treating.

Treating the nasal passages

1 If your doctor has prescribed nose drops to treat your nasal passages, lie on your back and position the dropper as shown below. This will help the drops flow down the back of your nose, not your throat.

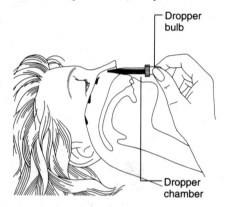

Dropper bulb

Dropper chamber

2 Squeeze the dropper bulb to release the correct number of drops.

3 Repeat the process in the other nostril, if indicated.

4 Breathe through your mouth so that you don't sniff the drops into your sinuses or lungs.

Treating the ethmoid and sphenoid sinuses

1 To treat a problem in these areas, lie on your back with a pillow under your shoulders and your head tilted backward, as shown below.

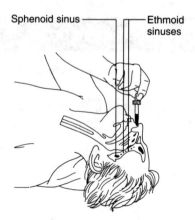

Sphenoid sinus

Ethmoid sinuses

2 Position the dropper above one nostril, and squeeze the bulb to release the prescribed number of drops.

3 Breathe through your nose. This will help the medication move through your sinuses.

Treating the frontal and maxillary sinuses

1 To treat a problem in these areas, lie on your back with a pillow under your shoulders and your head tilted to one side, as shown below.

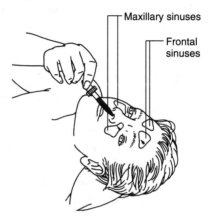

Maxillary sinuses

Frontal sinuses

2 Position the dropper above one nostril, and squeeze the bulb to release the prescribed number of drops.

3 Breathe through your nose. This will help the medication move through your sinuses.

Taking precautions

• Follow your doctor's orders exactly. Don't overuse your nose drops.

• Because nose drops are easily contaminated, don't buy more than you'll use in a short time. Discard discolored nose drops and drops that contain sediment.

• Don't share your nose drops with anyone. Doing so may spread germs.

Using medicated bath products

Your doctor may prescribe a medicated bath to help treat your skin problem. A medicated bath can do the following:
• clean, soften, and lubricate your skin
• relieve itching
• soften scales and crusts (for easier removal).

Preparing the bath
Before you begin, make sure your bathroom is warm and draft-free and that the bathtub is clean.

Adding the medication
The method will vary depending on the product your doctor has prescribed.

If you're using a colloidal preparation such as oatmeal, mix 1 measuring cup of oatmeal with a small amount of cool water to form a paste. Then begin filling the tub with warm water. Gradually swirl in the paste as the tub fills.

If you're using an oil preparation such as mineral oil (with a surfactant), fill the bathtub two-thirds full with warm water. Then add 2 ounces of the oil preparation and stir the water to distribute the oil.

Or you may find it more effective to mix ¼ teaspoon of bath oil with ¼ cup of water and apply it directly to your skin as you would a lotion.

If you're using a soda preparation such as baking soda, first fill the bathtub to the correct level with warm water. Then add the powder, stirring until it dissolves.

If you're using a starch preparation such as cornstarch, fill the bathtub to the appropriate level with warm water. While the tub is filling, slowly dissolve the powder in a small container of water. Then, when the water reaches the prescribed level, pour in the starch solution.

Bathing and drying off
Before immersing yourself in the bathwater, make sure the temperature feels warm enough. Then get in the tub carefully and soak for about 20 minutes.

When you've finished soaking, step out carefully; the slippery tub surface can be dangerous. Pat yourself dry with a clean, soft towel, removing excess medication in the process.

Keep in mind that a skin problem can cause you to lose body heat rapidly, so try not to become chilled. Once you're warm and dry, clean the tub so that it's ready for your next bath.

Inserting a rectal suppository

You can learn to insert a suppository quickly and easily. Be cautious, though. Only use rectal suppositories or other laxatives under your doctor's orders; routine use can lead to dependence.

If the doctor has directed you to use a rectal suppository, just follow these simple steps.

Getting ready **1** Wash your hands. Then gather the items you'll need: the suppository, a disposable glove, and a tube of water-soluble lubricating gel.

2 Put the glove on your right hand (or on your left if you're left-handed). Then remove the foil wrapper on the suppository.

If you have trouble doing this, the suppository may be too soft to insert. Hold it under cold running water until it becomes firm or put it in the freezer for a minute or two before inserting it — just don't let it get too cold and hard. (It's best to store your suppositories in the refrigerator.)

Inserting the **1** Once you've removed the foil wrapper, put a gener-
suppository ous dab of lubricating gel on the rounded end of the suppository. Hold the lubricated suppository in your gloved hand.

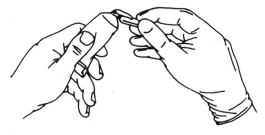

2 Lie on your side with your knees raised toward your chest. Take a deep breath as you gently insert the suppository — rounded end first — into the anus with your gloved hand. Push the suppository in as far as your finger will go to keep the suppository from coming back out.

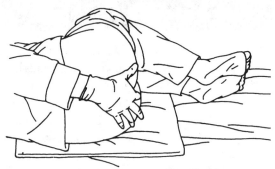

3 Once the suppository is in place, you'll feel an immediate urge to have a bowel movement. Resist the urge by lying still and breathing deeply a few times.

Try to retain the suppository for at least 20 minutes so your body has time to absorb it and get the maximum effect from the medication. After you have a bowel movement, discard the glove and wash your hands.

Inserting a vaginal medication

Plan to insert a vaginal medication after bathing and just before bedtime to ensure that it will stay in the vagina for the appropriate amount of time. Follow these instructions.

Getting ready **1** Collect the equipment you'll need: the prescribed medication (suppository, cream, ointment, tablet, or jelly), an applicator, water-soluble lubricating jelly, a towel, a hand mirror, paper towels, and a sanitary pad.

2 Empty your bladder, wash your hands, and place the towel on the bed. Sit on the towel, and open the medication wrapper or container.

3 Using the hand mirror, carefully inspect the area around the insertion site. If you see signs of increased irritation, don't insert the medication. Notify the doctor, who may want to change your medication.

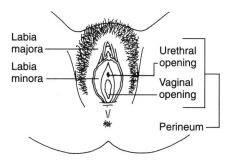

Labia
majora
Labia
minora
Urethral
opening
Vaginal
opening
Perineum

Inserting the medication

1 Place a vaginal suppository or tablet in the applicator or fill it with cream, ointment, or jelly according to package or label directions.

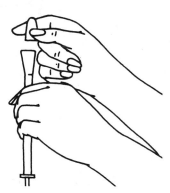

2 To make insertion easier, lubricate the suppository or applicator tip with water or water-soluble lubricating jelly.

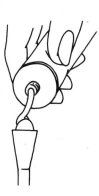

3 Now lie down on the bed with your knees flexed and legs spread apart.

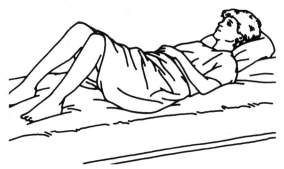

4 Use one hand to spread apart the outer vaginal opening and the other to insert the applicator tip into the vagina. Advance the applicator about 2 inches (5 centimeters), angling it slightly toward your tailbone.

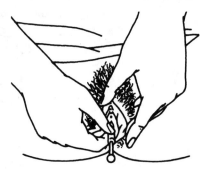

5 Push the plunger to insert the medication. It may feel cold.

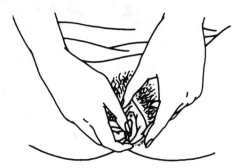

6 Remove the applicator, and discard it if it's disposable. If it's reusable, wash it thoroughly with soap and water, dry it with a paper towel, and return it to its container.

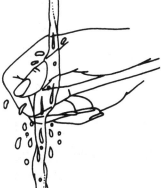

7 If your doctor prescribes it, apply a thin layer of cream, ointment, or jelly to the vulva (the area around the opening of the vagina).

8 Remain lying down for about 30 minutes so the medication won't run out of your vagina. If you like, apply the sanitary pad to avoid staining your clothes or bed linens.

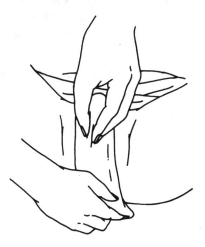

9 Then remove the pad and check your vagina for signs of an allergic reaction. If the area seems unusually red or swollen, contact your doctor.

Giving yourself a subcutaneous injection

A subcutaneous injection inserts medication into the tissue directly below your skin so that it can be absorbed quickly into your bloodstream. The needle does not penetrate deeply, and the injection is easy to administer. Before you can administer your injection, you must transfer the correct amount of medication from the bottle to the syringe. Follow these guidelines.

Getting ready

1 Wash your hands. Then assemble this equipment in a clean area: a sterile syringe and needle, the medication, and alcohol pads (or rubbing alcohol and cotton balls).

2 Check the label on the medication bottle to make sure you have the right medication. As an extra precaution, check the expiration date as well.

3 Clean the top of the medication bottle with an alcohol pad.

4 Select an appropriate injection site. Pull the skin taut; then, using a circular motion, clean the skin with another alcohol pad or with a cotton ball soaked in alcohol.

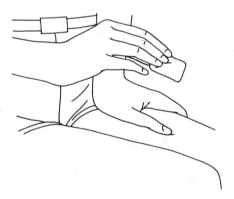

5 Remove the needle cover. *To prevent possible infection, don't touch the needle;* touch only the barrel and plunger of the syringe. Pull back the plunger to the prescribed amount of medication. This draws air into the syringe.

Insert the needle into the rubber stopper on the medication bottle, and push in the plunger. This pushes air into the bottle and prevents a vacuum.

6 Hold the bottle and syringe together in one hand; then turn them upside down so the bottle is on top. You can hold the bottle between your thumb and forefinger and the syringe between your ring finger and little finger, against your palm. Or you can hold the bottle between your forefinger and middle finger, while holding the syringe between your thumb and little finger, as shown below.

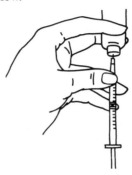

7 Pull back on the plunger with your other hand until the top black portion of the barrel aligns with the mark that indicates you have withdrawn the correct amount of medication. Then remove the needle from the bottle.

8 If air bubbles appear in the syringe after you fill it with medication, tap the syringe and push lightly on the plunger to remove them. Draw up more medication if necessary.

Injecting the medication
1 Using your thumb and forefinger, pinch the skin at the injection site. Then quickly plunge the needle (up to its hub) into and below the skin at a 90-degree angle. Push the plunger down to inject the medication.

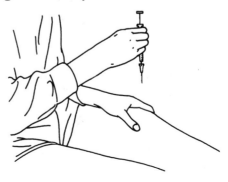

2 Place an alcohol pad over the injection site and press down on it lightly as you withdraw the needle. Don't rub the injection site while you're withdrawing the needle.

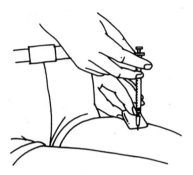

3 Snap the needle off the syringe and properly dispose of both.

Using an anaphylaxis kit

If you're severely allergic to insect stings or to certain foods or drugs, your doctor will prescribe an anaphylaxis kit for you to keep on hand for emergencies. The kit contains everything you need to treat an allergic reaction, including:

• a prefilled syringe containing two doses of epinephrine (a drug that helps open your airways)
• alcohol pads
• a tourniquet
• antihistamine tablets.

When an allergic emergency occurs, use the kit as follows; then call your doctor immediately or ask someone else to call him.

Getting ready **1** Take the prefilled syringe from the kit and remove the needle cap.

2 Hold the syringe with the needle pointing up. Then push in the plunger until it stops, as shown at the top of the next page. This will expel any air from the syringe.

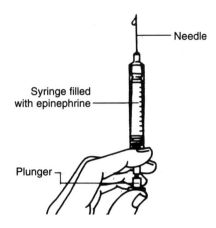

Needle

Syringe filled with epinephrine

Plunger

3 Clean about 4 inches (10 centimeters) of the skin on your arm or thigh with an alcohol pad. (If you're right-handed, you should clean your left arm or thigh. If you're left-handed, clean your right arm or thigh.)

Injecting the
epinephrine **1** Rotate the plunger one-quarter turn to the right so that it's aligned with the slot.

2 Insert the entire needle — like a dart — into the skin.

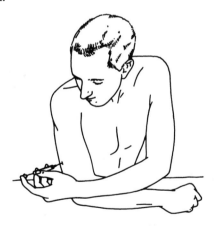

3 Push down on the plunger until it stops. It will inject 0.3 ml of epinephrine, a dose designed for an adult or a person over age 12. Withdraw the needle.

Note: The dose and procedures for babies and for children under age 12 must be directed by the doctor.

Removing the stinger

If you've been stung by an insect, quickly remove the insect's stinger if you can see it. Use your fingernails or tweezers to pull it straight out. Don't pinch, scrape, or squeeze the stinger; this may push it farther into the skin and release more poison.

If you can't remove the stinger quickly, stop trying and go on to the next step.

Applying the tourniquet to the sting

1 If you were stung on your *neck, face,* or *body,* skip this step and go on to the next one.

2 If you were stung on an *arm* or a *leg,* apply the tourniquet between the sting site and your heart. Tighten the tourniquet by pulling the string.

3 After 10 minutes, release the tourniquet by pulling on the metal ring.

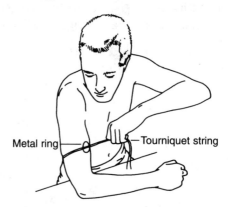

Metal ring — Tourniquet string

Applying ice to the sting

Apply ice packs — if available — to the area of the insect sting.

Taking the antihistamine tablets

For all types of allergic reaction, if your doctor has advised you to take antihistamine tablets, *chew and swallow* the tablets now. (For children age 12 and under, follow the dosage and administration directions supplied by your doctor or provided in the kit.)

What to do next

Important: If you don't notice an improvement within 10 minutes, give yourself a second injection by following the directions in your kit. If your syringe has a preset second dose, don't depress the plunger until you're ready to give the second injection. Proceed as before, following the instructions for injecting the epinephrine.

Avoid exertion, keep warm, and get to a doctor or a hospital immediately.

Taking precautions
• Keep your kit handy so you're always ready for an emergency.

• Ask your pharmacist for storage guidelines. Can the kit be stored in a car's glove compartment or do you need to keep it in a cooler place?

• Periodically check the epinephrine in the preloaded syringe. A pinkish brown solution needs to be replaced.

• Make a note of the kit's expiration date, and renew the kit just before that date occurs.

• When the crisis is over, dispose of the used needle and syringe safely and properly.

Giving an intramuscular injection

To give yourself or someone else an intramuscular injection, you need the right training from your doctor or a nurse. Follow their directions exactly. The guidelines below will act as a review for you until the process becomes routine.

Selecting the site
First choose the injection site. You can use the thigh, hip, buttock, or upper arm. If you're giving yourself the injection, use the front or side of the thigh. If you're giving someone else the injection, you can use the hip, buttock, or upper arm. If possible, though, you should avoid using the upper arm because the muscle there is small and very close to the brachial nerve.

If a series of injections is necessary, rotate the sites. To reduce pain and improve drug absorption, don't use the same site twice in a row.

Thigh
To find the target, place one hand at your knee and the other at your groin. As shown at the top of the next page, use the area marked by solid lines for adult injections and

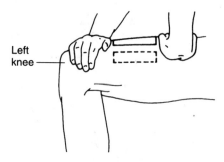

the area marked by dotted lines for injections for infants and children.

Hip   To find this site, place your right hand on the person's left hip (or your left hand on the person's right hip). Then spread your index and middle fingers to form a V. Your middle finger should be on the highest point of the pelvis, known as the iliac crest. The triangular area shown in the illustration below is the injection site.

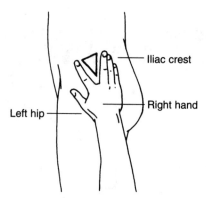

Buttock   Imagine lines dividing each buttock into four equal parts. Give the injection in the upper outermost area near the iliac crest, as shown below. Don't give it in the sciatic nerve area.

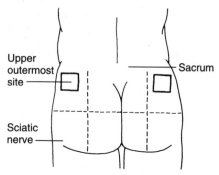

Upper arm   Locate the injection site by placing one hand at the top of the person's shoulder and extending your thumb down the person's upper arm. Place the other hand at armpit level, as shown below. The triangular space shown between the hands is the injection area.

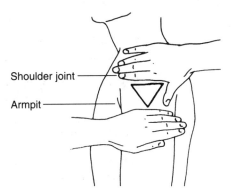

Shoulder joint

Armpit

Getting ready   **1** Wash your hands and gather the medication, alcohol pads, syringe, and needle. Make sure you have the right medication. As an extra precaution, check the expiration date.

2 Remove the top of the medication bottle, and wipe the rubber stopper with an alcohol pad. Unwrap the syringe and remove the needle cover.

3 Pull back on the plunger of the syringe until you've drawn air into it in an amount equal to the medication you'll be injecting. Insert the needle into the bottle through the rubber stopper. Then inject the air in the syringe into the bottle without withdrawing the needle. This will prevent formation of a vacuum and will make withdrawing the medication easier.

4 Invert the medication bottle. With the needle positioned below the fluid level, draw the medication into the syringe by pulling back on the plunger while you measure the correct amount by checking the markings on the side of the syringe. Then withdraw the needle from the bottle.

5 Check for air bubbles in the syringe. If you see any, hold the syringe with the needle pointing up, and tap the syringe lightly so that the bubbles rise to its top. Then push the plunger to get rid of the air and, if necessary, draw up more medication to obtain the correct amount.

Again hold the syringe with the needle pointing up, and pull back on the plunger just a little bit more. This will cause a tiny air bubble to form inside the syringe; when you inject the medication, this bubble will help clear the needle and keep the medication from seeping out of the injection site. Replace the needle cover.

6 Check the injection site for any lumps, depressions, redness, warmth, or bruising on the skin. Then gently tap the site to stimulate nerve endings and reduce the initial pain of injection.

7 Clean the site with an alcohol pad, beginning at the center and wiping outward in a circular pattern (as shown below) to move dirt particles away from the site.

Let the skin dry for 5 to 10 seconds. If it's not dry, the injection might push some of the alcohol into the skin, causing a burning sensation.

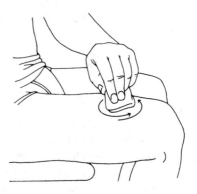

Injecting the medication

1 Remove the needle cover. Then, with one hand, stretch the skin taut around the injection site, as shown at the top of the next page. This makes inserting the needle easier and helps disperse the medication after the injection.

With your other hand, hold the syringe and needle at a 90-degree angle to the injection site. Then insert the needle with a quick thrust.

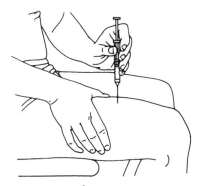

2 Holding the syringe firmly in place, remove the hand stretching your skin and use it to pull back slightly on the plunger.

If blood appears in the syringe, you've entered a blood vessel. Take the needle out and press an alcohol pad over the site. Then discard everything and start again.

If no blood appears, inject the medication slowly, keeping the syringe and needle at a 90-degree angle. Never push the plunger forcefully.

3 When you've injected all the medication, press an alcohol pad around the needle and injection site, and withdraw the needle at the same angle at which you inserted it.

Using a circular motion (extending from the center outward), massage the site with the alcohol pad to help distribute the medication and promote its absorption.

4 Dispose of the used syringe and needle by returning the cover to the needle. Then, holding the syringe, unscrew or snap off the needle and cover. Put both in a covered container used only for disposal of needles and syringes. Keep the container in a safe place until you can dispose of it; then dispose of it properly.

Giving injections through an implanted port

Giving yourself injections through an implanted port is not difficult but it does require close attention to procedure and careful maintenance to prevent infection. Here are some guidelines that may help.

Getting ready

1 Gather together the equipment you'll need: an extension set with a special needle (called a Huber needle), a clamp, a 10-milliliter syringe filled with saline solution, a syringe containing the prescribed medication, a sterile needle filled with heparin flush solution, a povidone-iodine pad, and two alcohol pads.

2 Wash and dry your hands. Attach the 10-milliliter syringe filled with saline solution to the end of the extension set. Gently push on the plunger of the syringe until the extension tubing and needle are filled with the solution and all of the air is removed. Make sure all the air is removed by flicking the tubing of the extension set.

3 Locate the port by feeling for the small bump on your skin. (The site is over a bony area, usually on the upper chest.) Hold the port between two fingers, and clean the site with an alcohol pad. Allow the site to air-dry; then wipe it with a povidone-iodine pad.

Injecting the medication

1 Again, hold the site between two fingers, as shown below.

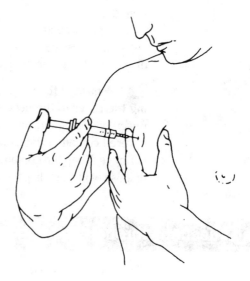

Insert the Huber needle through the skin and port septum until it hits the bottom of the port's chamber. Make sure the needle is inserted at a 90-degree angle, as shown below.

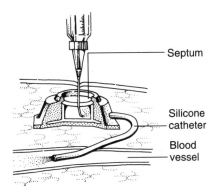

Septum

Silicone catheter

Blood vessel

2 Check for a blood return by pulling back on the syringe that's attached to the extension set. The appearance of blood tells you that the needle is in the proper position in the port and that the port's catheter hasn't slipped out of place inside you.

3 Flush the port with 5 milliliters of the saline solution by pushing down halfway on the plunger of the syringe containing the saline solution.

4 Clamp the extension set and remove the saline-filled syringe.

5 Connect the medication-filled syringe to the extension set. Open the clamp and inject the medication, as ordered by your doctor.

6 Check the skin around the needle for swelling and tenderness. If you notice either of these signs, stop the injection and call your doctor.

7 When the injection is complete, clamp the extension set and remove the medication syringe.

8 Attach the saline-filled syringe to the extension set. Then open the clamp and flush the port again with the remaining 5 milliliters of saline solution by pushing down on the plunger of the syringe. Remember to flush the port before and after each injection; this minimizes medication interactions. Clamp the extension set and remove the syringe. Put a protective cap on the end of the extension set.

9 Tape the needle in place and apply a gauze dressing.

Taking precautions
• To keep your implanted port trouble-free, flush it according to your doctor's instructions (usually monthly).
• Check with the doctor if you develop a fever or if you observe redness, pain, swelling, or pus at the port site.

Checking Pulse and Blood Pressure

When the doctor prescribes a drug, particularly one for your heart, you may need to check your pulse rate or blood pressure before taking a drug dose. If you're giving medication to someone else, you may need to check that person's pulse or blood pressure.

Depending on the results, you may go ahead and take — or give — the drug. Or you may need to contact the doctor for a change in the dosage.

This section of *Taking Your Medications Safely* shows you the right way of taking the pulse rate and blood pressure.

Taking your pulse

Your pulse rate tells you the number of times your heart beats in a minute. If you have heart or blood pressure problems, your doctor may want you to check your pulse rate on a regular basis.

Getting ready   You'll need to find a quiet time — not after you've just finished exercising or eating a big meal. You'll also need a watch or a clock with a second hand.

Taking the pulse   **1** Begin by sitting down and relaxing for 2 minutes.

2 Place your index and middle fingers on your wrist, as shown here.

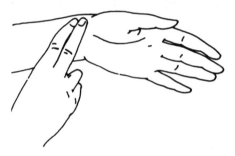

3 Count the pulse beats for 30 seconds and multiply by 2. (Or count for 60 seconds, but do not multiply. Your doctor may instruct you to use the 60-second method if you have an irregular heart rhythm.)

4 Record this number and the date.

Taking your own blood pressure

To take your own blood pressure, your best resource is a digital blood pressure monitor. (You can also use a standard blood pressure cuff and stethoscope, but you'll probably need help from someone else to do so.)

Before you begin, review the instruction booklet that comes with the blood pressure monitor. Steps vary with different monitors, so follow the directions carefully.

Start by taking your blood pressure in both arms. Readings can differ by as much as 10 points from arm to arm. If the readings stay similar consistently, the doctor will probably suggest that you use the arm with the higher reading. Here are some guidelines.

Getting ready **1** Sit down and relax for 2 minutes. Rest your arm on a table, level with your heart. (Use the same arm in the same position each time you take your blood pressure.)

2 Wrap the cuff securely around your upper arm, above the elbow. Make sure that you can slide only two fingers between the cuff and your arm. Turn on the monitor.

Taking the pressure **1** Inflate the cuff as the instructions direct. When the digital scale reads 160, stop inflating. The numbers will start changing rapidly. When they stop changing, your blood pressure reading will appear on the scale.

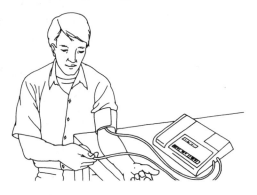

2 Record this reading, the date, and the time. Then deflate and remove the cuff, and turn off the machine.

Taking another person's blood pressure

You can use a standard blood pressure cuff and stethoscope to take the blood pressure of the person in your care. If you're using an aneroid model, you may need to have it adjusted every 6 months. Follow these steps.

Getting ready **1** Ask the person to sit comfortably and relax for about 2 minutes. Tell him to rest his arm on a table so it's level with his heart. (Use the same arm in the same position each time you take his blood pressure.)

2 Push up the person's sleeve, and wrap the cuff around his upper arm (just above the elbow) so you can slide only two fingers between the cuff and his arm.

Taking the pressure

1 Using your middle and index fingers, feel for a pulse in the person's wrist.

When you find this pulse, turn the bulb's screw counterclockwise to close it; then squeeze the bulb rapidly to inflate the cuff. Note the reading on the gauge when you can no longer feel the pulse. (This reading, called the palpatory pressure, is your guideline for inflating the cuff.)

Now deflate the cuff by turning the screw clockwise.

2 Place the stethoscope's earpieces in your ears. Then place the stethoscope's disk over the pulse in the crook of the person's arm, as shown below.

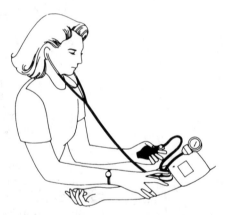

3 Inflate the cuff 30 points higher than the palpatory pressure. Then loosen the bulb's screw to allow air to escape from the cuff. When you hear the first beating sound, record the number on the gauge: This is the systolic pressure (the top number of a blood pressure reading).

4 Slowly continue to deflate the cuff. When you hear the beating stop, note and record the number on the gauge: This is the *diastolic* pressure (the bottom number of a blood pressure reading).

5 Deflate and remove the cuff. Record the blood pressure reading, the date, and the time.

Medications

This section of *Taking Your Medications Safely* describes the drugs most commonly prescribed for home use and offers directions and tips on taking them. These drugs are listed alphabetically by brand name and the information about each one is organized under several easy-to-spot headings.

An introductory paragraph explains what the drug is used for and gives its generic name. The generic name, which is sometimes called the drug's public name, usually describes the drug's chemical structure. For instance, one of the most widely used generic drugs is acetaminophen. While many people don't recognize this name, just about everyone recognizes one of its brand names. In fact, dozens of different pharmaceutical companies manufacture this drug, which is sold under the brand names Tylenol, Panadol, Anacin-3, Genapap, and others. When you buy any of these brand names, you are buying the same drug.

Following the generic name are simple instructions on how to take or administer the medication, what to do if you miss a dose, and how to manage any side effects. Next, you'll learn the danger of combining this drug with certain other drugs, alcohol, or foods and the special directions you must follow when using this drug (such as what other medical conditions you should report to your doctor).

A final paragraph gives important reminders for pregnant and breast-feeding women, athletes, older people, and others who may be particularly affected by the medication.

A

Accutane

Accutane helps treat acne. The generic name for this drug is isotretinoin.

How to take Accutane

Take Accutane capsules exactly as prescribed, either with a meal or shortly afterward.

What to do if you miss a dose

Take the missed dose as soon as you can. But if it's almost time for your next dose, skip the missed dose and take the next one at the scheduled time. Don't take a double dose.

What to do about side effects

Call your doctor if you develop headache, nausea, vomiting, or vision problems. Also call if your eyes burn, itch, or get red.

Dry, itchy skin should go away after you've taken Accutane for a while as should pain, soreness, or stiffness in your muscles, bones, or joints. If these symptoms persist, check with your doctor.

When you start taking Accutane, you may find that your acne worsens temporarily. If it becomes severe, check with your doctor.

Relieve mouth dryness with sugarless hard candy or gum, ice chips, mouthwash, or a saliva substitute. If the dryness continues for more than 2 weeks, check with your doctor or dentist for further measures.

If the medication interferes with your night vision, avoid driving and other potentially dangerous activities. Notify your doctor.

Accutane leaves your skin extra sensitive to light, so when you first start taking it, limit your sun exposure.

What you must know about alcohol and other drugs

Limit your intake of alcoholic beverages when taking Accutane because alcohol can increase the triglyceride (fat) level in your blood.

Preparations that tend to dry your skin — medicated soaps, acne preparations that contain skin-peeling agents, and alcohol-based products (cosmetics, after-shave, cologne) — can increase the skin-drying and irritation caused by Accutane. Vitamin A and tetracycline antibiotics can also increase these side effects, so check with your doctor before taking them.

Special directions
• Before taking Accutane, tell your doctor about any other medical problems you have. Some conditions might affect your use of the medication.

• Don't donate blood for at least 30 days after you stop taking Accutane.

Important reminders
Don't take this drug if you're pregnant or think you may be, and don't take it if you're breast-feeding.

Children are especially prone to side effects.

If you have diabetes, be aware that Accutane can alter your blood sugar level. If you notice any change, tell your doctor.

Achromycin

Achromycin helps treat infection. The drug's generic name is tetracycline.

How to take Achromycin
Take it 1 hour before meals or 2 hours after them, because food can decrease your body's ability to absorb the drug. Don't take it with milk or other dairy products. To help prevent stomach irritation, drink a full glass of water with each dose.

What to do if you miss a dose
Take the missed dose as soon as possible. But if it's almost time for your next dose, adjust your schedule as follows:

If you're taking one dose a day, you can make up a missed dose the following day provided you leave a 12-hour space between dosages. (For example, take your regularly scheduled dose at 7 a.m. and a makeup dose at 7 p.m.)

If you're taking two doses a day, space the missed dose and the next dose 5 to 6 hours apart.

If you're taking three or more doses a day, space the missed dose and the next dose 2 to 4 hours apart.

Once you have taken the missed dose, resume your regular dosing schedule.

What to do about side effects

Call your doctor if you develop a sore throat, diarrhea, reddened skin, a rash, or hives — or if you notice skin changes after being in the sun.

Also tell your doctor if you have trouble swallowing, or if you have indigestion, loss of appetite, or nausea. You should also report any vaginal infection.

Because Achromycin may make your skin more sensitive to sunlight, limit your exposure to the sun.

What you must know about other drugs

Because of possible absorption problems, don't take Achromycin with antacids (such as Maalox), iron preparations (such as multivitamins containing iron), or sodium bicarbonate (such as Alka-Seltzer).

Achromycin may keep birth control pills from working properly. To be safe, use another method of birth control while you're taking Achromycin.

If you have diabetes, let your doctor know about it before beginning a course of Achromycin. The drug could make your diabetes worse. The doctor should also be advised if you have liver or kidney disease, which may leave you at greater risk of developing side effects from Achromycin.

Important reminder

If you're pregnant, don't take Achromycin. It could stain your baby's teeth or cause other problems.

Achromycin drops or ointment

This drug comes as eyedrops or eye ointment for treating eye infections. It's an *ophthalmic* (eye) form of the generic drug tetracycline.

How to use Achromycin drops

First wash your hands. If you're using a suspension, shake the bottle well. Then tilt your head back, and pull your lower eyelid away from your eye to form a pouch below your eye. Without touching your eye with the applicator, squeeze the prescribed number of drops into the pouch. Then gently close your eye and don't blink. Keep your eye closed for 1 to 2 minutes to give the medication time to saturate the eye area.

How to use Achromycin ointment

Wash your hands. Pull your lower eyelid away from your eye to form a pouch. Without touching your eye with the applicator, squeeze a thin strip of ointment, about ⅓ inch (1 centimeter) long, into the pouch. Gently close your eye. Keep your eye closed for 1 to 2 minutes to give the medication time to saturate the eye area. Wipe the tip of the ointment tube with a clean tissue. Keep the tube tightly closed.

After you finish using the medication, wash your hands again. Use all of the medication as prescribed by your doctor, even if your eye seems better after a few days.

What to do if you miss a dose

Give yourself the missed dose as soon as possible. However, if it's almost time for your next dose, skip the missed dose and give yourself the next dose at the regularly scheduled time.

What to do about side effects

Achromycin may cause your vision to blur for a few minutes after you apply it. However, this is to be expected.

You shouldn't develop any bothersome side effects while using this medication. But if any unusual symptoms occur, tell your doctor.

Special directions

• Because Achromycin may make certain medical problems worse, tell the doctor if you have any type of kidney problem. Also tell the doctor if you've ever had an allergic reaction to tetracycline.
• While you're using the medication, your skin may be more sensitive to sunlight, so limit your exposure to the sun.
• If your symptoms don't go away after a few days or if they become worse, call your doctor.

Important reminders

Don't use Achromycin if you're pregnant. Also, don't give it to children younger than age 8; it could stunt their growth or stain their teeth.

Actifed

Actifed contains a decongestant (the generic name is pseudoephedrine) and an antihistamine (the generic name is triprolidine). It's used to relieve a stuffy nose caused by colds or hay fever.

How to take Actifed

Actifed comes in tablets, capsules, extended-release capsules, and a syrup. Follow your doctor's directions exactly. If you bought the medication without a prescription, read the package instructions carefully before using it. If the medication irritates your stomach, take it with food or a full glass (8 ounces) of milk or water.

You should swallow the extended-release capsules whole. If they're too big to swallow easily, mix the contents of a capsule with applesauce and swallow without chewing.

If Actifed gives you trouble sleeping, take your last dose a few hours before bedtime.

What to do if you miss a dose

Take the missed dose as soon as possible. But if it's almost time for your next dose, skip the missed dose and take your next dose on schedule. Don't take a double dose.

What to do about side effects

Check with your doctor if this medication makes you feel anxious, nervous, or restless — or if it causes palpitations or sleeping problems.

The antihistamine in Actifed may make you feel drowsy, dizzy, or less alert than normal. Tell your doctor if these symptoms continue or become bothersome.

What you must know about alcohol and other drugs

Avoid alcoholic beverages while taking Actifed because the combination may cause drowsiness. For the same reason, avoid medications that slow down the central nervous system, such as sleeping pills, tranquilizers, and other medications for colds, flu, and allergies.

Check with your doctor or pharmacist before you take any other medications, especially those for appetite control, high blood pressure, stomach cramps, and depression. Actifed may affect the way other drugs work, or they may affect the way Actifed works.

Special directions
• Tell your doctor if you have other medical problems, especially asthma, diabetes, an enlarged prostate, glaucoma, high blood pressure, an overactive thyroid, or heart or blood vessel disease. These problems may affect how and if you use Actifed.
• Because Actifed can make you drowsy, make sure you know how you react to it before you drive or perform other activities that require you to be alert.

Important reminders
If you're pregnant, check with your doctor before using this medication. Don't use it if you're breast-feeding.

Children and older adults may be especially prone to side effects.

If you're an athlete, you should know that the U.S. Olympic Committee tests for pseudoephedrine, one of Actifed's ingredients. Athletes may be disqualified if amounts of this drug in their urine exceed certain limits.

Adalat

Usually, doctors prescribe Adalat to treat angina (chest pain). The drug can also be prescribed to treat Raynaud's disease, a condition in which the blood supply to the fingers or toes sporadically diminishes. This drug's generic name is nifedipine. Another brand name is Procardia.

How to take Adalat
This medication comes in capsules and sustained-release tablets. Check the prescription label carefully and take only the prescribed amount.

Take Adalat exactly as your doctor has directed. Swallow capsules whole; don't break, crush, or chew them.

What to do if you miss a dose
Take the missed dose as soon as you remember it. But if it's almost time for your next dose, skip the missed dose and resume your regular schedule. Don't take a double dose.

What to do about side effects
Call your doctor if you have any of these symptoms: ankle swelling, a very fast or very slow heartbeat, shortness of breath, a severe headache, or fainting.

If swelling occurs, the doctor may want you to drink less fluid and limit your salt intake.

Chest pain may occur when you first start taking Adalat. Although such pain is usually temporary, report it to the doctor *immediately*.

Constipation, dizziness, flushing, headache, and nausea can also occur. These side effects usually go away over time as your body adjusts to the medication. Check with your doctor if they persist or become bothersome.

If constipation occurs, drink more fluids and add more bulk to your diet. If the problem persists, consult your doctor about taking a bulk laxative.

Because Adalat can make you dizzy or light-headed, avoid potentially hazardous activities, such as driving a car, while taking it.

To help prevent dizziness, get up slowly from a sitting or lying position.

What you must know about other drugs

Check with your doctor before taking other drugs, including nonprescription medications. Heart failure or very low blood pressure may occur if you take Adalat with another angina medication or with drugs used to treat blood pressure or heart rhythm problems.

Special directions

• Make sure your doctor knows about your medical history, especially if you've had heart failure or constriction of the aorta.

• Call your doctor if the medication doesn't relieve your chest pain.

• Schedule your activities so you can get enough rest.

• Don't stop taking this medication suddenly, even if you feel better. The doctor may need to reduce your dosage by degrees.

Important reminders

If you're pregnant, check with your doctor before taking this medication.

If you're an older adult, you may be especially prone to side effects from Adalat.

Adapin

Your doctor has prescribed Adapin to help relieve your depression. The generic name for this drug is doxepin. Another brand name is Sinequan.

How to take Adapin This medication is available in capsules or as an oral solution. Follow your doctor's instructions exactly. Don't take more than you have been directed to take, and don't take the drug more often or longer than prescribed. Take Adapin with food, even for a daily bedtime dose, unless your doctor has told you to take it on an empty stomach.

If you're using the *oral* solution, use the dropper provided to measure the dose accurately. Just before you take each dose, dilute it in about 4 ounces of water, milk, or juice. Don't use grape juice or carbonated beverages because these liquids may decrease the drug's effectiveness.

Don't stop taking Adapin suddenly; check with your doctor first.

What to do if you miss a dose If you miss a dose, adjust your schedule as follows:

If you take one dose a day at bedtime, check with your doctor about what to do. Don't take the missed dose in the morning because it may cause disturbing side effects during waking hours.

If you take more than one dose a day, take the missed dose as soon as possible. But if it's almost time for your next dose, skip the missed dose and take your next dose on schedule. Don't take a double dose.

What to do about side effects Check with your doctor if Adapin makes you feel drowsy, dizzy, or faint, especially when you get up suddenly from a sitting or lying position. Also call if you experience blurred vision, dry mouth, a fast pulse rate, constipation, difficulty urinating, or unusual sweating.

Because drowsiness and dizziness are potential side effects of this drug, avoid activities that require you to be fully alert — driving, for example — until you are sure you know how it affects you.

What you must know about alcohol and other drugs

Don't drink alcoholic beverages while taking Adapin unless your doctor okays it. Adapin may increase the depressant effect of alcohol.

Your medication may not work well if you take it with barbiturates (found in some sleeping pills and seizure medications).

Taking Adapin with the ulcer drug Tagamet (cimetidine) may cause unwanted side effects.

While you're taking Adapin, your doctor may recommend that you avoid certain medications used to treat psychological disorders.

Special directions

• Tell your doctor if you have other medical problems, especially heart disease.

• Before you have medical tests, tell the doctor you're taking Adapin; the drug may affect some test results.

Important reminders

If you're pregnant or breast-feeding, check with your doctor before taking Adapin.

If you have diabetes, be aware that Adapin can affect your blood sugar levels. If you notice a change in the results of your blood sugar tests, call your doctor.

Advil

Advil relieves mild to moderate pain and reduces fever. Its generic name is ibuprofen. Another brand name is Motrin.

How to take Advil

Advil comes in tablets, caplets, and an oral liquid. Dosages up to 200-mg strength are available over the counter; stronger dosages must be prescribed by a doctor.

If your doctor has prescribed Advil, follow his instructions for taking it. If you purchased it over the counter, follow the package instructions.

Advil is generally taken with food or an antacid to reduce stomach upset. However, your doctor may instruct you to take the first few doses either 30 minutes before or 2 hours after meals to speed its effect on your system.

When taking the tablet or caplet form, drink a full glass (8 ounces) of water. To prevent irritation that may cause trouble swallowing, avoid lying down for 15 to 30 minutes after taking the medication.

What to do if you miss a dose
Take the missed dose as soon as you remember it. But if it's almost time for your next dose, skip the missed dose and take the next one at the regular time.

What to do about side effects
If your throat feels like it's closing and you have trouble breathing, get emergency medical care *immediately.*

Advil may also cause dizziness, drowsiness, head-ache, heartburn, and nausea. Less common side effects include swelling of your ankles and feet or ringing in your ears. If these problems persist or worsen, tell your doctor.

Because this drug can cause drowsiness, make sure you know how you respond to it before driving or performing other activities that require you to be fully alert.

What you must know about other drugs
Avoid taking Advil with Lasix (furosemide) or with thia-zide diuretics (water pills); it can reduce the effects of these drugs. Avoid taking it with oral anticoagulants (blood thinners) and Lithane (lithium) for the opposite reason—it can increase the effects.

Special directions
• Don't take Advil if you're allergic to aspirin. If you have other allergies, check with your doctor before taking Advil.

• If you're on a special low-salt or diabetic diet, check with your doctor before taking Advil oral liquid.

• If you're using nonprescription Advil and your symptoms don't disappear, or if they worsen, contact your doctor.

• If you're taking Advil to reduce fever, call your doctor if your fever lasts for more than 3 days. If you're taking it for pain, call the doctor if the injured area becomes or stays red or swollen.

• Before undergoing surgery or dental work, tell your doctor or dentist that you're taking Advil.

Important reminders
If you're pregnant, check with your doctor before taking Advil.

If you're an older adult, you may be especially suscep-tible to Advil's side effects.

Aldactazide

The doctor has prescribed this medication to treat your high blood pressure. It works by decreasing the amount of water in your body. This drug is a combination of the generic products hydrochlorothiazide and spironolactone.

How to take Aldactazide

Take Aldactazide exactly as prescribed. If you're on just one dose a day, take it in the morning after breakfast. If you're on more than one dose a day, take the last dose before 6 p.m. so the need to urinate won't disturb your sleep. If necessary, take the medication with milk or meals to prevent stomach upset.

What to do if you miss a dose

Take the missed dose as soon as possible. However, if it's almost time for your next dose, skip the missed dose and take your next dose as scheduled. Don't take a double dose.

What to do about side effects

If you develop persistent fever, sore throat, joint pain, or easy bleeding or bruising, stop taking this medication and call your doctor *immediately*.

Aldactazide may cause dehydration, low blood sugar level, fatigue, anxiety, irritability, muscle cramps, numbness, "pins and needles" sensation, weakness, increased urination and thirst, and weak, irregular pulse. If these effects persist, call your doctor.

Because Aldactazide can decrease your body's potassium level, your doctor may suggest that you eat foods high in potassium (for example, uncooked dried fruits, fresh orange juice), take a potassium supplement, and cut down on salt.

Contact your doctor if you experience persistent or severe diarrhea or vomiting, which can cause excessive potassium and water loss and severely decrease blood pressure.

Because this medication may make you sensitive to sunlight, limit your sun exposure, wear protective clothing and sunglasses, and use a sunblock.

What you must know about other drugs

Check with your doctor before taking prescription or nonprescription drugs while you're on this medication. Other drugs can increase or decrease the effects of Aldactazide.

Special directions

• Before taking Aldactazide, let your doctor know if you're allergic to sulfa drugs or other medications.

• If you're already on a special diet, such as one for diabetes, let your doctor know about it.

Important reminders

If you're pregnant or breast-feeding, check with your doctor before taking Aldactazide.

Older adults are especially sensitive to this medication and should monitor side effects closely.

If you're an athlete, be aware that the National Collegiate Athletic Association and the U.S. Olympic Committee ban the use of diuretics (water pills) such as Aldactazide.

Aldactone

Aldactone helps treat high blood pressure and a condition called hyperaldosteronism. Because it's used as a diuretic (water pill), it makes you urinate more while also increasing the amount of potassium in your body. The generic name for Aldactone is spironolactone.

How to take Aldactone

Aldactone comes in tablets, which are better absorbed when taken with meals. Take it exactly as directed.

What to do if you miss a dose

Take the missed dose as soon as possible. However, if it's almost time for your next dose, skip the missed dose and take your next dose on schedule. Don't take a double dose.

What to do about side effects

Call your doctor if you experience abdominal cramps, diarrhea, loss of appetite, or nausea; confusion, drowsiness, fatigue, headache, loss of coordination, or weakness; a rash; or excessive thirst. Men on this medication should advise the doctor if they notice any breast enlargement; women should call if they experience breast soreness, deepening voice, increased facial hair, or menstrual irregularities.

Aldactone can cause you to retain too much potassium. Don't use salt substitutes (which contain a lot of potassium) or eat potassium-rich foods (for example, bananas, carrots, and nonfat dry milk) without first checking with your doctor.

Because Aldactone can make you drowsy, make sure you know how it affects you before you drive or perform other activities that might be dangerous if you're not fully alert.

What you must know about other drugs

Tell your doctor about other medications you're taking, and check with him before you take any new medications.

Don't take aspirin or aspirin-containing drugs; Aldactone may not work well if you do. Your doctor also needs to know if you take the heart medication Lanoxin (digoxin), potassium pills, or other water pills.

Special directions

• Tell your doctor if you have other medical problems, especially diabetes, urinary problems, and kidney or liver disease. Such problems may affect the use of this medication.
• Keep all appointments for follow-up examinations so that your doctor can check your progress.
• The doctor may direct you to take a higher dose of Aldactone at first and then to reduce the amount as your body adjusts.

Important reminders

If you're pregnant, don't use Aldactone unless your doctor tells you to do so.

If you're an athlete, you should know that diuretics such as spironolactone are banned and tested for by the U.S. Olympic Committee and the National Collegiate Athletic Association.

Aldomet

Aldomet is usually prescribed to treat high blood pressure. It controls impulses along certain nerve pathways, which relaxes blood vessels. The generic name for this medication is methyldopa.

How to take Aldomet

Aldomet is available in tablets and in an oral suspension. Check the label carefully. Take only the prescribed amount.

What to do if you miss a dose

Take the missed dose right away. However, if it's almost time for your next dose, skip the missed dose and resume your regular schedule. Don't take a double dose.

What to do about side effects

Call your doctor *immediately* if you develop a fever shortly after you start taking this medication.

Contact your doctor *as soon as possible* if you experience swelling of the feet or lower legs, depression, anxiety, nightmares, stomach pain or cramps, pale stools, diarrhea, nausea, vomiting, fever, chills, joint pain, troubled breathing, fast heartbeat, weakness, a rash, itching, dark or amber urine, or yellow eyes or skin.

Drowsiness, dry mouth, and headache may occur, and you may feel dizzy or light-headed when getting up from a lying or sitting position. Check with your doctor if these side effects persist or become bothersome.

Avoid potentially hazardous activities, such as driving a car or using dangerous tools, until you know how the drug affects you. Aldomet can make you drowsy or less alert.

What you must know about other drugs

Check with your doctor or pharmacist before taking Aldomet with either Larodopa or Dopar (levodopa). The combination may lower your blood pressure too much and cause other problems.

Contact your doctor or pharmacist before taking a tricyclic antidepressant or monoamine oxidase (MAO) inhibitor (drugs for depression) or a phenothiazine (used for anxiety, nausea and vomiting, or psychosis). Combining Aldomet with one of these drugs may cause high blood pressure.

Consult your doctor or pharmacist before taking Aldomet with any nonprescription remedies (such as those used for colds, hay fever, or cough). This, too, could increase your blood pressure.

Special directions
- Make sure your doctor knows about your medical history, especially if you're taking diuretics (water pills) or other drugs to reduce your blood pressure. Also tell the doctor if you have Parkinson's disease, kidney or liver problems, or mental depression — or if you've ever had liver problems when taking Aldomet in the past.
- Follow any special diet the doctor prescribes such as a low-salt diet.
- Don't stop taking this medication suddenly, even if you think it's not working or if unpleasant side effects occur. Instead, contact your doctor.

Important reminder
If you're an older adult, you may be especially sensitive to Aldomet's side effects.

Aldoril

Aldoril is usually prescribed to treat high blood pressure. It works by relaxing blood vessels and helping reduce the amount of water in the body. The drug is a combination of two generic products, methyldopa and hydrochlorothiazide.

How to take Aldoril
Take only the amount prescribed.

What to do if you miss a dose
Take the missed dose as soon as you remember it. However, if it's almost time for your next dose, skip the missed dose and resume your regular dosage schedule. Never take a double dose.

What to do about side effects
Call your doctor *right away* if you develop a fever shortly after you start taking this medication.

Contact your doctor promptly if you have symptoms of too much potassium loss. These symptoms include an irregular heartbeat, muscle pain or cramps, nausea or vomiting, increased thirst, or unusual weakness or fatigue.

You may experience drowsiness, dry mouth, or a headache. You may also feel dizzy or light-headed when rising from a sitting or lying position. Check with your doctor if these effects persist.

Avoid potentially hazardous activities such as driving a car until you know how Aldoril affects you. This drug can make you drowsy or less alert.

Aldoril may also increase your sensitivity to sunlight, so stay out of direct sunlight, wear sunglasses and protective clothing, and apply a sunblock.

What you must know about alcohol and other drugs

Limit alcoholic beverages. They increase the chance for dizziness and light-headedness.

Check with your doctor before taking other medications, especially nonprescription drugs such as those taken for colds, cough, hay fever, asthma, or appetite control. And check before taking prescription products such as Lithane (lithium), Urex (methenamine), an adrenocorticoid (one of a family of cortisone-like drugs), a digitalis glycoside (heart medication), or a monoamine oxidase (MAO) inhibitor (an antidepressant). These drugs affect the way Aldoril works.

Special directions

• Make sure your doctor knows your medical history, especially if you have or have had angina (chest pain), diabetes, gout, kidney or liver disease, lupus, depression, inflammation of the pancreas (pancreatitis), Parkinson's disease, or pheochromocytoma. Also tell him if you've ever had liver problems when taking Aldoril in the past.

• Keep taking this medication exactly as directed, even if you feel well.

• Follow any special diet the doctor prescribes such as a low-salt diet.

Important reminders

If you're pregnant or breast-feeding, check with your doctor before taking Aldoril.

If you're an older adult, you may be especially sensitive to the drug's side effects.

If you have diabetes, be aware that Aldoril can increase your blood sugar level. Test your blood sugar regularly.

Alupent

Alupent is usually prescribed to treat asthma. It's also used to treat bronchospasm (wheezing or difficulty breathing) associated with chronic bronchitis, emphysema, or other lung diseases or to prevent bronchospasm caused by exercise. This drug's generic name is metaproterenol. Another brand name is Metaprel.

How to take Alupent

This medication is available as an inhalation aerosol, an inhalation solution, or an oral tablet or syrup. You may need to take it as many as 12 times daily if you're using the inhalation aerosol, every 4 hours if you're using the inhalation solution in a nebulizer, or every 6 to 8 hours if you're taking it orally.

Check the label carefully to find out how much to take at each dose. Take only the amount prescribed.

To take the *aerosol* form, shake the container, and then exhale through your nose completely. Put the mouthpiece into your mouth, sealing your lips around it tightly. Now inhale deeply through your mouth as you push down on the container to release a dose of the medication. Hold your breath for 10 seconds; then exhale slowly. Don't take more than two inhalations at a time unless prescribed. After the first inhalation, wait 1 to 2 minutes to see if you need a second.

If you're using Alupent in a *nebulizer* or a *combination nebulizer and respirator*, make sure you understand how to take it correctly. Ask your doctor or pharmacist if you have any questions.

What to do if you miss a dose

If you're using this medication regularly, take the missed dose as soon as you remember it. If you have any more doses left that day, take them at regularly spaced intervals. Never take a double dose.

What to do about side effects

If you think you may have taken an overdose, get emergency medical help *immediately*. Symptoms of an overdose include severe dizziness, light-headedness, headache, chills, fever, nausea, vomiting, severe muscle cramps, severe weakness, blurred vision, severe shortness of breath or troubled breathing, or unusual anxiety or restlessness.

Trembling, nervousness, and restlessness may occur. These side effects usually go away over time as your body adjusts to the medication. But you should check with your doctor if they persist or become bothersome.

If you're using an oral inhaler, you may notice an unusual or unpleasant taste. This symptom will go away when you stop using the medication.

If your mouth and throat feel dry after taking Alupent, try rinsing your mouth with water after each dose.

What you must know about other drugs

Check with your doctor if you're taking a beta blocker; it may prevent Alupent from working properly. Beta blockers are drugs prescribed to treat high blood pressure or angina. Some examples are Tenormin (atenolol), Normodyne (labetalol), and Inderal (propranolol).

Notify your doctor or pharmacist if you're taking Hydergine (ergoloid mesylates), Ergomar (ergotamine), Ludiomil (maprotiline), or a tricyclic antidepressant (a drug for depression). These drugs can increase Alupent's effects on the heart and blood vessels.

Check with your doctor or pharmacist if you're taking a digitalis glycoside (a drug used to treat an abnormal heart rhythm). When taken with Alupent, a digitalis glycoside increases the possibility of an irregular heartbeat.

If you're taking a monoamine oxidase (MAO) inhibitor (a drug for depression), check with your doctor or pharmacist. Alupent may increase the effects of the MAO inhibitor if the two drugs are taken within 2 weeks of each other.

Special directions

• If you have an unusually rapid heartbeat, don't take Alupent. It may aggravate this condition.

• Make sure your doctor knows your medical history, especially if you have brain damage, seizures, diabetes, an underactive thyroid, heart disease, or blood vessel disease. Alupent may make these conditions worse.

• Call your doctor *right away* if you still have trouble breathing or if your condition gets worse after you start using this medication.

• If you're using the *aerosol* form, keep the spray away from your eyes to avoid irritation.

• If you're using the *aerosol* form and are also using an adrenocorticoid aerosol, or if you are using Atrovent (an ipratropium aerosol), take Alupent at least 5 minutes before taking the other aerosol (unless your doctor tells you otherwise). Adrenocorticoids available in aerosol form include Beclovent (beclomethasone), Decadron Respihaler (dexamethasone), and Aerobid (flunisolide).

• Save the applicator; you may be able to get refills.

• Don't use more of the drug or use it more often than recommended (except under doctor's orders). This could cause serious side effects.

• If you have been using this medication for a long time and find that its effects don't last as long as they did when you first started using it, contact your doctor.

Important reminders

If you're pregnant or breast-feeding, check with the doctor before taking Alupent.

If you're an older adult, you may be especially sensitive to the effects of this medication.

If you have diabetes, the doctor may need to adjust the dosage of your insulin or other diabetes medication while you're taking Alupent.

Amoxil

This drug treats bacterial infections. Its generic name is amoxicillin. Another brand name is Trimox.

How to take Amoxil

Take Amoxil on a full or an empty stomach at evenly spaced times during the day and night. This medication works best when you have a constant amount in your blood.

Take the *liquid form* straight or mixed with other liquids. To get the full dose, take it immediately after mixing and drink all the liquid.

Don't break, chew, or crush the *capsule* form of the drug. Swallow it whole. The *chewable* tablet form should be chewed or crushed before swallowing.

What to do if you miss a dose

Take the missed dose as soon as possible. If you take two doses a day and it's almost time for your next dose, space the missed dose and your next dose 5 to 6 hours apart. If you're taking three or more doses a day, space the missed dose and the next dose 2 to 4 hours apart. Then go back to your regular schedule.

What to do about side effects

Contact your doctor *immediately* and stop taking this medication if you develop difficulty breathing, a rash, hives, itching, or wheezing. Such symptoms may indicate an allergic reaction.

Common side effects of Amoxil include nausea and diarrhea. If these side effects persist or become severe, notify your doctor.

What you must know about other drugs

Tell your doctor about any other medications that you're taking. Taking Zyloprim (allopurinol) with Amoxil may make you more likely to develop a rash. On the other hand, Probalan (probenecid) increases blood levels of Amoxil — a beneficial side effect.

Special directions

• Tell your doctor if you're allergic to other penicillins or to cephalosporins, Fulvicin (griseofulvin), or Cuprimine (penicillamine). If you're allergic to Amoxil, carry medical identification that describes your allergy.

• Before taking Amoxil, inform your doctor if you have kidney, stomach, or intestinal disease or infectious mononucleosis. These problems may increase the risk of side effects.

• If your symptoms don't improve within a few days, or if they become worse, check with your doctor.

• If you develop severe diarrhea, check with your doctor before taking diarrhea medication. It may make your diarrhea worse or make it last longer.

• Finish all your medication, even when you feel better. If you stop it too soon, your symptoms may return.

Important reminders

If you have diabetes and test your urine for glucose, be aware that Amoxil may cause false test results with some urine glucose tests. If your glucose levels appear to be fluctuating, call your doctor before changing your diet or the dosage of your diabetes medication.

If you're breast-feeding, discuss with your doctor whether you should continue to do so while taking Amoxil.

Anaprox

Anaprox is usually prescribed to reduce joint pain, swelling, and stiffness caused by arthritis. The generic name for this drug is naproxen. Another brand name is Naprosyn.

How to take Anaprox

This medication is available in regular and extended-release tablets as well as in an oral suspension. Check the label carefully and take only the prescribed amount.

Take each dose with a full glass (8 ounces) of water. Stay upright for about 30 minutes afterward.

If you're taking the *extended-release tablets,* be sure to swallow them whole. Don't crush or break them.

If you're taking the *regular tablets* and they give you heartburn, check with your doctor to see whether you can take them with food or an antacid.

If you're taking the *oral suspension,* don't mix it with an antacid.

What to do if you miss a dose

Take the missed dose as soon as you remember it. However, if it's almost time for the next dose, skip the missed dose and resume your regular schedule. Don't take a double dose.

What to do about side effects

Call your doctor *right away* if you see blood in your urine, if you start urinating less often, or if you have diarrhea, black stools, sore throat, wheezing, dizziness, drowsiness, light-headedness, ringing in your ears, vision changes, swollen ankles, or a rash.

Headache, heartburn, indigestion, nausea, or vomiting may occur as well as stomach or abdominal cramps or pain. Call your doctor if these side effects persist or become bothersome.

Avoid potentially hazardous activities such as driving a car until you know how you react to Anaprox; it may make you drowsy.

What you must know about alcohol and other drugs Avoid drinking alcoholic beverages while taking this medication. Alcohol may increase the depressant effects of Anaprox.

Check with your doctor before taking other drugs. Many drugs increase the potential of Anaprox to cause serious side effects. In particular, avoid aspirin and steroids; these drugs increase the risk of gastrointestinal side effects.

Special directions • Don't take this medication if you're allergic to aspirin.

• Make sure your doctor knows about your medical history, especially if you've had stomach or intestinal disease, ulcers, kidney disease, or heart or blood vessel disease.

• Take all doses at the prescribed times. Don't postpone a dose to make the drug last longer than intended.

• Keep taking the medication even if your symptoms don't get better right away. It may take a month for Anaprox to achieve its effect.

• If you're taking this medication on a long-term basis, go for regular checkups so the doctor can evaluate your progress.

Important reminders If you're pregnant, check with your doctor before taking this medication.

If you're an older adult, you may be especially vulnerable to stomach upset.

Ansaid

Your doctor has prescribed Ansaid to relieve the inflammation, swelling, stiffness, and joint pain of arthritis. The generic name for this drug is flurbiprofen.

How to take Ansaid Take your medication exactly as directed. Ansaid tablets should be taken with food or an antacid plus a full glass (8 ounces) of water. To prevent possible swallowing problems, remain upright for 15 to 30 minutes after taking it.

What to do if you miss a dose

If you are only an hour or two overdue, take the missed dose as soon as you remember it. If the time lag is greater than that, skip the missed dose and take your next regularly scheduled dose. Don't take a double dose.

What to do about side effects

Sometimes serious side effects, including ulcers and bleeding, may occur with or without warning. Stop taking Ansaid and seek medical attention *at once* if you experience severe abdominal cramps, pain, or burning; if you have have severe, continuing nausea, heartburn, or indigestion; or if you vomit blood or material that looks like coffee grounds.

Ansaid may also cause headache, fluid retention, heartburn, nausea, diarrhea, stomach pain, burning and frequent urination, drowsiness, and dark, tarry stools. If these symptoms persist or become severe, tell your doctor.

What you must know about alcohol and other drugs

Don't drink alcoholic beverages while taking Ansaid; stomach problems are more likely to occur. Also, don't combine Ansaid with Tylenol (acetaminophen), aspirin, or another salicylate for more than a few days; this increases your risk of unwanted effects. Aspirin can also decrease Ansaid's effectiveness.

Taking Ansaid with anticoagulants (blood thinners) may increase your risk of bleeding. And taking it with diuretics (water pills) may make it less effective.

Special directions

• Be sure to tell your doctor about other medical problems you have. They may affect the use of this medication.

• Schedule regular medical checkups so your doctor can monitor your progress and check for unwanted side effects.

• Before undergoing a dental or surgical procedure, tell the dentist or doctor that you're taking Ansaid.

• Until you know how you react to Ansaid, don't drive or perform activities that require you to be totally alert.

• Protect yourself from excessive sun.

Important reminders

Consult your doctor if you're breast-feeding or become pregnant while taking Ansaid.

If you're an older adult, you may be especially prone to side effects from Ansaid.

Antivert

Antivert is usually prescribed to prevent and treat the nausea, vomiting, and dizziness caused by motion sickness. Your doctor may also prescribe it to treat dizziness caused by other medical problems. The generic name for this drug is meclizine. Another brand name is Bonine.

How to take Antivert   This medication comes in both regular and chewable tablets and in capsules.

Some preparations of the drug are available only by prescription; others are available without a prescription. If you're treating yourself, read the label instructions carefully to find out how much to take and how often to take it. If your doctor prescribed the drug or gave you special instructions on how to use it and how much to take, follow his instructions.

What to do if you miss a dose   Take the missed dose as soon as possible. However, if it's almost time for your next dose, skip the missed dose and resume your regular dosage schedule. Never take a double dose.

What to do about side effects   Drowsiness may occur. If it persists or becomes bothersome, call your doctor.

Because Antivert can make you drowsy, avoid potentially hazardous activities, such as driving a car, until you know how it affects you.

If you've been vomiting a lot, be sure to drink plenty of fluids to prevent dehydration.

If the drug makes your mouth dry, try using sugarless gum or hard candy or ice chips. If the condition lasts for more than 2 weeks, see your doctor or dentist for further evaluation.

<table>
<tr><td>What you must know about alcohol and other drugs</td><td>Avoid alcoholic beverages, sedatives (such as drugs that relax you and make you feel sleepy), antihistamines (such as Benadryl), and other depressant drugs while taking Antivert. They could increase the sedative effects of the drug.</td></tr>
</table>

Special directions

• Don't take Antivert if you're allergic to similar medications, such as Bucladin-S Softabs (buclizine), Marezine (cyclizine), or Dramamine (dimenhydrinate).

• Tell your doctor about other medical problems you may have, especially narrow-angle glaucoma, asthma, an enlarged prostate, or a blockage of the genitourinary or gastrointestinal tract. Antivert may aggravate these conditions.

• Take this medication 1 hour before starting your trip, and continue to take it regularly every travel day during the trip.

Important reminders

If you're pregnant or breast-feeding, check with your doctor before taking Antivert or other brands of meclizine.

If you're an athlete, you should know that the U.S. Olympic Committee bans meclizine; using it can lead to disqualification in biathlon and pentathlon events.

Apresoline

Your doctor has prescribed Apresoline to lower your blood pressure or to treat your heart condition. The generic name for this drug is hydralazine.

How to take Apresoline

Take it exactly as prescribed and at the same time each day, preferably at mealtimes. Continue it for as long as the doctor has ordered, even after you begin to feel better. Apresoline doesn't cure high blood pressure; it helps to control it and reduces the risk of complications caused by high blood pressure.

What to do if you miss a dose

Take the missed dose as soon as possible. But if it's almost time for your next dose, skip the missed dose and resume your normal schedule. Don't take a double dose.

What to do about side effects

A rare but possibly serious side effect of Apresoline is an irregular heartbeat. If this occurs, call your doctor *immediately*. Also call him if you develop chest pain, swelling of the feet or lower legs, weight gain, sore throat, fever, muscle and joint pain, or a rash.

Apresoline may cause headaches, dizziness, rapid heartbeat, nausea, vomiting, diarrhea, or loss of appetite. These effects may go away as your body adjusts to the medication; check with your doctor if they continue or are bothersome, but don't suddenly stop taking the medication.

Because Apresoline can cause dizziness, make sure you know how you react to it before driving or performing other activities that require you to be totally alert.

To minimize dizziness, rise slowly from a sitting or lying position.

What you must know about other drugs

Check with your doctor before taking any other prescription or nonprescription medications; certain drugs can interfere with Apresoline's action or can cause side effects.

Special directions

• Tell your doctor about other medical problems you may have, especially kidney, heart, or blood vessel disease, including stroke.

• Follow a low-salt diet if your doctor has prescribed it.

• If your doctor has instructed you to take your blood pressure at home, follow the directions closely and notify your doctor of any significant change.

Important reminders

If you're pregnant or think you may be, check with your doctor before taking Apresoline.

Older adults may be especially sensitive to side effects.

Asacol

Asacol is usually prescribed to treat ulcerative colitis and other inflammatory diseases of the bowel. The generic name of this drug is mesalamine. Another brand name is Rowasa.

How to take Asacol This medication is available in a rectal suspension and in rectal suppositories. Check the label carefully and take only the amount prescribed.

If the doctor has prescribed the *suspension* form, take it once a day as an enema, preferably at bedtime. You may need to continue the routine for up to 6 weeks. Just before taking the enema, empty your bowels. Then shake the suspension well and administer the enema. Be sure to retain the medication for at least 8 hours.

What to do if you miss a dose If you remember the same night, take the missed dose as soon as possible. If you don't remember until the next morning, skip the missed dose and resume your regular dosage schedule.

What to do about side effects Stop taking the medication, and contact your doctor *immediately* if you develop a rash, wheezing, itching, hives, severe stomach or abdominal pain or cramps, fever, bloody diarrhea, or severe headache. These symptoms may indicate an intolerance to the medication or a sensitivity to sulfites.

Call your doctor as soon as possible if you suddenly have rectal pain, bleeding, burning, itching, or other symptoms of rectal irritation after you start using this medication.

You may experience a mild headache, mild stomach or abdominal pain or cramps, nausea, diarrhea, bloating, and flatulence (gas). These side effects usually go away as your body adjusts to the medication. Check with your doctor if they persist or become bothersome.

Special directions • Don't take this medication if you're allergic to any of its contents (including sulfites).

• Make sure your doctor knows your medical history, especially if you've had kidney disease, because Asacol may further damage your kidneys. Also let your doctor know if you're allergic to Azulfidine (sulfasalazine), Dipentum (olsalazine), or aspirin.

• Continue to take Asacol for the full treatment time prescribed by your doctor, even if you feel better within several days. Don't miss any doses.

• Have regular medical checkups so the doctor can evaluate your progress.

Asendin

Your doctor has prescribed Asendin to help treat your depression. The generic name for this drug is amoxapine.

How to take Asendin

Take it with food, unless the doctor directs you otherwise.

What to do if you miss a dose

If you usually take one dose daily at bedtime, don't take the missed dose in the morning because it may cause disturbing side effects during the day. Call your doctor for instructions.

If you take more than one dose daily, take the missed dose as soon as possible. But if it's almost time for your next dose, skip the missed dose and go back to your regular schedule. Don't take a double dose.

What to do about side effects

If your urine output drops and your hands, ankles, and feet swell, stop taking Asendin and notify your doctor *immediately*.

Other side effects include drowsiness, dizziness, dry mouth, light-headedness (especially when you stand up), irregular or fast pulse, blurred vision, constipation, and sweating. Notify your doctor if these effects persist or become severe.

Get up slowly to help prevent dizziness.

For temporary relief of mouth dryness, use sugarless gum or hard candy, ice chips, or a saliva substitute.

Asendin may increase your sensitivity to light. Avoid direct sunlight if possible. Wear protective clothing and use a sunblock with a skin protection factor (SPF) of 15 or higher. If you have a severe sun reaction, check with your doctor.

What you must know about alcohol and other drugs

Check with your doctor about drinking alcoholic beverages or using nonprescription medications while you're on Asendin.

Tell your doctor if you're taking other prescription medications. Barbiturates (antianxiety medications) may decrease Asendin's effectiveness; Tagamet (cimetidine) and Ritalin (methylphenidate) may increase it.

Combining Asendin with Adrenalin (epinephrine), a drug used to treat breathing problems, may raise your blood pressure.

Combining Asendin with monoamine oxidase (MAO) inhibitors (drugs used for depression) may cause severe excitation, high fever, or seizures.

Special directions
• Tell your doctor of any other medical problems you may have. They could affect the use of Asendin.
• Until you know how Asendin affects you, don't drive or perform other activities that require you to be totally alert.
• Before you have medical tests, surgery, dental work, or emergency treatment, advise the doctor that you're taking Asendin.

Important reminders
This medication may affect your blood sugar levels. If you have diabetes, contact your doctor if you notice a change in your blood test results.

Let your doctor know if you're breast-feeding or if you become pregnant while taking Asendin.

Children and older adults may be especially vulnerable to side effects.

Aspirin

Aspirin is used to relieve pain and reduce fever. It can also be used to relieve some symptoms caused by arthritis (rheumatism) and to lessen the chance of heart attack, stroke, or other problems that may occur when blood clots block a blood vessel. Don't take aspirin for any of these secondary purposes unless your doctor has ordered you to; the medication has blood-thinning properties that may increase your chance of serious bleeding. Aspirin is the generic name for this drug, which is available under many brand names.

How to take Aspirin
This time-tested pain reliever is available in capsules, tablets, chewable tablets, chewing gum tablets, delayed-

release (enteric-coated) tablets, extended-release tablets, and suppositories.

Take it after meals or with food (except for enteric-coated tablets and suppositories) to lessen stomach irritation. Take the *tablets* and *capsules* with a full glass (8 ounces) of water. To prevent irritation that may lead to trouble swallowing, remain upright for 15 to 30 minutes after taking the medication.

Chewable tablets can be chewed, dissolved in liquid, crushed, or swallowed whole. *Enteric-coated tablets* must be swallowed whole. Check with your pharmacist about how to take *extended-release tablets;* some can be broken into pieces (but not crushed) before swallowing; others must be swallowed whole.

If you're using a *suppository* and it's too soft to insert, chill it in the refrigerator for 30 minutes or run cold water over it before you remove the foil wrapper. To insert the suppository, first wash your hands, and then remove the foil wrapper. Lie on your side and draw your knees up toward your chest. With your index finger, push the suppository rounded end first into your rectum as far as you can.

What to do if you miss a dose

If you're taking this medication regularly and you miss a dose, take the missed dose as soon as you remember it. However, if it's almost time for your next dose, skip the missed dose and go back to your regular schedule. Don't take a double dose.

What to do about side effects

Call your doctor *immediately* and stop taking this medication if you experience difficulty breathing; wheezing; flushing, redness, or other changes in skin color; hives; itching; or swelling of eyelids, face, or lips. These effects may mean that you're allergic to the drug.

Call your doctor *immediately* and stop taking the medication if you experience ringing in your ears or hearing loss; this may indicate that there is too much aspirin in your system (a condition called aspirin toxicity).

You may also experience nausea, stomach problems, or easy bruising. If these symptoms persist or become severe, notify your doctor.

If you have rectal irritation from using suppositories, contact your doctor.

It's also important to call the doctor if you're taking aspirin to relieve pain and the pain lasts for more than 10 days (5 days for children) or gets worse, if new symptoms occur, or if redness or swelling occurs.

If you're taking aspirin to reduce a fever and the fever lasts for more than 3 days, returns, or gets worse; if new symptoms occur; or if redness or swelling occurs, call the doctor.

If you're taking aspirin for a sore throat and your throat is very painful or if the pain lasts for more than 2 days or occurs with or is followed by fever, headache, rash, nausea, or vomiting, you should also notify your doctor.

What you must know about alcohol and other drugs

Check with your doctor about drinking alcoholic beverages while taking aspirin; this combination may cause stomach problems.

If you're taking other medications, check with your doctor before taking aspirin. Ammonium chloride, for example, increases blood levels of aspirin, which can lead to aspirin toxicity.

Antacids in high doses make aspirin less effective. So can corticosteroids, such as prednisone, which cause aspirin to be eliminated from the body quickly.

Combining anticoagulants (blood thinners) with aspirin medication may increase your risk of bleeding problems.

Aspirin may also increase the effect of oral diabetes medication, causing low blood sugar reactions.

Check the labels of all nonprescription and prescription medications and skin products (shampoo, for example) for aspirin, other salicylates, or salicylic acid. Count these products as part of your total aspirin dosage for the day. Pepto-Bismol (bismuth subsalicylate) is an example of a commonly used nonprescription medication that contains salicylates. Using salicylate-containing products while you're taking aspirin can lead to overdose.

Special directions

• Tell your doctor if you have other medical problems. They may affect the use of an aspirin medication.

• Don't give aspirin to children or teenagers who have fever or other symptoms of a viral infection; it may put them at risk of developing a serious disorder called Reye's syndrome. Check with the doctor.

• Don't use any aspirin product if it has a strong, vinegar-like odor. This odor means the medication is breaking down and is no longer effective.

• Don't take aspirin for 5 days before surgery (including dental surgery) unless otherwise directed by your doctor or dentist. Taking aspirin during this time may cause bleeding problems.

• Don't use the chewable forms of aspirin for 7 days after having your tonsils removed, a tooth pulled, or other dental or mouth surgery.

• Don't place aspirin directly on a tooth or gum surface because it may cause a burn and erode the tooth enamel.

• See your doctor at regular intervals if you're taking aspirin for more than 10 days (5 days for children) or if you're taking large amounts of it.

• If you're taking aspirin to lessen the chance of heart attack, stroke, or other problems caused by blood clots, take only the amount ordered by your doctor. Talk to your doctor if you need medication to relieve pain, fever, or the symptoms of arthritis; the doctor may not want you to take extra aspirin.

Atarax

Atarax helps treat many different problems. It helps relieve anxiety and tension as well as rashes and itching, and may even be given to children to treat hyperactivity. The drug's generic name is hydroxyzine. Another brand name is Vistaril.

How to take Atarax Follow your doctor's instructions exactly. Atarax comes in tablets, capsules, a syrup, and an oral liquid. Take it with food or a glass of water or milk to reduce stomach upset.

What to do if you miss a dose Take the missed dose as soon as possible. But if it's almost time for the next regular dose, skip the missed dose and take the next dose at the scheduled time. Never take two doses at once.

What to do about side effects

If you think you've taken an overdose of Atarax or you're experiencing symptoms of an overdose — including seizures, clumsiness or unsteadiness, severe drowsiness, trouble breathing, extreme mouth dryness, and hallucinations — get emergency medical care *immediately*.

Common side effects include drowsiness and dry mouth. These problems should subside as your body adjusts to the medication; if they persist or worsen, tell your doctor.

Relieve mouth dryness with sugarless hard candy or gum, ice chips, mouthwash, or a saliva substitute. If dryness continues for more than 2 weeks, tell your doctor or dentist; it can increase your risk of tooth and gum problems.

What you must know about alcohol and other drugs

Don't drink alcoholic beverages while taking Atarax. This combination can result in an overdose.

For the same reason, check with your doctor before taking other prescription or nonprescription medications with Atarax.

Special directions

• Tell your doctor about other medical conditions you may have and let him know if you're on a special diet, such as low-salt or low-sugar.

• Make sure you know how you react to Atarax before you drive or perform other activities that require you to be totally alert.

• Atarax may mask the signs of appendicitis or overdose. If you develop symptoms of appendicitis (such as stomach pain, cramping, or tenderness) or if you think you may have taken an overdose of another medication, let your doctor know you're taking Atarax.

Important reminders

If you're pregnant or think you may be, check with your doctor before starting this medication, and don't take it while you're breast-feeding.

Children and older adults are especially vulnerable to side effects.

Ativan

Ativan may be prescribed to treat anxiety, tension, agitation, irritability, or insomnia (difficulty sleeping). Its generic name is lorazepam.

How to take Ativan

Ativan comes in tablets. Check the label carefully and take only the amount prescribed.

What to do if you miss a dose

If you are only an hour off schedule, take the missed dose right away. If you don't remember it within an hour, skip the missed dose and resume your regular dosage schedule. Never take a double dose.

What to do about side effects

If you think you've taken an overdose, get emergency help *immediately.* Symptoms of an overdose include confusion, staggering, slurred speech, extreme drowsiness, and weakness.

Drowsiness, light-headedness, dizziness, and clumsiness may occur. These side effects usually go away over time as your body adjusts to the medication. But you should check with your doctor if they persist or become bothersome.

Because Ativan can make you drowsy or less alert, avoid potentially hazardous activities, such as driving a car, until you know how it affects you.

What you must know about alcohol and other drugs

Avoid alcoholic beverages, sedatives (such as drugs that relax you and make you feel sleepy), antihistamines such as Benadryl (diphenhydramine), and other depressants while taking Ativan because of the risk of added sedation.

Special directions

• Don't take Ativan if you have glaucoma.
• Make sure your doctor knows your medical history, particularly of psychosis (mental illness), myasthenia gravis, Parkinson's disease, respiratory problems, liver problems, drug addiction, or drug abuse.
• Take the medication only as directed. Extended use may cause drug dependence and withdrawal symptoms.
• Don't stop taking Ativan without your doctor's approval.

Important reminders   If you're pregnant or breast-feeding, be sure to tell your doctor before taking Ativan.

Older adults are especially likely to become dizzy, drowsy, light-headed, clumsy, and less alert when taking this drug.

If you're an athlete, you should know that the U.S. Olympic Committee and the National Collegiate Athletic Association ban lorazapam for athletes participating in shooting events.

Atromid-S

Your doctor has prescribed Atromid-S to lower the levels of cholesterol and triglycerides (fatty substances) in your blood. The generic name for this drug is clofibrate.

How to take Atromid-S   Atromid-S comes in capsules. Take it exactly as your doctor prescribes. Don't break, chew, or crush the capsules; swallow them whole. Taking Atromid-S with food or right after meals may help minimize potential stomach upset.

Don't stop taking the medication abruptly; check with your doctor first.

What to do if you miss a dose   Take the missed dose as soon as possible. But if it's almost time for your next dose, skip the missed dose and take your next dose on schedule. Don't take a double dose.

What to do about side effects   Call your doctor *immediately* if you develop flulike symptoms, such as fever or aches and pains.

Check with your doctor if you gain weight or experience diarrhea, heartburn, increased appetite, nausea, or vomiting.

What you must know about other drugs   Tell your doctor about any other medications you're taking; Atromid-S can increase the effects of certain drugs, including water pills, blood thinners, and diabetes medication.

Atromid-S should not be used with cholesterol-lowering drugs such as Mevacor (lovastatin).

Atromid-S may not work properly if taken with birth control pills or Rifadin (rifampin), a tuberculosis medication.

Taking Atromid-S with Probalan (probenicid), a gout medication, may cause serious side effects.

Special directions
• Tell your doctor if you have any other medical problems, especially kidney or liver disease or peptic ulcers.
• When you stop using Atromid-S, your blood fat levels may rise again. To prevent this, your doctor may recommend a special diet.
• Keep all appointments for follow-up visits, and have your blood cholesterol and triglyceride levels measured regularly.

Important reminders
If you're pregnant or think you may be, check with your doctor before taking this medication. And don't use Atromid-S if you're breast-feeding; it can cause unwanted side effects in the breast-feeding infant.

Don't give this medication to children under age 2; they need cholesterol for normal development.

Atropisol

Atropisol is prescribed for the relief of stomach and intestinal cramps or spasms. It's also used with antacids or other medications to treat peptic ulcers. Atropisol eyedrops and ointment are used to dilate (enlarge) the pupil and to treat certain eye inflammations. The generic name for Atropisol is atropine.

How to take Atropisol
Atropisol is available in tablet (oral) form and also as an ophthalmic (eye) solution and an ophthalmic ointment. Check your prescription label and follow the directions exactly.

Take the *tablets* 30 minutes to 1 hour before meals, unless your doctor instructs otherwise.

If you're using the *eyedrops,* wash your hands first. Right-handers: Begin with your left eye. With the middle finger of your left hand, apply pressure to the inner corner of the eye, tilt your head back and, with the index finger of the same hand, pull the lower eyelid away from the eye to form a pouch. Squeeze the drops into the pouch and gently close the eye. Don't blink. Keep the eye closed for 1 or 2 minutes while continuing to apply pressure to the inner corner with your middle finger. Repeat the process in the right eye, using the index finger of your left hand to apply pressure to the corner of the eye and the middle finger of the same hand to pull down the lower lid. Left-handers: follow the same process, but hold the medication in your left hand and start with your right eye.

If you're applying the *eye ointment*, wash your hands, and then follow the process just described, squeezing a thin strip of ointment into the pouch instead of drops.

Wash your hands immediately after using eyedrops or ointment. If you gave the medication to an infant or a child, be sure to wash his hands too, as well as any other place the medication may have touched. Don't let any eye medication enter the child's mouth.

To keep the medication germfree, don't let the applicator tip touch any surface. Also keep the container tightly closed.

What to do if you miss a dose

Take the missed dose as soon as you remember. But if it's almost time for your next dose, skip the missed dose and resume your normal schedule. Don't take or apply a double dose.

What to do about side effects

Oral Atropisol:
Make sure family members know to contact the doctor immediately if you become so sleepy that you can't be roused.

More common side effects from Atropisol tablets include difficulty sleeping, dizziness, rapid pulse rate, palpitations, chest pain, dry mouth, constipation, and blurred vision. If these symptoms persist or worsen, call your doctor.

Because Atropisol can make you dizzy or lightheaded, make sure you know how you react to it before driving or performing activities that require you to be alert.

If you feel dizzy, light-headed, or faint when getting up from a bed or chair, try rising slowly and see if that relieves the problem.

To relieve mouth dryness, use sugarless hard candy or gum, ice chips, or a saliva substitute. If dryness persists for more than 2 weeks, check with your doctor or dentist. Continued mouth dryness increases the risk of dental disorders.

Because it can decrease perspiration, oral Atropisol can increase your body temperature. Hot baths or saunas may make you feel dizzy or faint. Take extra care not to become overheated during exercise or in hot weather; you may end up with heatstroke.

Ophthalmic Atropisol:

The most common side effects associated with the eye medication are blurred vision and sensitivity to light. These symptoms may last for several days after you stop using the medication. If they persist beyond that, notify your doctor.

Protect light-sensitive eyes by wearing sunglasses and avoiding bright lights.

Because ophthalmic Atropisol may temporarily affect your level of alertness and your ability to see clearly, avoid driving a car or performing other tasks that require alertness and clear vision.

What you must know about other drugs

Tell the doctor about other medications you're taking. Atropisol taken with Levoprome (methotrimeprazine) can cause involuntary body movements, such as twitching, changes in muscle tone, and abnormal posture.

Don't take oral Atropisol within 2 to 3 hours of taking antacids or diarrhea medications. Taking these medications too close together can prevent Atropisol from working properly.

Special directions

• If you think you may have taken an overdose of oral Atropisol, get emergency help immediately.

• Check with your doctor before you begin using new medications (prescription or nonprescription) or if you develop new medical problems while taking Atropisol tablets.

• Also check with the doctor before you stop using oral Atropisol. Abrupt withdrawal from this drug can cause unpleasant side effects such as vomiting, sweating, and dizziness. The doctor may want you to reduce your dosage gradually.

Important reminders   If you're breast-feeding, be aware that oral Atropisol can reduce milk flow and that ophthalmic Atropisol can cause rapid pulse rate, fever, or dry skin in breast-feeding infants. Discuss these possibilities with your doctor.

Children (especially those with blond hair and blue eyes) and older adults are especially sensitive to ophthalmic Atropisol and prone to its side effects.

Augmentin

Augmentin combines the generic drugs amoxicillin and clavulanate potassium. It's used to treat certain bacterial infections.

How to take Augmentin   Take this medication on a full or an empty stomach at evenly spaced times during the day and night. This medication works best when you have a constant amount in your blood. Finish all of the medication prescribed.

If you're taking the *chewable* tablets, crush or chew them well before swallowing.

If you're taking the *oral suspension,* use the dropper that comes with the bottle to measure the correct amount. If your medication doesn't have a dropper, use a specially marked measuring spoon.

What to do if you miss a dose   Take the missed dose as soon as possible. But if it's almost time for your next dose and you usually take two doses daily, space the missed dose and the next one 5 to 6 hours apart. If you take three or more doses daily, space the missed dose and the next one 2 to 4 hours apart. Then go back to your regular schedule.

What to do about side effects   Call your doctor *immediately* and stop taking this medication if you experience difficulty breathing, itching, a rash, hives, or wheezing. These effects may indicate that you're allergic to Augmentin.

You may also have nausea and diarrhea. Call the doctor if these symptoms persist or become severe.

What you must know about other drugs Tell your doctor about other medications you're taking. Zyloprim (allopurinol) taken with this medication may increase your chances of developing a rash. Probalan (probenecid) increases blood levels of Augmentin, a beneficial side effect.

Special directions • Inform your doctor if you have kidney, stomach, or intestinal disease or infectious mononucleosis. They may increase the risk of side effects.

• Tell your doctor if you're allergic to other penicillins or cephalosporins, griseofulvin (Fulvicin), or penicillamine (Cuprimine). If you're allergic to Augmentin, carry medical identification that describes your allergy.

• If you develop severe diarrhea, don't take diarrhea medication without checking with your doctor. Diarrhea medications may make your diarrhea worse or last longer.

Important reminders If you have diabetes and test your urine for glucose, be aware that this medication may cause false test results with some urine glucose tests. Call your doctor before changing your diet or the dosage of your diabetes medication.

If you're breast-feeding, discuss with your doctor whether you should continue taking this medication.

Axid

Your doctor has prescribed Axid to treat your duodenal ulcers or to prevent their return. The generic name for this drug is nizatidine.

How to take Axid Axid comes in capsules. Follow the directions on the prescription label exactly. If you're taking one capsule daily, take it at bedtime unless your doctor gives you other instructions. If you're taking two capsules, take one in the morning and one at bedtime.

What to do if you miss a dose

Take the missed dose as soon as possible. However, if it's almost time for your next dose, skip the missed capsule and take your next dose as scheduled. Don't take a double dose.

What to do about side effects

Call your doctor *at once* if you start to bleed or bruise easily or if you become unusually tired. Also tell him right away if you develop rashes or other skin problems.

Axid may make you sleepy or sweaty. In rare cases it may cause irregular heartbeat. Check with your doctor if such symptoms persist or are troublesome.

Don't smoke while taking this medication; cigarette smoking reduces Axid's effectiveness. If you can't stop smoking completely, at least hold off until after you've taken your last dose for the day.

What you must know about other drugs

Tell your doctor if you're taking other medications and check with him before taking new medications. In particular, let him know if you take aspirin regularly in high doses; Axid may increase aspirin's side effects.

If you take an antacid to relieve stomach pain, wait 30 minutes to 1 hour before taking Axid.

Special directions

• Continue to take the medication even after you begin to feel better. If you stop too soon your ulcer may not heal completely.

• Axid may aggravate certain medical conditions, so it's important that you tell your doctor if you have other medical problems, especially kidney or liver disease.

• If you plan to have testing done—skin tests for allergies, for example, or tests to measure how much acid is in your stomach—let your doctor know you're taking Axid. It could affect the test results.

• Avoid foods and other substances that irritate your stomach, such as alcohol, carbonated soft drinks, and citrus products.

• Keep appointments for follow-up examinations so your doctor can check your progress.

Important reminders

If you're pregnant or breast-feeding, check with your doctor about using Axid.

If you're an older adult, you may be especially vulnerable to this medication's side effects, particularly dizziness and confusion.

Azactam

Azactam helps treat bacterial infections. It comes in a vial and must be given by intramuscular injection. The generic name for this drug is aztreonam.

How to inject Azactam The label on your prescription vial tells you how much Azactam to inject and when to inject it. Read the label carefully and follow the directions exactly. If you don't know how to give yourself an intramuscular injection, arrange for a visiting nurse or another skilled person to give it to you.

Inject the drug deeply into a large muscle mass, such as the upper outside part of your buttock or the outside area of your thigh.

To help clear up your infection completely, you must complete the entire course of prescribed Azactam therapy — even if you begin to feel better after a few days.

For this medication to be most effective, it must be administered at evenly spaced times as directed.

What to do if you miss a dose If you miss a dose of your medication, contact your doctor for instructions.

What to do about side effects Tell the doctor *immediately* if you develop pain, swelling, or redness at the injection site.

Stop using this medication and tell the doctor *immediately* if you experience difficulty breathing, wheezing, a tight feeling in your chest, difficulty swallowing, hives, a rash, or itching. These symptoms indicate that you may have an allergic reaction to the drug.

Some common side effects of Azactam include abdominal or stomach cramps, nausea, vomiting, and diarrhea. If these symptoms persist or become severe, notify your doctor.

What you must know about other drugs
Tell your doctor about other medications you're taking. Lasix (furosemide) can raise the amount of Azactam in your blood, as can Benemid, Benn, Probalan, or Robenecid (all forms of probenecid).

Special directions
• Tell your doctor if you have other medical problems, especially liver or kidney disease. Some medical problems can affect your use of Azactam.
• Check with your doctor before you begin taking any new medication — either prescription or nonprescription.
• Contact your doctor if you develop new medical problems while using Azactam.

Azulfidine

Your doctor has prescribed Azulfidine to help treat your bowel condition by reducing inflammation and other symptoms. The generic name for Azulfidine is sulfasalazine.

How to take Azulfidine
Take each dose with a full (8-ounce) glass of water and drink several more glasses of water during the day. This will help prevent certain side effects.

Because Azulfidine may upset an empty stomach, take the drug after meals or with food.

Follow your doctor's directions exactly. Take the entire prescription — even if you feel better after a few days.

What to do if you miss a dose
Take the missed dose as soon as possible. But if it's almost time for your next dose, skip the missed dose and take your next dose as scheduled.

What to do about side effects
Call your doctor *right away* if you develop any of these side effects: aching joints and muscles; continuous headache; skin rash or blisters; red, peeling skin; itching; or difficulty breathing.

Also tell your doctor if you develop nausea, vomiting, diarrhea, dizziness, or increased sensitivity to sunlight.

Because the medication can make you dizzy, don't drive or operate any machinery until you know how you respond to it.

You may notice that the medication turns your urine or skin an orange-yellow color. Don't be concerned. This symptom will disappear after you've finished your medication.

Because Azulfidine may make your skin more sensitive to sunlight, limit your sun exposure while you're taking it.

What you must know about other drugs

Azulfidine may change the way your body responds to other drugs, in particular oral drugs for diabetes, birth control pills, blood thinners, and folic acid. If you're taking any of these medications, let your doctor or pharmacist know.

Special directions

• Tell your doctor if you've ever had an allergic reaction to a sulfa drug, a diuretic (a water pill, such as Lasix), or an oral drug for diabetes. Also mention if you've ever had an allergic reaction to aspirin or to an oral drug for glaucoma.

• Inform your doctor if you have a history of anemia, glucose-6-phosphate dehydrogenase deficiency, urinary or intestinal tract obstruction, kidney or liver disease, severe allergies, asthma, blood disorders, or porphyria.

Important reminder

Don't take this drug if you're pregnant or breast-feeding.

B

Bactocill

Bactocill is used to treat bacterial infections. This drug's generic name is oxacillin. Another brand name is Prostaphlin.

How to take Bactocill

This antibiotic, a form of penicillin, comes in capsules and in an oral solution. Take it exactly as directed. For best results, take Bactocill 1 hour before or 2 hours after meals.

Try to take the doses at evenly spaced times to keep a constant amount of medication in your blood or urine.

Take Bactocill for the full treatment period even after you feel better. If you stop too soon, your infection may return.

What to do if you miss a dose

Take the missed dose as soon as possible. However, if it's almost time for your next dose, adjust your schedule as follows:

If you take two doses daily, space the missed dose and the next dose about 5 hours apart.

If you take three or more doses daily, space the missed dose and the next dose 2 to 4 hours apart.

Then resume your regular dosing schedule.

What to do about side effects

Stop taking Bactocill *at once* and call for emergency medical help if you have symptoms of an allergic reaction. These symptoms include difficulty breathing, light-headedness, fever, chills, a rash, hives, itching, and wheezing.

Check with your doctor if you have diarrhea or other digestive troubles, especially if these side effects persist or become bothersome.

In rare instances, Bactocill may cause seizures. If you experience a seizure, a friend or family member must call for medical help *at once*.

What you must know about other drugs
Tell your doctor if you're taking Benemid (probenecid), a medication for gout, because this medication can increase blood levels of Bactocill.

Special directions
• Tell your doctor about your medical history, especially if you have allergies, bleeding problems, kidney disease, mononucleosis, or stomach or intestinal disease.
• If you're allergic to another form of penicillin, don't use Bactocill.
• If you're allergic to penicillin, carry a medical card or wear a medical bracelet stating this.
• Before you have medical tests done, tell the doctor that you're taking Bactocill; it may affect the test results.

Important reminder
If you're breast-feeding, check with your doctor before using this medication.

Bactrim

Bactrim combats bacterial infections. This drug's generic name is co-trimoxazole. Another brand name is Septra.

How to take Bactrim
Bactrim is available in tablets and in an oral suspension. Take either form with a full glass (8 ounces) of water.

If you have trouble swallowing the *tablet* form, you may crush it and take it with water. If you're taking the *oral suspension*, shake the bottle well first. Use a specially marked spoon or dropper, not a household teaspoon, to measure the correct dose.

Keep taking Bactrim even after you begin to feel better. If you stop too soon, the infection may return.

What to do if you miss a dose
Take the missed dose as soon as possible. However, if it's almost time for your next dose, adjust your schedule as follows:

If you're taking two doses a day, space the skipped dose and the next dose 6 hours apart.

If you're taking three or more doses a day, space the skipped dose and the next dose 2 to 4 hours apart.

Then resume your regular dosing schedule.

What to do about side effects

Get emergency help *at once* if you show signs of an allergic reaction, for example, wheezing, hives, or difficulty breathing.

Stop taking this medication and call your doctor *right away* if you have a persistent fever, a sore throat, or joint pain; feel extremely tired; notice unusual bleeding; or start to bruise easily.

Check with your doctor if you experience skin problems, nausea, vomiting, or diarrhea.

Drink extra water—up to 3 to 4 quarts (3 to 4 liters) daily—to prevent side effects such as kidney stones.

Bactrim may make you more sensitive to sunlight, so try to avoid exposure to direct sunlight while taking it.

What you must know about other drugs

Vitamin C can negate the effects of Bactrim, so avoid taking it while you are on the drug.

Bactrim can increase the effects of some medications, especially blood thinners and certain drugs for diabetes. It can also prevent birth control pills from working well.

Special directions

Tell your doctor about your medical history, especially if you have kidney or liver problems, porphyria, severe allergies, asthma, or AIDS. Also let him know if you're allergic to other sulfa drugs.

Important reminders

If you're pregnant or breast-feeding, talk to your doctor before beginning a course of Bactrim.

If you have diabetes, you may need to change your urine testing procedures while taking Bactrim. Copper sulfate tests may give false-positive results, so you'll need to rely on glucose enzymatic tests such as Clinistix or Tes-Tape.

Bactroban

Bactroban is usually prescribed to treat bacterial infections of the skin such as impetigo. The generic name of this drug is mupirocin.

How to apply
Bactroban

Bactroban comes in an ointment. In Canada, you can buy it without a prescription. If you're treating yourself, read the package instructions carefully to find out how much to use and when to use it.

If your doctor prescribed this medication or gave you special instructions on how to use it, follow his instructions exactly.

The doctor will probably instruct you to apply Bactroban to affected skin areas two or three times daily. Before applying it, clean the affected area with soap and water and dry it thoroughly. Then apply a small amount of the ointment and rub it in gently. You can cover the treated area with a gauze dressing if you wish.

What to do if you
miss a dose

Apply the missed dose as soon as possible. However, if it's almost time for your next dose, skip the missed dose and resume your regular dosage schedule.

What to do about
side effects

This medication may cause a rash, redness, or dryness. You may also notice itching, burning, pain, tenderness, or swelling at the place where you apply it. These side effects usually go away over time as your body adjusts to the medication. But you should check with your doctor if they persist or become bothersome.

Call your doctor if you have any other side effects.

Special directions

• Keep this medication out of your eyes.

• Don't use Bactroban on burns.

• To make sure your infection heals completely, continue to use the medication for the full treatment time prescribed, even if your symptoms disappear. Don't skip any doses.

• However, don't use this medication for a longer period than the doctor prescribes or the package instructions specify.

• Call you doctor or pharmacist if your condition doesn't improve within 3 to 5 days, or if it gets worse.

Beconase

This nasal aerosol or spray helps relieve the stuffy nose and irritation related to hay fever, other allergies, and other nasal problems. It also helps prevent nasal polyps from growing back after they've been surgically removed. Beconase's generic name is beclomethasone. Another brand name is Vancenase.

Beclomethasone also comes in an aerosol form for oral inhalation. It's known by the brand names Beclovent and Vanceril. The oral inhalant helps prevent asthma attacks. It cannot relieve an asthma attack that has already started.

How to take Beconase

Before using your medication, read the directions that come with the container. Follow them exactly. If you don't understand the directions or aren't sure how to use the medication, check with your doctor or pharmacist.

For this medication to work, you must take it every day at regular intervals as your doctor prescribes. Up to 4 weeks may pass before you feel the medication's full effects.

What to do if you miss a dose

Take the missed dose as soon as you remember. But if it's almost time for your next dose, skip the missed dose and resume your normal dosing schedule. Don't take a double dose.

What to do about side effects

Beconase may cause mild, transient nasal burning and stinging. If this persists or becomes severe, contact your doctor.

Special directions

• Tell your doctor if you have other medical problems, particularly lung disease or infections of the mouth, nose, sinuses, throat, or lungs.

For the *nasal* form:

• If you're taking Beconase for more than a few weeks, see your doctor regularly.

• Check with your doctor if you develop signs of a nasal, sinus, or throat infection; if your symptoms don't improve within 3 weeks; or if your condition worsens.

For the *oral* form:

• Notify your doctor if you experience unusual stress; if you have an asthma attack that doesn't improve after you take a bronchodilator; if signs of mouth, throat, or lung infection occur; if your symptoms don't improve; or if your condition worsens.

• Carry a medical card stating that you're taking Beclovent and may need additional medication in an emergency situation, during a severe asthma attack or other illness, or when you're under unusual stress.

• Before surgery (including dental surgery) or emergency treatment, tell the doctor or dentist that you're taking Beclovent.

• If you're using a bronchodilator inhalation aerosol (Proventil, for example) in conjunction with the Beclovent aerosol, use the bronchodilator first and then wait about 5 minutes before taking Beclovent unless your doctor gives you other instructions.

Benadryl

Benadryl is used to relieve symptoms of hay fever, stuffy nose, insomnia, motion sickness, nonproductive cough, and other conditions. The drug's generic name is diphenhydramine. It has more than 45 other brand names.

How to take Benadryl

Benadryl is available without a prescription in the form of capsules, tablets, elixir, and syrup. Check the medication label carefully, and follow the directions exactly. You may take your dose with food or a glass of milk or water to lessen stomach irritation.

If you're taking Benadryl to prevent motion sickness, take it at least 1 to 2 hours before traveling. If that's not possible, take it at least 30 minutes before departing.

What to do if you miss a dose

If you're taking this medication regularly and you miss a dose, take the missed dose as soon as possible. However, if it's almost time for your next dose, skip the missed dose and take your next dose on schedule. Don't take a double dose.

What to do about side effects

While taking this medication, you may feel drowsy or nauseated or experience dry mouth. Check with your doctor if these side effects bother you or become severe.

To relieve dry mouth or throat symptoms, try sugarless hard candy or gum, ice chips, or a saliva substitute.

What you must know about alcohol and other drugs

Avoid drinking alcoholic beverages while taking Benadryl; the combination may make you overly drowsy.

For the same reason, avoid simultaneous use of other medications that slow down the nervous system, including narcotic painkillers, tranquilizers, and many cold and flu remedies.

If you take certain antidepressants, your doctor may advise against taking Benadryl because of the increased risk of unwanted side effects.

If you regularly take large doses of aspirin for arthritis, be aware that Benadryl can cover up signs of aspirin overdose such as ringing in your ears.

Special directions

• Tell your doctor if you have other medical problems, especially asthma, glaucoma, bladder conditions, heart disease, high blood pressure, or an overactive thyroid gland.

• Before you schedule skin tests for allergies, let the doctor know you're taking Benadryl. The drug may affect test results.

• Make sure you know how you react to this medication before you drive or perform other tasks that require you to be fully alert.

Important reminders

If you're pregnant or breast-feeding, check with your doctor before taking Benadryl.

Children and older adults are especially vulnerable to side effects from this medication.

Bentyl

Your doctor has prescribed Bentyl to relieve your digestive cramps or spasms. The drug is often used in treating stomach ulcers. Its generic name is dicyclomine.

How to take Bentyl   Bentyl comes in capsule, syrup, and tablet forms. Read the instructions on the prescription label carefully and follow them exactly. Take this medication 30 minutes to 1 hour before meals, unless your doctor directs otherwise.

If you're taking Bentyl in the *capsule* form, don't break, chew, or crush it; swallow it whole.

Check with your doctor before you stop using Bentyl; he or she may want to reduce your dosage gradually to prevent unwanted effects.

What to do if you miss a dose   Take the missed dose as soon as possible. But if it's almost time for your next dose, skip the missed dose and take your next dose on schedule. Don't take a double dose.

What to do about side effects   Check with your doctor if you have any of the following side effects: headache, dizziness, palpitations, constipation, difficulty urinating, or impotence.

If this medication makes your mouth feel dry, use sugarless hard candy or gum, ice chips, or a saliva substitute. If the dryness lasts for more than 2 weeks, check with your doctor or dentist.

What you must know about other drugs   Don't take Bentyl within 2 to 3 hours of taking antacids or diarrhea medication; these medications may make Bentyl ineffective.

Special directions   • Tell your doctor if you have other medical problems, especially gastrointestinal, heart, liver, or kidney disease; glaucoma; or an overactive thyroid gland. Also mention if you have a history of urinary problems.

• Because you may not sweat as much while taking Bentyl, your body temperature may increase. Hot baths or saunas will make you dizzy or faint. To prevent heat stroke, take care not to become too hot during exercise or in hot weather.

• Make sure you know how you react to Bentyl before you drive or perform other tasks that require you to be fully alert.

Important reminders   If you're pregnant or breast-feeding, check with your doctor before taking this medication.

If you're an older adult, realize that you may be especially vulnerable to this drug's side effects.

Betapace

Your doctor has prescribed Betapace to help steady your irregular heartbeat. This drug's generic name is sotalol.

How to take Betapace

Betapace comes as a tablet. Take this medication on an empty stomach 1 hour before or 2 hours after a meal. Carefully follow the label directions.

Be sure to take all of the medication, even if you feel well. And don't stop taking this drug suddenly.

What to do if you miss a dose

Take the missed dose as soon as you remember. If it's almost time for your next dose, skip the missed dose, and return to your regular schedule. Don't take a double dose.

What to do about side effects

Betapace may make you feel dizzy, weak, or tired and may give you a headache. It can also cause irregular heartbeat and other heart problems such as congestive heart failure. You may experience nausea, vomiting, or diarrhea as well as chest pain or difficulty breathing. If any of these side effects persists or becomes severe, call your doctor.

What you must know about other drugs

Inform your doctor if you're taking other medications to control your heartbeat or to control your blood pressure, such as Sandril (reserpine) or Ismelin (guanethidine). Calcium channel antagonists, such as Calan (verapamil), shouldn't be taken with Betapace. Tell your doctor if you're taking Catapres (clonidine). If you're told to stop taking Catapres, your dosage of Betapace should be stopped first.

If you take insulin or oral diabetes drugs, the dosage may need to be adjusted because Betapace may increase blood sugar.

Special directions
• Tell the doctor if you have asthma or any other heart problems such as congestive heart failure. Also inform him if you have kidney problems or diabetes.
• Be aware that Betapace may mask symptoms of low blood sugar and may affect liver test results.
• Keep in mind that you may have to be hospitalized when you start taking Betapace (and again if your dosage is adjusted) so that your heart can be monitored.
• Your doctor will probably check your blood regularly (especially if you take a diuretic, or water pill) to make sure that the levels of minerals and salts (electrolytes) in your blood remain normal.

Important reminders
Tell your doctor if you're pregnant and discuss whether you should stop taking Betapace if you plan to breastfeed.

Bicillin

Bicillin treats bacterial infections. This drug's generic name is penicillin G. Another brand name is Pfizerpen.

How to take Bicillin
Bicillin comes in both tablet and oral liquid forms. Take it exactly as your doctor directs.
If you're taking the *tablets*, don't drink acidic beverages, such as fruit juices, within 1 hour of taking a dose.
If you're taking the *oral liquid*, use a specially marked measuring spoon (not a household teaspoon) or dropper to measure each dose.
Try to take your medication at evenly spaced times, day and night. Continue to take it as directed, even if you start to feel better. If you stop too soon, your infection may return.

What to do if you miss a dose
Take the missed dose as soon as possible. But if it's almost time for your next dose, follow these guidelines:
If you take two doses a day, space the missed dose and the next dose 5 to 6 hours apart.
If you take three or more doses a day, space the missed dose and the next dose 2 to 4 hours apart.
Then resume your regular dosing schedule.

What to do about side effects Call for emergency help *at once* if you have an allergic reaction to Bicillin. Symptoms include difficulty breathing, light-headedness, a rash, hives, itching, or wheezing.

Call the doctor *right away* if you have severe abdominal or stomach cramps, bloody or decreased urine, seizures, severe diarrhea, fever, joint pain, sore throat, or unusual bleeding or bruising.

Check with your doctor if Bicillin causes mild diarrhea, nausea, vomiting, or sore mouth or tongue.

What you must know about other drugs Tell the doctor about any other medications you're taking. Benemid (probenecid), a gout medication, may increase the level of Bicillin in your blood.

Check with your doctor before taking diarrhea medication; severe diarrhea may be a sign of a serious side effect.

Special directions • Tell your doctor if you have other medical problems, especially asthma, bleeding disorders, mononucleosis, or kidney, stomach, or intestinal disease. Also mention if you're allergic to penicillin or to any other medication.
• Before you have medical tests done, tell the doctor you're taking Bicillin; it may affect the test results.
• If you're allergic to penicillin, your doctor may want you to carry a medical card or wear a bracelet stating this.

Important reminder If you're breast-feeding, check with your doctor before using this medication.

Bleph-10

Bleph-10 is prescribed to treat eye infections. This drug's generic name is sulfacetamide. Another brand name is Cetamide.

How to use Bleph-10 This drug comes in two forms: eyedrops and eye ointment.

If you're using Bleph-10 *eyedrops,* follow these steps: First wash your hands. Then tilt your head back and pull your lower eyelid away from your eye to form a pouch. Squeeze the prescribed amount of medication into the pouch (without letting the applicator touch your eye). Close your eye gently and hold it closed for 1 to 2 minutes. Don't blink. If you think you didn't get the drops into your eye properly, repeat the process.

If you're using Bleph-10 *eye ointment*, follow these steps: Wash your hands; then pull your lower eyelid away from your eye to form a pouch. Now squeeze a thin strip of ointment, about ½ to 1 inch (1 to 2.5 centimeters) long, into the pouch (without letting the applicator touch your eye). Close your eye gently and keep it closed for 1 to 2 minutes.

After you finish using the medication, wash your hands again.

Use all of the medication prescribed by your doctor, even if your symptoms subside after a few days.

What to do if you miss a dose

Take the missed dose as soon as possible. However, if it's almost time for your next dose, skip the missed dose and take the next dose on schedule.

What to do about side effects

You may notice that your eyes sting or burn for a few minutes after you use the drops or ointment. This is to be expected. Also expect your vision to blur briefly after applying eye ointment.

You may be sensitive to the medication, in which case your eyelids may swell, itch, and burn constantly. If this happens, notify your doctor.

Also call your doctor if you develop a rash, if blisters form in your mouth or on your eyelids, or if your skin turns red and starts to peel.

What you must know about other drugs

Bleph-10 is not compatible with any type of silver eye preparation, such as silver nitrate or a mild silver protein for the eye. If you're using such a product, let your doctor or pharmacist know.

Special directions

• Tell your doctor if you've ever had an allergic reaction to any type of sulfa medication.
• Don't share your medication with anyone. If someone in your family develops the same symptoms you have, call your doctor.

Brethaire

Intended to help treat your breathing problem, Brethaire is available in oral and aerosol forms. This medication opens the air passages in your lungs, which will help you breathe easier. The generic name for this drug is terbutaline. Another brand name is Brethine.

How to take Brethaire

If you are taking the *oral* form of the medication, follow your doctor's instructions exactly.

If you are taking the *aerosol* form, follow these steps: Blow your nose and clear your throat. Breathe out, emptying your lungs as much as possible. Hold the medication canister in an upright position. Place the mouthpiece well inside your mouth and close your lips around it. Press down on the top of the medication canister. At the same time, breathe in deeply. Hold your breath for several seconds. Remove the mouthpiece from your mouth and breathe out slowly.

If your doctor has ordered more than one inhalation, wait at least 2 minutes before taking the second dose. Never use the inhaler more than twice in a row.

What to do if you miss a dose

If you're using Brethaire regularly, take your missed dose as soon as you remember it. Then take any remaining doses that day at regularly spaced intervals. Don't take two doses at once.

What to do about side effects

If your wheezing gets worse or your breathing becomes more difficult after you take Brethaire, stop the drug and call your doctor *immediately.*

You may feel nervous, develop a tremor, or get a headache while taking this medication. These symptoms are common, but if they become bothersome, call your doctor.

What you must know about other drugs

Don't take Brethaire with a monoamine oxidase (MAO) inhibitor (a type of antidepressant). The combination could cause severe high blood pressure.

If you're taking Tenormin or Lopressor (beta blockers, used to treat some heart conditions), tell your doctor or pharmacist. These medications could keep Brethaire from working properly.

Also tell your doctor if you're taking a digitalis glycoside, a heart medication.

Special directions Because Brethaire can make certain medical problems worse, make sure your doctor is aware of any history of seizures, brain damage, diabetes, mental illness, heart disease, high blood pressure, an overactive thyroid, or Parkinson's disease.

Important reminder If you're an athlete, you should know that the U.S. Olympic Committee bans and tests for the oral form of terbutaline. However, Olympic athletes are permitted to use aerosol or inhalation forms of the drug.

Bronkosol

Bronkosol is prescribed to relieve the symptoms of asthma, bronchitis, and emphysema and to prevent the wheezing and troubled breathing caused by exercising. This drug's generic name is isoetharine.

How to take
Bronkosol Bronkosol comes as an aerosol spray and as a solution used in a nebulizer. Take it exactly as prescribed. Overuse can cause serious side effects or decrease the medication's effectiveness.

To use the *aerosol spray,* first clear your nose and throat. Then breathe out, exhaling as much air as you can. Put the mouthpiece in your mouth, release the spray, and inhale deeply. Hold your breath for a few seconds; then remove the mouthpiece and exhale slowly.

Wait 1 to 2 minutes before using it again. You may not need another spray.

If you're taking a second inhaled medication in conjunction with Bronkosol, take the Bronkosol first and wait 5 minutes before taking the other medication.

If you're using the *solution form in a nebulizer,* follow your doctor's, nurse's, or pharmacist's instructions exactly.

What to do if you miss a dose

Take the missed dose as soon as you can. Then space out the day's remaining doses evenly. Never take a double dose.

What to do about side effects

If you think you may have taken an overdose or if you develop symptoms of an overdose, such as chest pain, seizures, chills, fever, severe muscle cramps, nausea, vomiting, fast or slow heartbeat, shortness of breath, or severe trembling or weakness, seek emergency care *immediately.*

Also seek emergency care if your skin develops a bluish color and you experience severe dizziness, continuous facial flushing, increased difficulty breathing, a rash, and swelling of your face or eyelids.

Bronkosol may cause tremor, headache, or rapid or pounding heartbeat. These side effects should disappear after you use the medication for a while. If they don't, tell your doctor.

What you must know about other drugs

Tell your doctor about any other prescription and nonprescription medications you're taking, especially beta blockers, such as propranolol, atenolol, metoprolol, or nadolol.

Special directions

• Tell your doctor if you have other medical problems. They may affect the use of this medication.
• Don't use medication that's cloudy or discolored.
• If you don't breathe easier after using Bronkosol, call your doctor immediately.
• Avoid caffeine-containing food and drink, such as coffee, tea, cola, and chocolate.

Important reminders

If you're pregnant or think you may be or if you're breast-feeding, check with your doctor before taking Bronkosol.

If you're an athlete, be aware that the U.S. Olympic Committee bans and tests for isoetharine.

Bumex

Bumex stimulates urination and reduces water in your body. The drug's generic name is bumetanide.

How to take Bumex Read your medication label carefully and follow the directions exactly. So that the urge to urinate doesn't interrupt your sleep, take your single daily dose in the morning after breakfast. If you're taking more than one dose a day, take the last dose before 6 p.m. unless the doctor advises you differently.

What to do if you miss a dose Take the missed dose as soon as you remember, unless it's almost time for your next dose. Then you should skip the dose you missed and resume your normal dosing schedule. Don't take a double dose.

What to do about side effects Common side effects include fatigue, dizziness, light-headedness, and fainting. If these symptoms persist or become severe, contact your doctor.

To help relieve dizziness or light-headedness, get up slowly from a bed or chair, limit the amount of alcoholic beverages you drink, and take care not to get overheated. If the problem persists or worsens, tell your doctor.

Because Bumex can reduce electrolytes needed by your body (such as potassium, chloride, sodium, calcium, and magnesium), have your blood tested regularly while you are taking it.

To replace lost potassium, eat foods and drink beverages containing potassium (for example, citrus fruits and orange juice) or take a potassium supplement or another medication prescribed by your doctor to minimize potassium loss.

To prevent excessive water and potassium loss, call your doctor if you experience persistent vomiting or diarrhea.

What you must know about other drugs Tell your doctor about other medications you're taking. Taking Bumex with certain antibiotics can increase your risk of hearing problems. Taking it with Probalan (probenecid), Indocin (indomethacin), and some pain relievers may decrease its effects.

Special directions • Before taking Bumex, let your doctor know of any other medical problems you might have.

• Before surgery (including dental surgery) or emergency treatment, inform the doctor or dentist that you're taking Bumex.

Important reminders If you have diabetes, check your blood sugar levels carefully and notify your doctor of any changes.

If you become pregnant while taking Bumex, tell your doctor promptly.

Older adults are especially sensitive to this medication and prone to side effects.

If you're an athlete, be aware that the National Collegiate Athletic Association and the U.S. Olympic Committee ban and test for bumetanide.

BuSpar

BuSpar is used to treat certain anxiety disorders and to relieve anxiety symptoms. Its generic name is buspirone.

How to take BuSpar Read your medication label carefully and follow the directions exactly. You may not feel the drug's full effects until 1 to 2 weeks after you begin taking it.

What to do if you miss a dose Take the missed dose as soon as you remember. But if it's almost time for your next dose, skip the dose you missed and resume your regular dosing schedule. Never take a double dose.

What to do about side effects Common side effects include drowsiness and dizziness. If these symptoms persist or worsen, notify your doctor.

What you must know about alcohol and other drugs Tell your doctor about other medications you're taking. BuSpar can cause drowsiness when taken with alcoholic beverages and other central nervous system depressants, such as sleeping pills, some cold or allergy medications, and tranquilizers. When taken with monoamine oxidase (MAO) inhibitors, such as Marplan (isocarboxazid), BuSpar can raise your blood pressure.

Special directions • Inform your doctor about your medical history, especially of any drug abuse or dependency or of kidney or liver disease. These and other medical problems may affect the use of BuSpar.

• If you're taking this medication regularly for a long time, schedule regular checkups to monitor your progress and the drug's side effects.

• Make sure you know how you react to this medication before you drive, operate machinery, or perform other activities that require you to be well coordinated and alert.

• If you think you may have taken an overdose of BuSpar, get emergency help at once.

Important reminder If you're an athlete, be aware that the National Collegiate Athletic Association and the U.S. Olympic Committee ban the use of buspirone in certain competitions.

C

Cafergot

The doctor has prescribed this combination medication to relieve your headaches. It contains ergotamine, which narrows your blood vessels, and caffeine, which helps ergotamine to be absorbed by the body. Another brand name for this combination is Wigraine.

How to take Cafergot

This medication is available in tablet and suppository forms. Carefully read the label on your medication bottle and follow the directions exactly. Use no more than 6 tablets or 2 suppositories for each attack or 10 tablets or 5 suppositories a week. If your headache isn't relieved, call your doctor. Don't increase the dose.

For best results, take Cafergot at the first sign of a headache. Rest in a dark, quiet room for about 2 hours after taking it.

To use the *suppository* form, remove the foil wrapper and moisten it with cold water. Lie on your side and use your middle or index finger to push the suppository into your rectum. If the suppository is too soft to insert, place it in the refrigerator for 30 minutes before removing the foil wrapper.

If you have been using Cafergot regularly, don't stop it abruptly. Doing so may increase the frequency and duration of headaches. Your doctor may want to reduce the dosage gradually.

What you must know about alcohol and other drugs

Avoid drinking alcoholic beverages because they can worsen your headache.

Don't use Cafergot if you're also taking a beta blocker such as Inderal (propranolol). This combination may be hazardous because it could cause excessive narrowing of the blood vessels.

Special directions

• Tell your doctor if you have other medical problems, especially diseases of the blood vessels, kidney, or liver.

Also tell your doctor if you have high blood pressure or severe skin itching.

• Cafergot may make you sensitive to cold temperatures. Wear warm clothes during cold weather, and be careful if you participate in winter activities that prolong your exposure to cold.

Important reminders   If you're pregnant or breast-feeding, don't take this medication.

If you're an older adult, you may be especially prone to side effects from ergotamine with caffeine.

If you're an athlete, you should know that high levels of caffeine are banned and sometimes tested for by the National Collegiate Athletic Association and the U.S. Olympic Committee.

Calan

This drug helps relieve chest pain, heart irregularities, and high blood pressure. Calan's generic name is verapamil. Other brand names include Isoptin and Verelan.

How to take Calan   Take Calan only as your doctor directs. If you're taking an *extended-release tablet*, swallow it whole, without crushing or chewing it.

Take Calan on an empty stomach. Taking extended-release tablets with food may decrease your body's ability to absorb the drug.

Take your medication even if you feel well. Stopping suddenly could cause your condition to worsen.

What to do if you miss a dose   Take the missed dose as soon as possible. However, if it's almost time for your next dose, skip the missed dose and take your next dose as scheduled.

What to do about side effects   Call your doctor *immediately* if you develop any of these side effects: breathing difficulty, coughing, or wheezing; irregular or rapid, pounding heartbeat; or swelling of the ankles, feet, or lower legs.

Also notify your doctor if you become constipated or faint, feel unusually tired, or continue to have chest pain.

Eat foods high in fiber and be sure to drink plenty of fluids (unless your doctor tells you otherwise) to help prevent constipation.

If fatigue is a problem, remember to allow yourself several rest periods during the day.

What you must know about other drugs
Some medications may affect how Calan works. At the same time, Calan may interfere with another drug's actions. Therefore, be sure to tell your doctor about any medications you're taking, particularly Eskalith (lithium) or heart medications, or medications for high blood pressure, seizures, tuberculosis, or glaucoma.

Special directions
Because Calan may cause certain medical conditions to worsen, tell your doctor if you have a history of kidney or liver disease or some other heart or blood vessel disorder.

Important reminder
If you're pregnant or breast-feeding, check with your doctor before taking Calan.

Calcium supplements

Your body needs calcium to keep your bones and teeth strong, to prevent excessive bleeding, and to keep your muscles, brain, and nerves functioning well. If your doctor recommends a nonprescription calcium supplement for you, here are some guidelines you need to know.

Choosing a supplement
• Read the bottle label to learn how much *elemental calcium* the supplement contains. Elemental calcium is the amount that's actually used by your body.
• Different supplements contain different amounts of elemental calcium. For example, calcium carbonate products, such as Caltrate 600, Os-Cal 500, Biocal, oyster shell calcium, and antacids (such as Tums), contain the most elemental calcium—about 40%.
• Other calcium products contain less: dibasic calcium phosphate (about 36%), tribasic calcium phosphate (about 29%), calcium citrate (about 24%), calcium lactate (about 13%), and calcium gluconate (about 9%).

• Don't take calcium supplements containing dolomite or bone meal. They may contain lead and cause lead poisoning.

• Calcium carbonate supplements may cause stomach pain due to gas and constipation. To relieve this pain, drink more liquids, such as juice or water, or eat more foods that are liquids at room temperature, such as ice cream, gelatin, or pudding. Eating more high-fiber foods, such as bran cereal or whole-wheat crackers, may also help. Just be sure to eat them between meals—extra fiber with meals interferes with your body's absorption of calcium.

Other calcium sources   Besides taking a calcium supplement, try to include calcium-rich foods in your daily diet. Good sources of calcium include collards, turnip greens, broccoli, dried peas and beans, sardines, salmon, tofu, and dairy products (milk, cheese, yogurt, and ice cream). Choose low-fat dairy products because they're lower in cholesterol.

If you have trouble digesting milk, most large grocery stores carry lactose-reduced milk or acidophilus milk. Or ask your pharmacist about products that can be added to milk to make it easier to digest.

More tips   These additional suggestions will help you get the most from the calcium you eat and take in vitamin form:

• Consume less red meat, chocolate, peanut butter, rhubarb, sweet potatoes, fatty foods, and caffeine-containing drinks.

• Calcium is most effective when your body has enough vitamin D. Spending just 15 minutes in sunshine every day will fill your daily requirement. Vitamin D is also present in egg yolks, saltwater fish, liver, and vitamin-fortified milk and cereals. But don't take vitamin D supplements unless your doctor prescribes them—too much of this vitamin can be harmful.

Capoten

Capoten helps control high blood pressure and congestive heart failure. This drug's generic name is captopril.

How to take Capoten   Carefully follow the label directions. Take Capoten 1 hour before meals unless your doctor directs otherwise.

What to do if you miss a dose   Take the missed dose as soon as you remember. But if it's almost time for your next scheduled dose, skip the dose you missed and take your next dose at the scheduled time. Don't take a double dose.

What to do about side effects   Contact your doctor *immediately* and stop taking this medication if you have a fever, chills, hoarseness, or sudden trouble swallowing or breathing or if your face, mouth, hands, or feet swell. These symptoms may indicate an allergic reaction.

A common side effect is a dry, continuing cough. If it persists or worsens, notify your doctor.

Dizziness, light-headedness, or even fainting may follow the first dose of this medication, especially if you have been taking a diuretic (water pill). These side effects may also follow heavy sweating, which depletes body water and lowers blood pressure. Avoid becoming overheated.

What you must know about other drugs   Tell the doctor about other medications you're taking. Some antacids and analgesics may decrease Capoten's effectiveness. Capoten taken with Lanoxin (digoxin) can increase the risk of toxic effects. And taking potassium supplements with Capoten increases your risk for having too much potassium.

Special directions   • See your doctor regularly to monitor Capoten's effectiveness and to check for side effects.

• Don't stop taking this medication on your own, even if you feel better. Although high blood pressure may not produce symptoms, you may still need ongoing treatment.

• Remember to follow any prescribed special diet that will help this medication lower your blood pressure.

• Don't take new medications (prescription or nonprescription) without first consulting your doctor.

• Notify your doctor promptly if you become sick while taking this medication, especially if you have severe or continuing vomiting or diarrhea, which can cause rapid body water loss and low blood pressure.

• Before medical tests, surgery (including dental surgery), or emergency treatment, tell the doctor or dentist that you're taking Capoten.

Important reminders   If you become pregnant while taking Capoten, tell your doctor, who may change your prescription to another blood pressure medication. If you're breast-feeding, discuss the use of Capoten with your doctor.

Carafate

Your doctor has prescribed Carafate to treat your stomach ulcer. This medication works by forming a barrier over your ulcer. This protects the ulcer from stomach acid and allows it to heal. This drug's generic name is sucralfate.

How to take Carafate   Take Carafate 1 hour before meals and at bedtime because Carafate works best on an empty stomach. For this reason, take the medication only with water.

If you have difficulty swallowing, try placing the Carafate tablet in an ounce of water. Let the tablet sit in the water at room temperature until it dissolves. Then drink the fluid.

Make sure that you continue taking the medication for as long as your doctor has prescribed, even after you've begun to feel better.

What to do if you miss a dose   Take the missed dose as soon as possible. But if it's almost time for your next dose, skip the missed dose and take the next one at the regular time. Don't take a double dose.

What to do about side effects   You may become constipated while you're taking this drug. If you do, call your doctor, who may prescribe a laxative to relieve the problem.

What you must know about other drugs   Antacids can keep Carafate from working properly, so don't take an antacid for a half hour before a scheduled dose of Carafate. Then, after taking a dose of Carafate, wait another half hour before you take an antacid.

Also, because Carafate can interfere with the way some other drugs work, check with your doctor or pharmacist if you're taking any other drugs while taking Carafate. In particular, be sure to tell your doctor if you're taking an antibiotic.

Special directions

• If you have a history of kidney failure or an intestinal obstruction, let your doctor know. He or she may want to change your medication.

• While you're taking Carafate, avoid activities that could worsen your condition. For example, don't smoke because smoking increases the production of acid in your stomach and could worsen your stomach ulcer. Also, don't drink alcoholic beverages, take aspirin, or eat foods that irritate your stomach.

• Store your medication in a cool, dry place—not in your bathroom medicine cabinet or near the kitchen sink. Protect the medication from direct light, and don't put it in the refrigerator.

• Don't take this medication for more than 8 weeks.

Important reminder

If you're pregnant or breast-feeding, check with your doctor before taking this medication.

Cardioquin

This medication is used to correct an irregular heartbeat or to slow an overactive heart. Cardioquin's generic name is quinidine. Other brand names include Quinaglute and Quinamm.

How to take Cardioquin

Cardioquin comes in the form of capsules, tablets, and extended-release tablets. Follow your doctor's directions for taking this medication exactly, even if you feel well.

To make sure your medication is well absorbed, take your dose with a full glass (8 ounces) of water on an empty stomach 1 hour before or 2 hours after meals. However, if you have an upset stomach, your doctor may want you to take your dose with food or milk.

If you're taking the *extended-release tablets*, swallow them whole—don't chew, crush, or break them.

Don't stop taking Cardioquin without first checking with your doctor.

What to do if you miss a dose

If you remember the missed dose within 2 hours, take it as soon as possible. However, if you don't remember until later, skip the missed dose and take your next dose on schedule. Don't take a double dose.

What to do about side effects

Call your doctor *at once* if you have blurred vision or other vision changes; dizziness, light-headedness, or fainting; fever; severe headache; hearing changes, such as buzzing in the ears; or wheezing, shortness of breath, or trouble breathing.

Check with your doctor if Cardioquin causes nausea, vomiting, or diarrhea.

What you must know about other drugs

Tell your doctor if you're taking other medications. Also check with him before you take new medications. In particular, your doctor needs to know if you use blood thinners, other heart medications, sedatives, seizure medications (for example, barbiturates), antacids, the ulcer drug Tagamet (cimetidine), and medications that make the urine less acidic such as Diamox (acetazolamide).

Special directions

• Tell your doctor if you have other medical problems, especially asthma, emphysema, blood diseases, myasthenia gravis, an overactive thyroid, psoriasis, and kidney or liver disease. Other medical problems may affect the use of this medication.

• Keep all appointments for follow-up visits so your doctor can check your progress.

• Before having surgery (including dental surgery), tell the doctor or dentist that you're taking Cardioquin.

Important reminder

If you're pregnant, check with your doctor before using Cardioquin.

Cardizem

This medication is used to relieve and control angina (chest pain) and high blood pressure. Cardizem's generic name is diltiazem. Another brand name is Dilacor.

Cardizem comes in both tablet form and sustained-release capsules. If you're taking the *sustained-release capsules,* the label may read Cardizem CD or Cardizem SR.

How to take Cardizem

Carefully follow the label directions.

If you're taking the *capsule* form, don't crush or chew it—swallow it whole.

If you're taking Cardizem regularly for several weeks, don't suddenly stop taking it. Your doctor may want to reduce your dose gradually before you stop completely.

If you have high blood pressure, you may not notice any symptoms of this disorder. Even so, it's essential that you take Cardizem exactly as directed.

What to do if you miss a dose

Take the missed dose as soon as possible. However, if it's almost time for your next dose, skip the missed dose and take your next dose on schedule. Don't take a double dose.

What to do about side effects

Check with your doctor if you feel nauseated, tired, or drowsy or have a headache or an irregular heartbeat. Also call if your feet and ankles become swollen or if you suddenly gain weight unexpectedly (more than 3 pounds [1.36 kilograms] in 1 week).

What you must know about other drugs

Tell your doctor about other medications you're taking, so harmful interactions can be avoided. For example, taking Cardizem with the ulcer medication Tagamet (cimetidine) can lead to toxic effects. If you take Lanoxin (digoxin) for a heart condition, Cardizem may cause an unwanted buildup of digoxin. Taking Inderal (propranolol) or other beta blockers (for high blood pressure) with Cardizem could lead to heart problems.

Special directions

• Tell your doctor if you have other medical problems, especially severe high blood pressure, heart disease, or a liver or kidney condition.

• Keep appointments for doctor's visits so your doctor can check your progress and adjust your dosage, if needed.

• Talk to your doctor about how to exercise safely, without overdoing it, to improve your condition.

• Ask your doctor how to measure your pulse rate. While you're taking Cardizem, check your pulse rate regularly. If it's much slower than your usual rate or less than 50 beats per minute, check with your doctor. A pulse rate that is too slow may cause circulation problems.

Important reminders If you're pregnant or breast-feeding, check with your doctor before using this medication. If you're an older adult, be aware that you may be especially sensitive to side effects from Cardizem.

Cardura

Cardura is prescribed to treat high blood pressure. The drug's generic name is doxazosin.

How to take Cardura This medication comes in tablet form. Carefully follow the label directions.

What to do if you miss a dose Take the missed dose as soon as you remember. However, if it's almost time for your next dose, skip the missed dose and resume your regular dosing schedule. Don't take a double dose.

What to do about side effects This medication may lower your blood pressure, causing you to feel dizzy, light-headed, or faint when you get up from a sitting or lying position. To reduce this problem try to get up slowly. Usually, this effect diminishes after the first dose, but it may recur if you stop taking your medication for a few days or if your dosage is adjusted. If this problem persists or becomes severe, call your doctor.

Check with your doctor if Cardura makes you feel sleepy or gives you a headache. Also call if you develop a rash, muscle or joint pain, or an irregular heartbeat.

Because Cardura can make you dizzy, make sure you know how you react to it before you drive, use machines, or perform other activities that could be dangerous if you're not fully alert.

What you must know about other drugs

Don't take Cardura with other medications to treat high blood pressure unless your doctor has directed you to do so. Taking this combination of medications may cause dangerously low blood pressure, possibly leading to loss of consciousness.

Special directions

• Tell your doctor if you have other medical problems, especially liver disease.

• Keep appointments for doctor's visits. You'll need to see your doctor at least every 2 weeks until your dosage is set properly, then at regular intervals so your progress can be checked.

• Your doctor may teach you how to take your blood pressure at home. If so, check your blood pressure at regular intervals and call your doctor if you detect any significant changes.

Important reminder

If you're pregnant or breast-feeding, check with your doctor before taking this medication.

Catapres

Catapres is designed to lower your high blood pressure. This drug's generic name is clonidine.

How to take Catapres

Catapres comes in tablet form and also as a patch. If you're taking the *tablets,* take them at the same times each day. Even if you feel well, continue to take Catapres exactly as directed.

If you're using the *skin patch,* apply it to a clean, dry, hairless area on your upper arm or chest. Change the patch every 7 days or as often as your doctor orders. Place the patch at a different site every week to prevent skin irritation. Be sure to read the instructions that come with the patches.

What to do if you miss a dose

Take the missed dose as soon as you remember. Then go back to your regular dosing schedule.

If you miss two or more tablet doses consecutively or if you miss changing the skin patch for 3 or more days, check with your doctor right away. If you go too long without Catapres, your blood pressure may rise, possibly causing unpleasant effects.

What to do about side effects

Call your doctor *at once* if you experience a severe headache, visual changes, or extreme dizziness. Also check with your doctor if you become drowsy or constipated or your mouth feels dry.

If you're using the skin patch, you may experience itching or a rash. If these symptoms persist or become severe, call your doctor.

Because Catapres may make you drowsy, make sure you know how you react to it before you drive, use machines, or perform other hazardous activities that require alertness.

What you must know about alcohol and other drugs

Don't drink alcoholic beverages, except in amounts permitted by your doctor, while taking Catapres because the combination may cause oversedation. Similarly, central nervous system depressants, such as sleeping pills and tranquilizers, may cause oversedation when used with Catapres.

If you're taking Catapres with Inderal (propranolol) or other drugs called beta blockers, these medications may raise your blood pressure when taken together. Also, Catapres may not work properly when taken with certain antidepressants.

Special directions

• Tell your doctor if you have other medical problems, especially heart or kidney disease, diabetes, or depression.
• Keep all appointments for follow-up visits so your doctor can check your progress.
• If you're using the skin patch, keep it on while showering, bathing, or swimming. If it loosens, cover it with the extra adhesive provided.

Important reminders

If you're pregnant or breast-feeding, check with your doctor before taking this medication. If you're an older adult, realize that Catapres may make you dizzy or faint. Take care to prevent falls.

Ceclor

Ceclor is used to treat infections caused by bacteria. This drug's generic name is cefaclor.

How to take Ceclor This drug comes in capsule and liquid forms. Carefully follow the label directions.

Take your daily doses at evenly spaced times over 24 hours as your doctor prescribes. If this medication upsets your stomach, you may take it with food.

If you're taking the *liquid*, shake the bottle well. Then use a medicine dropper or a measuring spoon to pour each dose accurately.

To help clear up your infection completely, take the medication for the full course of treatment, even if you begin to feel better after a few days. If you stop taking it too soon, your infection may recur.

What to do if you miss a dose If you forget to take your medication and your dosing schedule is one dose a day, space the missed dose and the next scheduled dose 10 to 12 hours apart. If you're taking two doses a day, space the missed dose and the next dose 5 to 6 hours apart. If you're taking three or more doses a day, space the missed dose and the next dose 2 to 4 hours apart. After taking the dose you missed, resume your normal dosing schedule.

What to do about side effects Common side effects include diarrhea, nausea, and a rash. If these persist or worsen, contact your doctor.

If you have mild diarrhea, you may take a diarrhea medication containing kaolin or attapulgite (Kaopectate or Diasorb) but no other type. Another type may increase or prolong the diarrhea.

Severe diarrhea is a serious side effect; if it occurs, check with your doctor before taking any more diarrhea medication.

What you must know about other drugs Tell your doctor if you're taking other medications. For example, Probalan (probenecid) may increase Ceclor's effects.

Special directions • Before starting to take Ceclor, inform your doctor if you have other medical problems. They may affect the use of this medication.

• If your symptoms don't improve within a few days or if you feel worse, notify your doctor.

Important reminders If you have diabetes and test your urine for glucose, be aware that Ceclor may cause false results on some urine glucose tests. Check with your doctor before changing your diet or the dosage of your diabetes medication.

If you're breast-feeding, consult your doctor before using Ceclor.

Ceftin

This medication is an antibiotic used to treat various infections, but not colds or flu. The drug's generic name is cefuroxime axetil.

How to take Ceftin This medication comes in tablet form. Carefully follow the label directions. Take the medication on a full stomach. If you can't swallow the tablet, you may crush it and mix it with a small amount of food.

To make sure that the infection clears up completely, take this medication for the entire time your doctor prescribes, even if your symptoms go away.

What to do if you miss a dose If you forget to take your medication, take the missed dose as soon as you remember. If it's almost time for your next dose and your dosing schedule is two times a day, space the dose you missed and the next scheduled dose 5 to 6 hours apart. Then resume your normal dosing schedule.

What to do about side effects Occasionally, this medication produces serious side effects, including allergic reaction, anemia, and colitis. If you have a fever, rash, itchy skin, restlessness, or difficulty breathing, stop taking the medication and *immediately* seek emergency medical care.

If you experience fatigue, weakness, pale skin, nausea, vomiting, appetite loss, or diarrhea, report these effects to your doctor promptly.

What you must know about other drugs

Tell your doctor about other medications you're taking. Probalan (probenecid) may increase the amount of Ceftin in your blood.

Special directions

• Tell your doctor if you're allergic to any antibiotics.
• Inform your doctor if you have other medical problems, particularly kidney disease.
• Avoid taking diarrhea medication without first consulting your doctor. Many diarrhea medications can increase diarrhea or make it last longer.
• Check with your doctor before taking new medications (prescription or nonprescription) or if you develop new medical problems.
• If your symptoms don't go away within a few days or if you feel worse, call your doctor.

Important reminder

If you're pregnant or breast-feeding, consult your doctor before taking this medication.

Chloromycetin

Chloromycetin treats specific severe infections. Because it may cause serious side effects, the doctor prescribes it only when other antibiotics are ineffective. This drug's generic name is chloramphenicol. Another brand name is Chloroptic.

How to take Chloromycetin

Chloromycetin comes in capsules, liquids, eardrops, eyedrops or eye ointment, and skin creams. Carefully follow the label directions.

Take *capsules* with a full glass of water on an empty stomach, either 1 hour before or 2 hours after a meal. Don't open the capsule because Chloromycetin has an unpleasant taste.

To take the *liquid* form, use a special measuring spoon to make sure you pour an accurate dose.

If you're using the *drops, ointment,* or *cream*, wash your hands before and after applying medication to your eyes, ears, or skin. Keep eye, ear, and skin medications as germfree as possible. Don't touch a dropper tip or let it touch anything, including your eye or ear. After using ointment, wipe the tip of the tube with a clean tissue. Keep all containers tightly closed.

To use the *eardrops*, lie down or tilt your head so the infected ear is up. Gently pull your earlobe up and back (down and forward for children) to straighten the ear canal; then squeeze the drops into the ear canal. Keep your head tilted for 1 to 2 minutes. Then put a sterile cotton ball into your ear opening to hold the medication in.

To use the *eyedrops* or *eye ointment*, gently clean any crusted matter from your eyes. Sit down, and if you're using eyedrops, tilt your head back. Gently pull down your lower lid to create a pocket. Carefully squeeze eyedrops or a thin strip of ointment into the pocket; then close your eyes gently. Don't blink. Keep your eyes closed for 1 to 2 minutes. After applying ointment, your vision may be blurred for a few minutes.

Before applying *skin cream,* wash the site with soap and water and dry it thoroughly.

To ensure that your infection clears up completely, take this medication for the entire time prescribed, even when your symptoms subside.

What to do if you miss a dose

If you forget to take your *capsule* or *liquid,* take the missed dose as soon as you remember. But if it's almost time for your next dose and your dosing schedule is two doses a day, space the missed dose and the next dose 5 to 6 hours apart. If you take three or more doses a day, space the missed dose and the next dose 2 to 4 hours apart. Then resume your normal dosing schedule.

If you miss a dose of *ear, eye,* or *skin medication,* apply the missed dose as soon as you remember. But if it's almost time for your next dose, skip the dose you missed and apply your next dose at the scheduled time.

What to do about side effects

Serious blood problems (such as severe anemia, infections, and abnormal bleeding) may occur, particularly with long-term use of the *capsule, liquid,* or *cream* forms. Promptly report fever, weakness, confusion, bleeding, sore throat, or mouth sores to your doctor.

If you develop signs and symptoms of an allergic reaction fever, rash, itching, restlessness, difficulty swallowing or breathing stop taking the medication and seek emergency medical care *immediately.*

Also stop using the medication and seek emergency medical care *immediately* if you're giving this medication to an infant who develops a swollen abdomen, breathing difficulties, extreme sleepiness, or grayish skin.

When using *eye medication,* be alert for itching, swelling, or persistent burning. With *ear medication,* be alert for ear pain or fever. With *skin cream,* watch for a rash, itching, or burning. If these effects occur, stop taking the medication and call your doctor.

What you must know about other drugs

Discuss other medications you're taking with your doctor. Tylenol (acetaminophen), for example, affects the amount of Chloromycetin circulating in the blood, which may increase the drug's effects.

Special directions

• Inform the doctor if you have other medical problems, especially kidney or liver disease, bleeding problems, porphyria, or glucose-6-phosphate dehydrogenase deficiency. Before using Chloromycetin eardrops, tell the doctor if you've ever had a punctured or ruptured eardrum. Also report any allergic reactions to Chloromycetin or other medications or food.

• Have regular checkups and blood tests (especially if you're taking capsules or liquid Chloromycetin) so your doctor can monitor the medication's effectiveness and check for complications.

• If you don't notice improvement in a few days or if your symptoms worsen, notify your doctor.

• Check with your doctor before taking new medications (prescription or nonprescription) or if you develop new medical problems.

• Because of possible bleeding problems, be careful when brushing and flossing your teeth. If possible, delay dental procedures until you stop taking this medication.

• Don't share this medication, including the eye, ear, or skin forms, with anyone. Also, use separate washcloths and towels to prevent spreading the infection.

Important reminder   If you're pregnant or breast-feeding, tell your doctor before taking Chloromycetin.

Chlor-Trimeton

Chlor-Trimeton can relieve or prevent hay fever and other allergy symptoms. This drug's generic name is chlorpheniramine.

How to take
Chlor-Trimeton

This medication comes in tablet, chewable tablet, timed-release tablet or capsule, and syrup forms. Carefully follow the label directions. To reduce possible stomach upset, you can take this medication with food or a full glass of milk or water.

If you're taking the *timed-release tablets* or *capsules*, swallow them whole—don't break, chew, or crush them. If you have trouble swallowing, consult your doctor, nurse, or pharmacist.

What to do if you
miss a dose

Take the missed dose as soon as you remember. However, if it's almost time for the next dose, skip the dose you missed, and take your next dose at the regular time. Don't take a double dose.

What to do about
side effects

You may feel jittery or drowsy, and your mouth may be dry. Relieve dry mouth with ice chips or sugarless gum or hard candy. If these symptoms persist or worsen, tell your doctor.

Make sure you know how you respond to this medication before you drive or perform other activities requiring alertness.

What you must know about alcohol and other drugs

Tell your doctor about other medications you're taking. Avoid taking Chlor-Trimeton with alcoholic beverages, medications that depress the nervous system (such as some allergy and cold remedies, seizure medications, and pain relievers), and monoamine oxidase (MAO) inhibitors (such as Marplan). Doing so increases unwanted side effects. Keep in mind, too, that Chlor-Trimeton may hide unwanted side effects of high-dose aspirin therapy (for arthritis, for example) such as ringing in the ears.

Special directions

Before you undergo allergy tests, tell the doctor that you're taking this medication. Chlor-Trimeton may affect test results.

Important reminders

If you're breast-feeding, tell your doctor before taking this medication.

Children and older adults are especially sensitive to this medication's side effects.

Chronulac

Your doctor has prescribed this laxative to relieve your constipation. This drug's generic name is lactulose. Another brand name is Cephulac.

How to take Chronulac

Take each dose of Chronulac in or with a full glass (8 ounces) of cold water or fruit juice. For the best effect, your doctor may recommend that you then drink another glass of water by itself.

What to do if you miss a dose

Take the missed dose as soon as you remember unless it's almost time for your next dose. If so, skip the missed dose and take the next dose at its scheduled time.

Special directions

• Before taking Chronulac, tell your doctor if you're allergic to laxatives or to another medication or substance.
• Don't use this or any other laxative if you have symptoms of appendicitis or an inflamed bowel — lower abdominal or stomach pain, bloating, cramping, soreness,

nausea, or vomiting. Instead, call your doctor *immediately.*

• If you notice a sudden change in your bowel habits or function that lasts longer than 2 weeks or that keeps returning periodically, contact your doctor before taking Chronulac.

• Keep in mind that you may have to wait 24 to 48 hours before Chronulac starts working.

• Because Chronulac contains large amounts of carbohydrates, sodium, and sugar, don't take this medication if you're on a low-calorie, low-salt, or low-sugar diet. Instead, check with your doctor or pharmacist.

Important reminder   Don't give this or any other laxative to a child under age 6 unless your doctor prescribes it.

Cinobac

This medication helps treat and prevent infections of the urinary tract. This drug's generic name is cinoxacin.

How to take Cinobac   Available in capsule form, Cinobac is typically taken in two to four doses daily. Follow your doctor's directions exactly. Take this medication with meals or snacks, unless otherwise directed by your doctor.

Take your doses at evenly spaced times, day and night, to keep a constant amount of Cinobac in your body.

Continue taking this medication for the full time of treatment, even if you start to feel better. If you stop taking it too soon, your infection might return.

What to do if you miss a dose   Take the missed dose as soon as possible. But if it's almost time for your next dose, adjust your dosing schedule as follows.

If you're taking two doses a day, space the missed dose and the next dose 5 to 6 hours apart.

If you're taking three or more doses a day, space the missed dose and the next dose 2 to 4 hours apart. Then resume your regular dosing schedule.

What to do about side effects This medication may make you dizzy or cause headache, nausea, vomiting, or abdominal pain. Check with your doctor if you have any of these side effects, especially if they persist or become severe.

What you must know about other drugs Tell your doctor about other medications you're taking. If you take Probalan (probenecid), a gout medication, you may be at special risk for Cinobac's side effects.

Special directions • Because certain medical problems may interfere with the use of Cinobac, tell your doctor if you have other medical problems, especially kidney disease.
• If your symptoms don't improve within a few days or if they get worse, check with your doctor.
• This medication makes some people dizzy. Make sure you know how you react to Cinobac before you drive, use machines, or perform other hazardous activities that require alertness.

Important reminders If you're pregnant or breast-feeding, don't take this medication without checking first with your doctor.
Don't give Cinobac to children under age 12 unless otherwise directed by your doctor because it may interfere with bone development.

Cipro

Your doctor has ordered Cipro to treat a bacterial infection in your body. This drug's generic name is ciprofloxacin.

How to take Cipro This medication is available in tablets. Carefully follow the label directions. Take your dose with a full glass of water. You may take it with meals or on an empty stomach. Take this medication at evenly spaced times, day and night, to keep a constant amount in your body.
Keep taking Cipro for the full time of treatment, even if you begin to feel better after a few days. If you stop taking it too soon, your symptoms may return.

What to do if you miss a dose Take the missed dose as soon as possible. But if it's almost time for your next dose, skip the missed dose and take your next dose on schedule. Don't take a double dose.

What to do about side effects Call your doctor *right away* if you experience a seizure while taking this medication. Check with your doctor if you have nausea, diarrhea, or a skin rash.

Cipro may make you more sensitive than usual to sunlight, so limit your exposure to direct sun.

This medication may make you dizzy or drowsy. Make sure you know how you react to it before you drive, use machines, or perform other activities that require full alertness.

What you must know about other drugs Tell your doctor about other medications you're taking. Antacids containing magnesium hydroxide or aluminum hydroxide may decrease the absorption of Cipro. Therefore, if you take these antacids, take them 2 hours before or 2 hours after taking Cipro. Probalan (probenecid), a gout medication, may increase the risk of side effects from Cipro. Cipro may increase the blood levels of Theo-Dur (theophylline), an asthma medication, which could lead to side effects.

Special directions • Before taking Cipro, tell your doctor if you have other medical problems, especially conditions that cause seizures. Also reveal if you've ever had an allergic reaction to Cipro or another medication.

• Drink several extra glasses of water every day while taking this medication, unless your doctor gives you other directions. Drinking extra water will help to prevent side effects.

• If your symptoms don't improve within a few days or if they become worse, check with your doctor.

Important reminders Don't take this medication if you're pregnant or breast-feeding unless instructed by your doctor. Also, don't give it to infants, children, or adolescents unless instructed by your doctor.

Cleocin

Your doctor has prescribed Cleocin to treat your bacterial infection. This drug's generic name is clindamycin.

How to take Cleocin This medication is available in capsule and oral solution forms and in gel, lotion, and topical solution forms. If you're taking *capsules,* take them with a full glass (8 ounces) of water or with meals. If you're using the *oral solution,* measure your dose with a specially marked measuring spoon, not a household teaspoon.

Before you apply *topical* Cleocin, wash the affected skin and pat it dry. If you're using the gel or lotion, apply a thin film of medication.

If you're using the topical solution, wait 30 minutes after washing or shaving before applying this medication because the alcohol it contains may sting.

Avoid getting this medication in your eyes, nose, or mouth.

Keep taking your medication for the full time of treatment, even if you start to feel better. Stopping too soon might allow your infection to return.

What to do if you miss a dose If you miss an *oral* dose, take the missed dose as soon as possible. But if it's almost time for your next dose (and you take three or more doses a day), space the missed dose and the next dose 2 to 4 hours apart. Then go back to your regular dosing schedule.

If you miss a *topical* dose, apply the missed dose as soon as possible. But if it's almost time for your next dose, skip the missed dose and apply your next dose on schedule.

What to do about side effects Call your doctor *right away* if you have: severe, bloody diarrhea; abdominal pain with vomiting; black, tarry, or bloody stools; signs of an allergic reaction (chest tightness, wheezing, hives, itching, or rash). Also check with your doctor if you have nausea, mild diarrhea, or difficulty swallowing.

What you must know about other drugs Tell your doctor about other medications you're taking. E-Mycin (erythromycin), another antibiotic, may prevent Cleocin from working properly. Also avoid the use of kaolin (an ingredient in some diarrhea medications) because it decreases the absorption of Cleocin.

Special directions • Tell your doctor if you have other medical problems, especially diseases of the liver, kidney, stomach, or intestines. Also reveal if you have asthma or allergies.

• Before having surgery (including dental surgery) with a general anesthetic, tell the doctor or dentist in charge that you're taking Cleocin.

Important reminder If you're pregnant or breast-feeding, check with your doctor before using this medication.

Clinoril

Clinoril helps control inflammation and relieve pain. This drug's generic name is sulindac.

How to take Clinoril Follow your doctor's instructions exactly. Take Clinoril with milk, meals, or an antacid. This will help prevent stomach upset, which could occur if you take the drug on an empty stomach.

Also drink a full (8-ounce) glass of water with each dose. Don't lie down for 15 to 30 minutes after taking the medication. This will help prevent irritation that could cause you to have difficulty swallowing.

What to do if you miss a dose If your doctor has prescribed this medication on a regular schedule and you miss a dose, take the missed dose as soon as you remember. But if it's almost time for your next dose, skip the missed dose and take your next dose as scheduled.

What to do about side effects Tell your doctor *immediately* if you notice any of these side effects: stomach pain or burning; bloody or black, tarry stools; easy bruising and bleeding; changes in vision; swelling in your face, feet, or lower legs; or persistent nausea.

Because this medication makes some people drowsy or dizzy, don't drive or operate machinery until you know how you react to the medication.

What you must know about other drugs

Because Clinoril may affect the action of other drugs, tell your doctor and pharmacist about any drugs you're taking at the same time. In particular, mention if you're taking aspirin, a blood thinner, or drugs for seizures, thyroid problems, or inflammation.

Special directions

• Tell your doctor if aspirin or another anti-inflammatory drug has ever caused you to have difficulty breathing, a tight sensation in your chest, a runny nose, or itching.
• Also tell the doctor if you have a history of gastrointestinal bleeding, liver or kidney disease, asthma, heart disease, or high blood pressure.

Important reminders

This drug can hide the symptoms of an infection. If you have diabetes, you need to be especially careful about your feet and watch for any problem, such as redness or sores.

Because Clinoril can cause you to retain fluid, have your blood pressure checked when your doctor recommends.

Cloxapen

Your doctor has prescribed Cloxapen (a form of penicillin) to treat your bacterial infection. This drug's generic name is cloxacillin. Another brand name is Tegopen.

How to take Cloxapen

This medication comes in capsules and an oral solution. If you're taking the *capsules,* don't break, chew, or crush them—swallow them whole. If you're taking the *oral solution,* use a dropper or specially marked measuring spoon to measure each dose accurately.

Take your dose with a full glass (8 ounces) of water on an empty stomach, either 1 hour before or 2 hours after meals, unless your doctor tells you otherwise. Don't take your dose with fruit juice or carbonated drinks; doing so may prevent Cloxapen from working.

Keep taking your medication, even after you start to feel better. Stopping too soon may allow your infection to return.

What to do if you miss a dose

Take the missed dose as soon as possible. But if it's almost time for your next dose, adjust your dosing schedule as follows:

If you take two doses a day, space the missed dose and the next dose 5 to 6 hours apart.

If you take three or more doses a day, space the missed dose and the next dose 2 to 4 hours apart.

Then resume your regular dosing schedule.

What to do about side effects

Call your doctor *at once* if you develop any symptoms of an allergic reaction to this medication, such as difficulty breathing, skin rash, hives, itching, or wheezing.

If you develop nausea, heartburn, or diarrhea, check with your doctor, especially if these symptoms persist or become severe.

What you must know about other drugs

Tell the doctor about other medications you're taking. If you're taking Probalan (probenecid), a gout medication, your blood levels of Cloxapen may increase. This may or may not be a beneficial effect; check with your doctor.

If you develop severe diarrhea, don't take any diarrhea medications without first checking with your doctor. Some of these medications may make your diarrhea worse.

Special directions

• Tell your doctor about your medical history, especially if you're allergic to other antibiotics, including penicillins, cephalosporins, and griseofulvin. Also reveal if you have kidney disease.

• If you become allergic to Cloxapen, you should carry medical identification stating this.

• Before you have medical tests, tell the doctor that you're taking Cloxapen because this medication may interfere with some test results.

Important reminder

If you're pregnant or breast-feeding, check with your doctor before using this medication.

Cogentin

Cogentin relieves symptoms of Parkinson's disease and controls reactions to medications that cause Parkinson-like symptoms. This drug's generic name is benztropine.

How to take Cogentin

Follow the label directions carefully. To lessen stomach upset, take Cogentin with meals, unless your doctor directs otherwise.

What to do if you miss a dose

Take the missed dose as soon as you remember. But if you remember within 2 hours of your next scheduled dose, skip the missed dose and resume your normal dosing schedule. Don't take a double dose.

What to do about side effects

Common side effects include constipation and dry mouth. To relieve dry mouth, use sugarless hard candy or gum, ice chips, or a saliva substitute. Consult your dentist if dryness persists because it increases the risk of tooth decay and other disorders. If these effects persist or worsen, contact your doctor.

If your eyes are sensitive to light, wear sunglasses and avoid bright lights.

Make sure you know how you react to Cogentin before performing activities that require clear vision and alertness.

If you feel dizzy or light-headed when arising, get up slowly.

Avoid becoming overheated because Cogentin may make you sweat less and thus increase your body temperature.

What you must know about alcohol and other drugs

Check with your doctor before drinking alcoholic beverages or taking nonprescription medications. Also tell your doctor about other medications you're taking. Symmetrel (amantadine); phenothiazines, such as Thorazine (chlorpromazine); and tricyclic antidepressants such as Tofranil (imipramine), may increase your risk of side effects from Cogentin.

If you take an antacid or medication for diarrhea, take it 1 hour before or 1 hour after taking Cogentin. Taking them closer together may reduce Cogentin's effectiveness.

Special directions
• Be sure to tell your doctor if you have other medical problems. They may affect the use of Cogentin.
• If you think you've taken an overdose of Cogentin, get help *at once.*
• Have regular checkups, especially during the first few months you're taking Cogentin, so that your doctor can adjust the dosage to meet your needs.
• Don't stop taking Cogentin abruptly. Check with your doctor, who may direct you to gradually reduce the dosage.

Important reminders
If you're breast-feeding, check with your doctor before taking Cogentin.

Children and older adults may be especially sensitive to Cogentin and more likely to experience side effects.

Cognex

Your doctor has prescribed Cognex to help relieve some of the symptoms of Alzheimer's disease. This drug's generic name is tacrine.

How to take Cognex
Cognex comes in capsules. Take your medication between meals when possible (at least 1 hour after eating). The doctor may want to check your progress and change your dosage, so be sure to follow his directions carefully.

Cognex won't cure your condition but it may help with some of the symptoms. To make your medication as effective as possible, take the right amount on time every day. If you need help remembering to take your medicine, ask a friend or relative to remind you or give it to you.

What to do if you miss a dose
Take the missed dose as soon as you remember. However, if it's within 2 hours of your next dose, skip the missed dose and go back to your regular dosing schedule. Don't take a double dose.

What to do about side effects

Cognex may cause headaches, tiredness, confusion, dizziness, or wakefulness. You may also feel clumsy, depressed, agitated or hostile, or shaky. This drug may also cause you to imagine things.

Cognex can also cause coldlike symptoms, such as a runny nose and coughing, and may cause upper respiratory infection or urinary tract infection. You may also experience flushing, rash, or chest pain.

If you have nausea, vomiting diarrhea, upset stomach, lack of appetite, abdominal pain, gas, or constipation, try taking Cognex with a meal. Taking this drug with a meal may make it less effective but could help with your stomach problems.

You may find you need to urinate more frequently or you may not be able to control your urine flow. Try to empty your bladder regularly. You may find an adult incontinence pad helpful (most drug stores carry them). Other side effects include weakness, muscle aches or pain, small hemorrhages (spots of blood) under your skin, and back pain.

Be sure to call your doctor if any of these side effects persists or becomes severe.

What you must know about other drugs

Cognex may interfere with anticholinergic medications, such as Atropisol (atropine) or Cogentin (benztropine). These drugs are sometimes prescribed for intestinal problems, irregular heartbeat, and Parkinson's disease.

Cognex can increase the effect of muscle relaxants such as Anectine (succinylcholine), or cholinesterase inhibitors such as Prostigmin (neostigmine), or cholinergic agonists such as Urecholine (bethanechol). Cognex also increase the action of Theo-Dur (theophylline), so your dosage may need adjustment. Tagamet (cimetidine) increases the amount of Cognex in your blood.

Special directions

• Tell your doctor if you have intestinal problems, liver disease, asthma, seizures, or heart problems.

• Cognex may affect liver and digestive test results. Be aware that you may need blood tests to check your liver enzymes during the first few months on Cognex.

• If you are to receive anesthesia for surgery make sure that your doctor and anesthetist know you're taking

Cognex. This drug may increase the muscle relaxation effect of certain types of anesthetics.

• Don't stop taking Cognex suddenly. Doing so could cause a sudden worsening of your symptoms.

Colace

This medication is a laxative used to treat constipation. Its generic name is docusate sodium.

How to take Colace Colace is available in tablet, capsule, oral liquid, and syrup forms. If your doctor prescribed this medication, follow his directions exactly. If you bought this medication without a prescription, carefully read the package directions before taking your first dose.

What to do if you miss a dose Check with your doctor or pharmacist for how to handle a missed dose.

What to do about side effects Although side effects aren't common, Colace may irritate your throat or leave a bitter taste in your mouth. You may also have mild abdominal cramping or diarrhea. If these symptoms persist or become severe, call your doctor.

What you must know about other drugs Don't take mineral oil while you're taking Colace because it may cause your body to absorb too much mineral oil, causing unwanted effects.

If you're taking other medications, take them at least 2 hours before or 2 hours after taking Colace because Colace may interfere with the desired actions of the other medications.

Special directions • Don't use Colace (or any other laxative) if you have symptoms of appendicitis or an inflamed bowel, such as stomach or lower abdominal pain, cramping, bloating, soreness, nausea, or vomiting. Instead, check with your doctor as soon as possible.

• Drink at least 6 to 8 glasses (8 ounces each) of water or other liquids daily. This will help soften your bowel movements and relieve constipation.

• Don't take Colace for more than 1 week unless your doctor has prescribed or ordered a special schedule for you. This is true even if you continue to be constipated.

• If you notice a sudden change in your bowel habits or function that lasts longer than 2 weeks, or that occurs from time to time, check with your doctor. Your doctor will need to find the cause of your problem before it becomes more serious.

• Don't overuse Colace. Otherwise, you may become dependent on this medication to produce a bowel movement. In severe cases, overuse of laxatives can damage the nerves, muscles, and other tissues of the bowel.

Important reminders　If you're pregnant, check with your doctor before taking Colace.

Don't give this medication to children under age 6 unless prescribed by a doctor.

Cold remedies

The only real cure for a cold is time. After 7 to 10 days, a cold and its symptoms have usually run their course. But during this period, a cold can make you feel miserable.

Cold remedies offer temporary relief from aches, sniffles, and sneezes. Learn about ingredients. Then pick your product carefully and use it as directed.

Safety first　You want to avoid undesirable side effects from any cold remedy, so take only one cold remedy at a time. Taking more than one could cause an overdose if the products contain the same ingredients. Also, don't take both a cold remedy and a prescription drug without asking your doctor if it's safe to combine them.

Pain relievers　Most cold remedies contain pain relievers, such as aspirin or Tylenol (acetaminophen), to decrease fever, muscle soreness, and headaches. Avoid taking these medications if you're taking painkillers for another condition.

Antihistamines   These drugs have a drying effect on your body's tissues. That's why they relieve a runny nose and watery eyes. But most of them also make you sleepy. If you take them, avoid activities that require alertness, such as driving or using power tools. Check the labels of any medications for insomnia or diarrhea. They may contain antihistamines, too. Taking both remedies increases your chances for such side effects as constipation, dry mouth, and blurred vision.

Decongestants   By narrowing the blood vessels in your nose, decongestants reduce stuffiness. If you use a decongestant, take only the amount directed because it can raise your blood pressure. Check the label for *phenylpropanolamine,* a stimulant and diet pill ingredient, which can produce unwanted side effects.

Consider using decongestant nasal sprays or drops. They're safer than liquids or tablets because little of the drug enters your bloodstream when applied directly into your nose. Don't overuse the spray, though. If you do, stuffiness may continue after your cold goes away.

Cough medicines   These products may contain a cough suppressant, an expectorant, or both. Use suppressants if you have a dry hacking cough. Don't use them if your cough brings up mucus. A "wet" cough helps clear your breathing passages.

Expectorants loosen mucus to produce a wet cough. Drink plenty of fluids to make your mucus easier to expel.

Other ingredients   Many liquid medications contain alcohol to dissolve the other ingredients and caffeine to neutralize the effects of alcohol or antihistamines. Avoid these medications if you can't tolerate them.

Colestid

Your doctor has prescribed Colestid to lower your blood cholesterol level. This drug's generic name is colestipol.

How to take Colestid   This medication comes in powder form.

Never take Colestid in its dry form because it might cause choking. Instead, follow these steps:

• Add the proper amount of Colestid to at least 3 ounces of your favorite drink. However, if you use a carbonated drink, slowly mix the powder in a large glass to prevent excess foaming.

• Stir until the medication is completely mixed (it won't dissolve). Then drink the solution.

• After drinking all the liquid, rinse the glass with a little more liquid and drink that also, to make sure you get all of the medication.

You may also mix Colestid with thin soups, milk in hot or cold cereals, or pulpy fruits, such as crushed pineapple, pears, or fruit cocktail.

What to do if you miss a dose   Take the missed dose as soon as possible. But if it's almost time for your next dose, skip the missed dose and go back to your regular dosing schedule. Don't take a double dose.

What to do about side effects   Constipation is the most common side effect of this medication. If constipation develops, eat more fiber-rich foods, such as fruits, vegetables, and whole-grain cereals. If it persists or becomes severe, check with you doctor about decreasing your dosage or using a stool softener.

What you must know about other drugs   Tell your doctor about other medications you're taking. Colestid may decrease the absorption of any medication that you take by mouth. Therefore, if you take another oral medication, take it least 1 hour before or 4 hours after you take Colestid. Also, certain drugs for diabetes may prevent Colestid from working properly.

Special directions   • Tell your doctor about your medical history, especially if you have problems with your liver, gallbladder, or digestive tract.

• Carefully follow the special diet your doctor has given you, which is necessary for Colestid to work properly.

• See your doctor regularly so that he or she can check your cholesterol level and decide if you should continue to take this medication.

• Don't stop taking Colestid without first checking with your doctor. When you stop taking it, your blood cholesterol level may rise again. Your doctor may want you to follow a special diet to help prevent this from happening.

Important reminders   If you're pregnant, check with the doctor before taking this medication. If you're an older adult, be aware that you may be especially sensitive to side effects from Colestid.

Compazine

Compazine is used to relieve or prevent nausea and vomiting. It's also used to manage some psychiatric problems. This drug's generic name is prochlorperazine.

How to take Compazine   This medication comes in several forms. Follow your doctor's directions exactly. If you're taking *oral* Compazine, take it with food, water, or milk. If you're taking the *extended-release capsules*, swallow them whole—don't crush, break, or chew them.

What to do if you miss a dose   If you take one dose a day, take the missed dose as soon as possible. But if you don't remember the missed dose until the next day, skip it and go back to your regular dosing schedule.

If you take more than one dose a day, take the missed dose right away if you remember within 1 hour or so. But if you don't remember until later, skip it and take your next dose on schedule. Don't take a double dose.

What to do about side effects   Call your doctor *right away* if you have fever, chills, headache, extreme tiredness, or skin problems.

Check with your doctor if you feel dizzy or have blurred vision, a rapid heartbeat, dry mouth, constipation, or difficulty urinating. Compazine also can cause a movement disorder called tardive dyskinesia, so be sure to report any uncontrolled movements of your mouth, tongue, or other body parts.

Because Compazine may make you dizzy, make sure you know how you react to it before you drive or perform other activities requiring alertness.

This medication may make you more sensitive to light, so cover up outdoors and limit your sun exposure.

What you must know about alcohol and other drugs

Don't drink alcoholic beverages while taking Compazine because the combination can cause oversedation. For the same reason, avoid medications that slow down the nervous system, including tranquilizers, sleeping pills, and cold and flu remedies.

Tell your doctor about other medications you're taking. In particular, your doctor may want to watch your progress closely if you're taking medications for Parkinson's disease or depression.

If you take antacids, take them at least 2 hours before or 2 hours after you take Compazine.

Special directions

Tell your doctor if you have other medical conditions, especially heart or blood disease, glaucoma, seizure disorders, Parkinson's disease, or kidney or liver problems. Other medical problems may affect the use of this medication.

Important reminders

If you're pregnant or breast-feeding, check with your doctor before taking this medication.

Children and older adults are especially prone to Compazine's side effects.

If you're an athlete, be aware that the U.S. Olympic Committee and the National Collegiate Athletic Association ban and may test for prochlorperazine.

Cordarone

Cordarone is prescribed to correct irregular heartbeats. This drug's generic name is amiodarone.

How to take Cordarone

Cordarone is available as a tablet. Carefully follow the label directions.

What to do if you miss a dose

Skip the missed dose completely and go back to your regular dosing schedule. Don't try to squeeze the missed dose in and don't take a double dose. If you miss two or more doses in a row, check with your doctor.

What to do about side effects

Check with your doctor *immediately* if you develop a cough, irregular heartbeat, shortness of breath, or painful breathing. Also check with him if you experience malaise, unusual fatigue, nausea, vomiting, increased sensitivity to sunlight, or visual disturbances.

Because Cordarone increases your skin's sensitivity to sunlight, avoid direct sunlight, wear protective clothing including a hat and sunglasses, and use a sunblock that contains zinc or titanium dioxide. Contact your doctor if you have a severe sun reaction. Keep in mind that your skin may continue to be sensitive to sunlight for several months after you stop taking this medication.

After you've taken this medication for a long time, your skin may turn blue-gray where it's been exposed to sunlight. This color usually fades after Cordarone treatment ends (although it may take several months).

What you must know about other drugs

Tell your doctor if you're taking an anticoagulant (blood thinner), other heart medication, or Dilantin (phenytoin). The effects of these medications may increase if taken with Cordarone.

Special directions

• Visit your doctor regularly to make sure the medication is working properly.
• Carry medical identification that states that you're taking Cordarone.
• Before surgery (including dental surgery) or emergency treatment, tell the doctor or dentist that you're taking Cordarone.

Important reminders

Tell the doctor if you're breast-feeding or if you become pregnant while taking Cordarone.

Older adults may be especially sensitive to side effects and more likely than younger adults to develop thyroid problems when taking Cordarone.

Cordran

This medication helps relieve redness, swelling, itching, and other skin discomfort. This drug's generic name is flurandrenolide.

How to apply Cordran

This medication is available as cream, lotion, ointment, and tape. Carefully follow the label directions. Apply Cordran exactly as prescribed and wash your hands after applying it. Don't bandage or wrap the skin being treated unless your doctor directs you to do so.

What to do if you miss a dose

Apply the missed dose as soon as possible. But if it's almost time for your next dose, skip the missed dose and apply the next scheduled dose.

What to do about side effects

Although side effects are uncommon, Cordran can cause such skin reactions as burning, itching, dryness, changes in color or texture, or a rash and inflammation (dermatitis). Tell your doctor if these effects occur.

Special directions

• If you have other medical problems, let your doctor know. They may affect the use of this medication.
• Don't get Cordran in your eyes. If you do, flush your eyes with water.
• If your doctor orders an occlusive dressing (an airtight covering, such as plastic wrap or a special patch) to be applied over this medication, make sure you understand how to apply it.
• Don't use leftover medication for other skin problems without first checking with your doctor.
• If you're applying Cordran to a child's diaper area, avoid using tight-fitting diapers or plastic pants. They could cause unwanted side effects.

Important reminders

Consult your doctor if you become pregnant while using Cordran.

Don't apply this medication to your breasts before breast-feeding.

Children and adolescents using this medication should have frequent medical checkups because this medication can affect growth and cause other unwanted effects.

If you're an older adult, you may be especially susceptible to certain side effects, such as skin tearing and blood blisters.

Corgard

This medication is usually prescribed to treat angina (chest pain) or high blood pressure. Its generic name is nadolol.

How to take Corgard
Carefully follow the label directions.

What to do if you miss a dose
Take the missed dose right away if you remember within an hour or so. However, if it's within 8 hours of your next dose, skip the missed dose and resume your regular schedule. Don't take a double dose.

What to do about side effects
Call your doctor *right away* if you start wheezing, have difficulty breathing, or experience confusion, hallucinations, a slow or irregular heartbeat, cold feet or hands, or swelling of the feet or ankles.

You may have trouble sleeping or experience drowsiness, dizziness, light-headedness, reduced sexual ability, or unusual fatigue or weakness. These side effects usually go away over time as your body adjusts to the medication. But you should check with your doctor if they persist or become bothersome.

Avoid hazardous activities, such as driving a car, because Corgard may make you drowsy or less alert.

What you must know about other drugs
Check with your doctor before taking other drugs, including nonprescription drugs. Some drugs may prevent Corgard from working properly.

Prescription drugs used to reduce blood pressure may increase the effects of Corgard on the heart. Other drugs used to treat angina may cause increased effects on your blood pressure when taken with Corgard.

Digitalis glycosides (heart medication) may cause an unusually slow heart rate when combined with Corgard.

Adrenalin (epinephrine) as well may constrict your blood vessels and slow your heart rate when taken with Corgard.

Special directions

• Make sure your doctor knows about your medical history, especially if you have heart or blood vessel disease, diabetes, kidney disease, liver disease, mental depression, asthma, hay fever, hives, bronchitis, emphysema, an unusually slow heartbeat, or an overactive thyroid gland.

• Ask your doctor about checking your pulse rate before each dose. Then while taking Corgard, check your pulse rate regularly. If it's slower than your usual rate, don't take the dose; call your doctor.

• The doctor may need to increase your dosage gradually to find the amount that causes the best response.

Important reminders

If you have diabetes, check with your doctor. This drug may cause your blood sugar level to drop and may mask signs of low blood sugar (such as a change in your pulse rate). Also, the dosage of your diabetes medication may need to be changed.

If you're pregnant or breast-feeding, check with your doctor before taking Corgard.

Also, be aware that older adults may be especially sensitive to the side effects of this medication.

Athletes should be aware that the U.S. Olympic Committee and the National Collegiate Athletic Association ban nadolol.

Cortaid

This medication helps relieve the itching, redness, swelling, and discomfort of your skin problem. The drug's generic name is hydrocortisone. Another brand name is Hytone.

How to apply Cortaid

Cortaid is available as an aerosol, cream, gel, lotion, ointment, or topical solution. Carefully follow the label directions. Wash your hands and skin before applying the medication. When applying the medication to hairy areas, part the hair and apply the medication directly to the skin.

If your doctor has prescribed an occlusive dressing (an airtight covering, such as plastic wrap or a special patch), apply a heavy layer of medication, cover the area with the occlusive dressing, and then secure the dressing to your skin with hypoallergenic tape.

If you're using the *aerosol* form, shake the can well. Direct the spray onto the area from a distance of 6 inches. To avoid freezing the tissues, spray for no more than 3 seconds. Apply to a dry scalp after shampooing; don't rub the medication into your scalp after spraying.

Avoid breathing in the spray and getting it in your eyes. If the medication accidentally gets in your eyes, promptly flush them with water.

What to do if you miss a dose

Apply the missed dose as soon as you can. But if it's almost time for your next regular dose, skip the missed dose and apply the next dose as scheduled.

What to do about side effects

Fever, skin tearing, painful reddened and inflamed skin with pus-filled blisters, thinning skin, reddish purple lines on the skin, or burning and itching skin with pinhead-size blisters may occur with the use of an occlusive dressing. If any of these problems occurs, remove the dressing and contact your doctor.

Special directions

• Before using Cortaid, tell your doctor if you're allergic to any medications or foods.

• For safety reasons, don't apply topical Cortaid near heat or open flame or while smoking.

• Don't use topical Cortaid more often or for a longer time than your doctor has instructed. Doing so increases the risk of side effects.

• Don't share your medication with others. Also, don't use any remaining medication to treat other skin problems without first consulting your doctor.

Important reminders

If you're pregnant or breast-feeding, check with your doctor before using this medication.

Don't use Cortaid for a child under age 2 without a doctor's order.

Children, adolescents, and older adults are especially prone to side effects and should be closely monitored by a doctor.

Cortisporin Otic

This medication helps to treat ear infections. It may also be used to relieve discomfort, irritation, and redness from other ear problems. This drug's generic name is hydrocortisone with neomycin and polymyxin B. Another brand name is Pediotic.

How to use Cortisporin Otic

Insert the eardrops, following the instructions you received from the nurse or doctor.

Before inserting the eardrops, warm them to body temperature (98.6° F [37°C]) by holding the bottle in your hand for a few minutes. Don't heat the bottle on the stove or in the microwave the medication won't work if it gets too warm.

Continue using this medication as ordered by your doctor, even after you feel better. Complete the full treatment to make sure the infection is completely cleared up.

What to do if you miss a dose

Insert the eardrops as soon as you remember unless it's almost time for your next regular dose. If so, skip the missed dose and insert the drops when next scheduled.

What to do about side effects

If you have itching, redness, swelling, or other signs of irritation, tell your doctor.

Special instructions

• Before using this medication, tell your doctor if you have other ear problems because using this medication could make some problems worse.

• Inform your doctor if you're allergic to any medications, particularly related antibiotics, such as Garamycin (gentamicin), streptomycin, or Nebcin (tobramycin).

• If your symptoms persist for more than 1 week or become worse, contact your doctor.

- Don't use this medication for more than 10 days in a row unless your doctor prescribes a longer course of treatment.

Coumadin

Your doctor has prescribed Coumadin to reduce your blood's ability to clot. This drug's generic name is warfarin.

How to take Coumadin

Take Coumadin only as your doctor directs. Don't take more or less, and don't take it more often or longer than directed. Take it at the same time each day.

What to do if you miss a dose

Take the missed dose as soon as possible. Then go back to your regular schedule.

If you miss a day, don't take the missed dose at all, and never take a double dose. This may cause bleeding.

What to do about side effects

Call your doctor *at once* if your gums bleed when you brush your teeth. Also call him if you have bruises or purplish marks on your skin, nosebleeds, heavy bleeding or oozing from cuts or wounds, excessive or unexpected menstrual bleeding, blood in your urine or sputum, vomit that looks like coffee grounds, or bloody or black, tarry stools.

Call your doctor if you have unusual pain or swelling in your joints or your stomach, unusual backaches, diarrhea, constipation, dizziness, or a severe or continuing headache.

What you must know about alcohol and other drugs

Avoid drinking alcoholic beverages on a regular basis because alcohol may interfere with Coumadin's effectiveness. An occasional drink is okay, but don't have more than one or two.

Check with your doctor before taking nonprescription drugs. Certain vitamins can reduce Coumadin's effectiveness, and aspirin and similar drugs can cause bleeding.

Also tell your doctor about other prescription medications you're taking. Some drugs, when taken with

Coumadin, could interfere with Coumadin's action or cause bleeding.

Special directions

• To reduce your risk of injuring yourself, always wear shoes, place a nonskid mat in your bathtub, shave with an electric razor, and use a soft toothbrush.

• Remember to keep your blood test appointments. If blood tests show that your blood isn't clotting at the correct rate, the doctor may decide to adjust your dosage.

• Be sure to let your other doctors and your dentist know you're taking Coumadin.

• Wear a medical identification tag identifying you as a Coumadin user.

• Check with your doctor before beginning any strenuous programs. And avoid risky activities—for example, roughhousing with children and pets.

Important reminder

If you're considering becoming pregnant, think about delaying pregnancy or discuss it with your doctor. Coumadin can impair your baby's development and cause placental bleeding.

Cytotec

This medication is usually prescribed to prevent stomach ulcers in patients who are taking anti-inflammatory medications (such as aspirin). This drug's generic name is misoprostol.

How to take Cytotec

This medication is available in tablets. You may need to take it four times a day.

Carefully follow the label directions.

To make the medication work better, take it with or after meals and at bedtime.

What to do if you miss a dose

Take the missed dose as soon as possible. However, if it's almost time for your next regular dose, skip the missed dose and resume your regular dosage schedule. Never take a double dose.

What to do about side effects

Diarrhea and abdominal or stomach pain may occur. These side effects usually go away over time as your body adjusts to the medication. But you should check with your doctor if diarrhea lasts more than 1 week or if abdominal or stomach pain persists or becomes bothersome.

Special directions

• Make sure your doctor knows about your medical history, especially if you have blood vessel disease or have had uncontrolled seizures. Cytotec may worsen blood vessel disease and may trigger seizures.

• Avoid smoking cigarettes because this may increase stomach acid secretion and make your ulcer worse.

• If the doctor has prescribed this medication to treat a duodenal ulcer, you may take an antacid to help relieve stomach pain (unless the doctor tells you not to). However, avoid antacids that contain magnesium because they may worsen diarrhea caused by Cytotec. Also, keep taking this medication for the full time of treatment, even if you start to feel better. However, don't take it for more than 4 weeks, unless the doctor wants you to continue treatment for another 4 weeks to make sure your ulcer heals completely.

Important reminders

If you're a woman of childbearing age, discuss the use of this medication with your doctor before starting treatment. You must have had a negative pregnancy test within 2 weeks before starting Cytotec. Also, you must begin taking this medication only on the second or third day of your next normal menstrual period, and you must use an effective birth control method during treatment.

If you become pregnant or even suspect you've become pregnant while taking this drug, stop taking it immediately and call the doctor. This drug may cause miscarriage, uterine contractions, and uterine bleeding.

If you're breast-feeding, check with your doctor before using Cytotec.

D

Dalmane

Dalmane is a drug that can help you sleep. This drug's generic name is flurazepam.

How to take Dalmane

Take Dalmane capsules exactly as directed. Don't increase your dose because overuse may lead to mental or physical dependence.

What to do about side effects

If you think you may have taken an overdose, seek emergency help *at once.* Overdose symptoms include continuous slurred speech or confusion, severe drowsiness, and staggering.

Dalmane may cause drowsiness, dizziness, headache, and poor coordination. If these symptoms persist or become severe, consult your doctor.

Don't drive or perform activities requiring alertness until you know how the medication affects you.

What you must know about alcohol and other drugs

Avoid alcoholic beverages, Tagamet (cimetidine), and medications that depress the nervous system (such as many allergy and cold remedies, narcotics, muscle relaxants, sleeping pills, and seizure medications). The combination of Dalmane and these medications may cause excessive drowsiness.

Special directions

• Tell your doctor about other medical problems you have. They may affect the use of this medication.
• See your doctor regularly to monitor your progress and check for side effects.
• Because Dalmane can affect some diagnostic test results, tell the doctor that you're taking this medication before you undergo any tests.
• Before you have dental work that requires an anesthetic, tell the dentist you're taking Dalmane.
• Don't stop taking Dalmane suddenly; doing so may cause unpleasant withdrawal symptoms. Consult your

doctor about gradually reducing your dosage before stopping the medication completely.

Important reminders If you're pregnant or breast-feeding, consult your doctor before taking this medication.

Children and older adults are especially prone to Dalmane's side effects.

If you're an athlete, be aware that the National Collegiate Athletic Association and the U.S. Olympic Committee ban the use of flurazepam.

Danocrine

Danocrine helps treat many medical problems, including endometriosis, breast cysts, and a rare condition called hereditary angioedema. This drug's generic name is danazol.

How to take Danocrine Carefully follow the label directions. For Danocrine to help you, you must take it regularly for the full time of treatment ordered by your doctor.

What to do if you miss a dose Take the missed dose as soon as possible. However, if it's almost time for your next dose, skip the missed dose and take your next dose on schedule. Don't take a double dose.

What to do about side effects If you're female, tell your doctor *right away* if you develop any masculinizing side effects while taking Danocrine. These effects include weight gain, increased hair growth on your body, a decrease in breast size, voice deepening, and oiliness of your skin or hair.

Danocrine may increase your sensitivity to sunlight, so limit your exposure to the sun.

Special directions • Tell your doctor if you have other medical problems, especially kidney, heart, or liver disease. If you're female, also reveal any history of abnormal vaginal bleeding.

• See your doctor for regular checkups to make sure that Danocrine doesn't cause unwanted side effects.

• If you're female, don't use birth control pills while taking Danocrine. Select a birth control method, such as a diaphragm, that doesn't contain hormones.

• If you're taking this medication for endometriosis or breast cysts, your menstrual period may be irregular, or you may not have a menstrual period while you're taking Danocrine. This is to be expected. However, if regular menstruation doesn't begin within 60 to 90 days after you stop taking this medication, check with your doctor.

• If you're taking Danocrine for breast cysts, examine your breasts regularly. Check with your doctor right away if you detect unusual changes in how your breasts feel.

Important reminders   If you're pregnant or think you may be, don't take Danocrine. Continued use of Danocrine during pregnancy may cause masculine changes in female babies. For the same reason, check with your doctor before you use this medication if you're breast-feeding.

If you have diabetes, be aware that Danocrine may affect your blood sugar levels. If you notice a change in the results of your blood or urine glucose test, call your doctor.

If you're an older male, you should know that taking Danocrine may increase your risk of developing prostate enlargement or prostate cancer.

If you're an athlete, you should know that the U.S. Olympic Committee bans the use of danazol.

Dantrium

This medication relieves muscle spasms, cramping, and tightness caused by multiple sclerosis, cerebral palsy, stroke, and other conditions. The drug's generic name is dantrolene.

How to take   If you're taking the *capsule* form, take your dose with
Dantrium   milk or meals to help prevent digestive upset.

If you have trouble swallowing the capsules, follow these steps:

• Empty the number of capsules needed for one dose into a small amount of fruit juice or other liquid.
• Stir gently to mix the powder with the liquid. Then drink it right away.
• Rinse the glass with a little more liquid and drink that also to make sure you've taken the entire dose.

What to do if you miss a dose

If you remember within 1 hour or so, take the missed dose right away. Then go back to your regular dosage schedule. But if you don't remember until later, skip the missed dose and take your next dose on schedule. Don't take a double dose.

What to do about side effects

Call your doctor *at once* if your skin or eyes start to turn yellow, if you develop a fever, or if your skin feels itchy. These symptoms could be signs of hepatitis, a liver disorder. Check with your doctor if you feel dizzy or drowsy or have muscle weakness. Also call if you have diarrhea or constipation.

Because Dantrium can make you drowsy or dizzy, make sure you know how you react to it before you drive, use machines, or perform other activities that could be dangerous if you're not alert.

What you must know about alcohol and other drugs

Don't drink alcohol while taking Dantrium because the combination may lead to oversedation. For the same reason, avoid other central nervous system depressants (medications that slow your nervous system), such as sleeping pills, tranquilizers, muscle relaxants, narcotic pain relievers, and many cold, flu, and allergy remedies.

Special directions

• Tell your doctor if you have other medical problems, especially lung, heart, or liver disease.
• See your doctor for regular checkups, especially if you're taking Dantrium for a long time. You may need to have certain blood tests to check for unwanted side effects.

Important reminders

If you're pregnant or breast-feeding, check with your doctor before using Dantrium.

If you're an athlete, you should know that the National Collegiate Athletic Association and the U.S. Olympic Committee ban the use of dantrolene.

Darvon

Darvon helps relieve pain. This drug's generic name is propoxyphene.

How to take Darvon

Darvon comes in three forms: tablets, capsules, and an oral suspension. Take Darvon exactly as the label directs. If you feel your medication isn't working well, don't take more than the prescribed dose. Check with your doctor instead. If you take too much of this medication or take it for too long, it could become habit-forming.

What to do if you miss a dose

Take the missed dose as soon as you remember. However, if it's almost time for your next dose, skip the missed dose and go back to your regular dosage schedule. Don't take a double dose.

What to do about side effects

The most common side effect from Darvon is dizziness. This medication may also make you feel drowsy or cause nausea or vomiting. Let your doctor know if these symptoms continue or become bothersome.

Because Darvon may make you dizzy, make sure you know how you react to it before you drive or perform other activities that might be dangerous if you're not fully alert.

If this medication makes your mouth feel dry, you may use sugarless hard candy or gum, ice chips, or a saliva substitute. If your dry mouth continues for more than 2 weeks, see your dentist.

What you must know about alcohol and other drugs

Avoid drinking alcoholic beverages while taking Darvon because the combination can cause oversedation. For the same reason, check with your doctor before using medications that slow down the central nervous system, such as sleeping pills, tranquilizers, sedatives, and many cold, flu, and allergy remedies.

Special directions

Tell your doctor if you have other medical problems, especially heart, liver, lung, or kidney disease. Also tell him if you have asthma, a seizure disorder, or a history of drug or alcohol abuse. Other medical problems may affect the use of this medication.

• Don't stop taking Darvon suddenly. Your doctor may want to reduce your dosage gradually to lessen the chance of side effects from withdrawal.

Important reminders   If you're pregnant or breast-feeding, check with your doctor before taking this medication.

If you're an older adult, you may be especially prone to Darvon's side effects.

If you're an athlete, you should know that the U.S. Olympic Committee bans and tests for propoxyphene.

DDAVP

The hormone DDAVP helps prevent or control symptoms associated with diabetes insipidus, such as frequent urination, increased thirst, and water loss. This drug's generic name is desmopressin.

How to take DDAVP   If you're using the *nasal solution*, first read the patient directions in the package. Before you administer your dose, gently blow your nose to clear your nasal passages.

If you're using the *injection* form, follow your doctor's instructions.

**What to do if you
miss a dose**   If you miss a dose, adjust your dosing schedule as follows:

If you take one dose a day, take the missed dose as soon as possible. Then go back to your regular dosing schedule. But if you don't remember the missed dose until the next day, skip the missed dose and go back to your regular dosing schedule.

If you take more than one dose a day, take the missed dose as soon as possible. Then go back to your regular dosing schedule. However, if it's almost time for your next dose, skip the missed dose and take your next dose on schedule. Don't take a double dose.

What to do about side effects

Generally, DDAVP causes few side effects. But check with your doctor if you experience any unwanted reactions, such as headache, runny nose, nausea, or skin flushing, especially if these symptoms persist or seem severe.

If you experience a mild headache from taking this medication, you may take aspirin or Tylenol (acetaminophen), unless your doctor gives you other instructions.

Special directions

• Tell your doctor if you have other medical problems, especially heart or blood vessel disease, high blood pressure, or a stuffy nose caused by a cold or an allergy.

• If you're using the *nasal solution*, check with your doctor if you develop a runny nose from a cold or an allergy. Nasal congestion can interfere with the absorption of this medication.

• Your doctor may ask you to check your weight daily to determine if your body is holding enough water.

Important reminders

If you're pregnant or breast-feeding, check with your doctor before taking this medication.

If you're an older adult, you may be especially prone to DDAVP's side effects.

Decadron (oral)

This oral medication treats inflammation, severe allergic reactions, and a wide variety of other conditions. Its generic name is oral dexamethasone.

How to take oral Decadron

Oral Decadron comes in tablet, oral solution, and elixir forms. Carefully check the label on your prescription bottle and follow the directions exactly. Don't take Decadron more often than ordered.

Take your medication with food to prevent stomach irritation. If you're taking only one dose daily, take it in the morning for best results.

Don't stop taking Decadron suddenly. Check with your doctor first. You may need to reduce your dosage gradually to prevent serious side effects.

What to do if you miss a dose
Take the missed dose as soon as possible. Then take any remaining doses for that day at regularly spaced intervals. But if it's almost time for your next dose, skip the missed dose and take the next dose on schedule. Don't take a double dose.

What to do about side effects
Call your doctor *at once* if you have trouble breathing or start to retain water because the medication may be causing a serious heart problem.

Check with your doctor if you experience mood changes or difficulty sleeping. Also call if you feel weak, are unusually thirsty, urinate frequently, or lose weight despite eating regularly.

What you must know about other drugs
Tell your doctor about other medications you're taking, including nonprescription drugs. Your doctor may want you to avoid certain pain relievers, such as aspirin, because they can increase the risk of stomach problems.

Your doctor also may need to adjust your Decadron dosage if you take barbiturates (found in some sleeping pills and medications for seizure disorders) or certain other drugs. Also, check with your doctor before you have any vaccinations.

Special directions
• Tell your doctor if you have other medical problems, especially a fungal infection, ulcers, high blood pressure, diabetes, or diseases of the kidney, liver, blood, bones, or other organs.
• Keep all appointments for follow-up visits.
• Your doctor may want you to carry a medical identification card stating that you're using Decadron and that you may need additional medication during an emergency, a severe asthma attack or other illness, or unusual stress.

Important reminder
If you're pregnant or breast-feeding, check with your doctor before using Decadron.

Decadron (topical)

Topical Decadron is a cream prescribed to treat skin and scalp problems. Its generic name is topical dexamethasone. Brand names for other forms of the drug are Decaspray (spray) and Decaderm (gel).

How to apply topical Decadron

Read the patient instructions provided in your medication package and follow the directions exactly.

Before applying your medication, wash the affected skin gently.

If you're using the *gel* or *cream*, apply a thin coat of medication to the affected area. Rub in the gel or cream gently to avoid injuring your skin. If you're treating a hairy area, part the hair and apply the medication directly to the affected area. Keep the medication away from your eyes, mouth, nose, and other mucous membranes.

If you're using the *spray*, shake the can well. Then spray while moving the nozzle over the affected area. Take care not to inhale the spray or get it in your eyes.

If you've used your fingers to apply your medication, be sure to wash your hands when you're finished.

Don't wrap the treated skin with a bandage or other tight dressing, unless your doctor has told you to do so.

What to do if you miss a dose

Apply the medication as soon as possible. But if it's almost time for your next application, skip the missed dose and apply the next one on schedule.

What to do about side effects

Check with your doctor if you experience skin reactions to topical Decadron, including a rash, itching, burning, redness, and dryness. Also report signs of skin infection, such as redness, oozing, and pain.

Special directions

• Tell your doctor if you have other medical problems, especially poor circulation.

• Keep all appointments for follow-up visits, so your doctor can check your progress and detect any unwanted side effects early.

• If you're using topical Decadron to treat diaper rash in a young child, don't cover the child's bottom with a tight-fitting diaper or plastic pants.

Decadron Phosphate Ophthalmic

This medication is prescribed to treat eye problems. Its generic name is ophthalmic dexamethasone.

How to use Decadron Phosphate Ophthalmic

This medication is available in cream and ointment forms. To use either, first wash your hands.

Pull your lower eyelid away from the affected eye to form a pouch. Squeeze the correct amount of cream or ointment into the pouch and gently close your eyes. Don't blink.

Keep your eyes closed for 1 to 2 minutes to allow the medication to be absorbed.

Repeat the procedure on the other eye, if directed.

Try to keep your medication as germfree as possible. Don't touch the applicator tip to any surface, including your eye. Keep the container tightly closed between uses.

What to do if you miss a dose

Apply the medication as soon as possible. Then apply any remaining doses for that day at regularly spaced intervals. But if it's almost time for your next application, skip the missed dose and go back to your regular schedule.

What to do about side effects

Stop using Decadron Phosphate Ophthalmic and call your doctor *right away* if you notice any changes in vision. Tell your doctor if you develop further problems with your eyes, such as blurred vision, burning, stinging, redness, or wateriness.

Special directions

• Tell your doctor if you have other medical problems with your eyes, such as a corneal abrasion or glaucoma. Also tell him if you're allergic to any medications.

• Once your eye infection is cured, don't save your medication and use it for a new eye infection. Always check with your doctor first.

• Don't share your medication with family members, even if they have symptoms that resemble yours. If a family member has the same symptoms, call the doctor.

• Don't rub or scratch around your eye while using Decadron Phosphate Ophthalmic. You might accidentally hurt your eye.

• Keep all appointments for follow-up visits with your doctor.

Demerol

Demerol is usually prescribed to treat moderate to severe pain. This drug's generic name is meperidine.

How to take Demerol   This drug is available in tablets and a syrup. Take only the amount prescribed.

If you're using the *syrup* form, take it with a full glass (8 ounces) of water to reduce numbness of the mouth and throat.

What to do if you miss a dose   If you're taking this medication on a regular schedule, take the missed dose as soon as possible. But if it's almost time for your next regular dose, skip the missed dose and resume your regular schedule. Never take a double dose.

What to do about side effects   Get emergency help *immediately* if you think you may have taken an overdose of this medication. Symptoms include cold, clammy skin; confusion; seizures; severe dizziness or drowsiness; slow heartbeat; slow or troubled breathing; and severe weakness.

Demerol may cause urine retention or constipation. These side effects and the others listed below usually subside as your body adjusts to the drug. But check with your doctor if they persist or become bothersome.

Demerol may cause nausea or vomiting for the first few doses. To reduce these problems lie down for a while after taking the dose. If nausea or vomiting persists, call your doctor.

Initially, this medication may make you feel faint, dizzy, or light-headed when rising from a lying or sitting position. To reduce this effect, get up slowly.

Avoid potentially hazardous activities, such as driving a car, because Demerol may make you drowsy or less alert.

What you must know about alcohol and other drugs Don't drink alcoholic beverages or take sleeping pills, sedatives, or antihistamines such as Benadryl (diphenhydramine) while taking Demerol because of the risk of additive sedative effects.

Check with your doctor if you're taking other prescription or nonprescription medications. Other drugs may change the way Demerol works.

Special directions • Tell your doctor about other medical problems you have, especially heart rhythm problems, a head injury, liver or kidney problems, asthma, respiratory problems, glaucoma, seizures, or drug abuse or addiction.
• If you've been taking Demerol regularly for several weeks or more, don't stop taking it suddenly because this could cause side effects from withdrawal. Check with your doctor for instructions on how to stop the drug gradually.

Important reminders If you're pregnant or breast-feeding, check with your doctor before taking Demerol.

Children and older adults are especially sensitive to Demerol's side effects.

If you're an athlete, you should know that the U.S. Olympic Committee bans the use of meperidine.

Depakene

This medication is prescribed to treat seizures. Its generic name is valproic acid. Another brand name is Depakote.

How to take Depakene This medication comes in tablets, capsules, and syrup. If you're taking a tablet or capsule, swallow it whole, without breaking or chewing it. To keep it from upsetting your stomach, take it with food or water. But don't take it with milk.

If you're taking the *syrup*, you may mix it with food or a beverage. However, don't mix it with a carbonated beverage like soda. Doing so may irritate your mouth and throat.

What to do if you miss a dose

If you take one dose a day, take the missed dose as soon as possible. But if you don't remember until the next day, skip the missed dose and take your next dose as scheduled.

If you take two or more doses a day and you remember the missed dose within 6 hours, take it right away. Then equally space your remaining doses for the day. Never take two doses at once.

What to do about side effects

Call your doctor *right away* if you develop any of the following side effects: unusual bleeding or bruising, extreme drowsiness, loss of appetite, continued nausea and vomiting, tiredness or weakness, yellow eyes or skin, trembling, or fever.

What you must know about alcohol and other drugs

Avoid drinking alcoholic beverages while taking Depakene. Alcohol may decrease the effectiveness of the medication while causing you to become overly sedated.

Don't take antacids or aspirin without first talking with your doctor. If taken while you're taking Depakene, these medications could cause undesirable side effects. Also tell the doctor if you're taking a blood thinner or other drugs to control seizures.

Special directions

• Let your doctor know if you have a history of liver disease because it may affect your body's ability to break down Depakene.
• Because the medication may make you drowsy, don't drive or do anything that could be dangerous if you're not alert until you know how you respond to the medication.
• Because Depakene may affect how quickly your blood can clot, take precautions to keep from cutting yourself. For example, use an electric razor and a soft toothbrush.
• Don't stop taking the medication suddenly. Doing so may cause seizures.

Important reminders If you have diabetes, be aware that this medication may make urine tests for ketones unreliable.

If you're pregnant or breast-feeding, don't take this medication until you talk with your doctor.

If you're an athlete, you should know that the U.S. Olympic Committee and the National Collegiate Athletic Association ban the use of valproic acid and sometimes test for it.

Desyrel

Your doctor has prescribed Desyrel to help treat your depression. This drug's generic name is trazodone.

How to take Desyrel Take your medication after a meal or light snack, even if you're taking a dose at bedtime. This will help your body absorb the medication better and will lessen your risk of becoming dizzy or developing an upset stomach.

Continue taking the medication, even if you don't feel any different. You need to take the medication for 2 weeks before you feel any effect at all and for 4 weeks before you feel the full effect.

What to do if you miss a dose Take the missed dose as soon as possible. However, if you don't remember until it's less than 4 hours until your next dose, skip the missed dose and take your next dose on schedule. Don't take two doses at once.

What to do about side effects If you're male, stop taking the medication and call your doctor *at once* if you develop a painful, inappropriate erection. For both sexes, call your doctor if you have confusion, muscle tremor, nausea and vomiting, loss of muscle coordination, or extreme drowsiness.

The most common side effects of Desyrel are drowsiness and dizziness. These should subside after a few weeks. Because the medication may make you drowsy or less alert than normal, don't drive or operate machinery. Also, to prevent dizziness and protect yourself against a fall, get up slowly after you've been lying down.

What you must know about alcohol and other drugs

Avoid drinking alcoholic beverages or taking central nervous system depressants because Desyrel will heighten their effects and place you at risk for oversedation. Examples of these drugs include cold or allergy medication, sleeping pills, pain medication, muscle relaxants, or anesthetics.

Desyrel may also alter how your body uses other medications. Before taking Desyrel, tell your doctor if you're taking blood pressure medicine, heart medication, medication for seizures, or a monoamine oxidase (MAO) inhibitor such as Marplan (isocarboxazid), an antidepressant.

Special directions

• Tell your doctor if you're allergic to any other medications used to treat depression.

• Because this drug can make certain medical conditions worse, inform your doctor if you have a history of heart, liver, or kidney disease or a problem with ejaculation.

• Don't stop taking this medication without first talking with your doctor, who may want you to reduce your dose gradually.

Important reminder

If you're pregnant or breast-feeding, don't take this medication until you talk with your doctor.

Diabinese

Because you have diabetes, your doctor has prescribed Diabinese to lower your blood sugar level. This drug's generic name is chlorpropamide.

How to take Diabinese

Diabinese comes in tablets. Carefully follow the label directions.

What to do if you miss a dose

Take the missed dose as soon as possible. But if it's almost time for your next dose, skip the missed dose and take the next one on schedule. Don't take a double dose.

What to do about side effects

Low blood sugar may occur while you use this medication. Watch for symptoms, such as cool pale skin, difficulty concentrating, shakiness, headache, cold sweats, or feelings of anxiety.

If your blood sugar level drops too low, eat or drink something sugary, such as glucose tablets or fruit juice. If you don't feel better within 15 minutes, eat or drink some more sugary food and call your doctor *right away.*

Tell your doctor if you experience nausea, vomiting, or heartburn or if you develop a rash or other allergic reactions.

This medication may increase your sensitivity to sunlight, so limit your exposure to the sun.

What you must know about alcohol and other drugs

Avoid drinking alcohol, except in amounts your doctor permits, because combined use of Diabinese and alcohol may make you ill or cause your blood sugar level to drop.

Talk to your doctor before taking any other prescription or nonprescription medications. Many medications can react with Diabinese to make your blood sugar too high or too low. In general, you need to avoid certain antidepressants, sulfa medications, Chloromycetin (chloramphenicol, an antibiotic), blood thinners, steroids, glucagon (a hormone), and diuretics (water pills).

Also, taking Diabinese with certain medications for high blood pressure may cover up symptoms of low blood sugar or make a bout of low blood sugar last longer. In addition, aspirin-containing products, appetite-control medications, and cough or cold medications may alter your blood sugar control.

Special directions

• Tell your doctor if you have other medical problems, such as a heart, liver, or kidney condition, or if you're taking insulin.

• Carefully follow your special meal plan because this is the most important part of controlling your diabetes. It's also necessary for Diabinese to work well.

• Test for sugar in your blood or urine as your doctor directs. Regular testing lets you know if your diabetes is under control — and warns you when it's not.

Important reminders

If you're pregnant, check with your doctor before taking this medication.

Don't use Diabinese if you're breast-feeding.

If you're an older adult, you may be especially prone to Diabinese's side effects.

Dialose

This medication is a laxative used to treat constipation. Its generic name is docusate potassium.

How to take Dialose

Dialose comes in capsule form. If this medication was prescribed, follow the doctor's directions exactly. If you bought this medication without a prescription, carefully read the package directions before taking your first dose.

What to do if you miss a dose

Check with your doctor or pharmacist for the best way to handle a missed dose.

What to do about side effects

Although side effects aren't common, Dialose may irritate your throat or leave a bitter taste in your mouth. You may also have mild abdominal cramping or diarrhea. If these symptoms persist or become severe, call your doctor.

What you must know about other drugs

Don't take mineral oil while you're taking Dialose because it may cause your body to absorb too much mineral oil, causing unwanted effects.

If you're taking other medications, take them at least 2 hours before or 2 hours after taking Dialose because Dialose may interfere with the desired actions of the other medications.

Special directions

• Don't use Dialose (or any other laxative) if you have symptoms of appendicitis or an inflamed bowel, such as stomach or lower abdominal pain, cramping, bloating, soreness, nausea, or vomiting. Instead, check with your doctor as soon as possible.

• Drink at least six 8-ounce glasses of water or other liquids daily. This will help soften your bowel movements and relieve constipation.

• Don't take Dialose for more than 1 week unless your doctor has prescribed or ordered a special schedule for you. This is true even if you continue to have constipation.

• If you notice a sudden change in your bowel habits or function that lasts longer than 2 weeks or that occurs from time to time, check with your doctor. Your doctor will need to find the cause of your problem before it becomes more serious.

• Don't overuse Dialose. Otherwise, you may become dependent on this medication to produce a bowel movement. In severe cases, overuse of laxatives can damage the nerves, muscles, and other tissues of the bowel.

Important reminders   If you're pregnant, check with your doctor before taking Dialose.

Don't give this medication to children under age 6 unless prescribed by a doctor.

Diamox

This medication helps control glaucoma, certain types of seizures, and heart failure. Diamox's generic name is acetazolamide.

How to take Diamox   This medication comes in tablet, long-acting capsule, and injectable forms.

Carefully follow the label directions. This medication increases urination, so if you take it once a day, take it in the morning with breakfast. If you take it more than once a day, take the last dose no later than 6 p.m. unless the doctor tells you otherwise.

Take Diamox with food or milk to minimize the chance of an upset stomach. If you have difficulty swallowing tablets, you can mix a tablet in 2 teaspoons of hot water and 2 teaspoons of honey or syrup. If you have trouble swallowing capsules, call the doctor.

What to do if you miss a dose   Take the missed dose as soon as you remember. But if it's almost time for your next dose, skip the missed dose and take the next dose at the regular time. Don't take a double dose.

What to do about side effects Notify the doctor as soon as possible if you start to bruise or bleed easily or if you develop a fever or sore throat.

Until you know how this medication affects you, avoid driving or any activity that requires alertness and coordination.

Special directions
• Inform your doctor about your medical history, especially if you have Addison's disease, diabetes, gout, or kidney, liver, or lung disease.
• Take only the amount of medication the doctor ordered. If you think you need more, consult your doctor.
• If this medication causes your body to lose potassium, your doctor may advise consuming potassium-rich foods and fluids, including bananas, potatoes, unsalted peanuts, and orange juice. Or the doctor may order a potassium supplement for you. Don't change your diet, however, without first consulting your doctor.
• If you're taking Diamox to control seizures, don't suddenly stop taking it.

Important reminders It you have diabetes, carefully monitor sugar levels in your blood and urine. This medication may increase sugar levels.

If you become pregnant while taking this medication, notify your doctor.

If you're an athlete, you should know that the National Collegiate Athletic Association and the U.S. Olympic Committee ban the use of acetazolamide.

Diflucan

Your doctor has prescribed Diflucan to treat your fungal infection. This drug's generic name is fluconazole.

How to take Diflucan Take Diflucan exactly as prescribed. To help clear up your infection completely, take it for the full course of treatment even if your symptoms subside. A fungal infection may require many months of treatment even after your symptoms are no longer bothersome.

What to do if you miss a dose Take a missed dose of medication as soon as you remember. If it's almost time for your next dose, skip the missed dose and take your next dose as scheduled. Don't take a double dose.

What to do about side effects Diflucan causes nausea in some people. If you experience persistent or severe nausea, contact your doctor.

What you must know about other drugs Combined with other medications, Diflucan may produce unwanted side effects. Be sure to tell your doctor about all the medications you take, especially Sandimmune (cyclosporine), Dilantin (phenytoin), INH (isoniazid), Rifadin (rifampin), Depakene (valproic acid), Coumadin (warfarin), and some oral medications used to lower blood sugar levels.

Special directions • Before taking Diflucan, tell your doctor about other medical problems you have, especially kidney or liver disease. They may affect the use of this medication.
• See your doctor regularly so he or she can monitor your progress and check for unwanted side effects.
• Check with your doctor if your symptoms don't disappear within a few weeks or if you feel worse.

Important reminders Consult your doctor if you become pregnant while taking Diflucan.

If you're breast-feeding, check with your doctor before taking Diflucan.

Dilantin

This medication is used to control seizures and treat several other medical problems. Dilantin's generic name is phenytoin.

How to take Dilantin Dilantin comes in capsules, chewable tablets, and an oral liquid. Don't take more or less than your doctor orders. Take Dilantin with meals to reduce stomach upset.

If you're taking the *liquid* form, use a specially marked measuring spoon (not a household teaspoon) to measure your dose.

If you're taking the *capsules,* be sure to swallow them whole.

What to do if you miss a dose

If you take one dose a day, take the missed dose as soon as possible. But if you don't remember until the next day, skip it and take your next dose on schedule.

If you take more than one dose a day, take the missed dose as soon as possible. However, if it's less than 4 hours until your next dose, skip the missed dose and take your next dose on schedule. Don't take a double dose.

What to do about side effects

Call your doctor *right away* if you have skin problems, palpitations, or difficulty breathing. Also call if you have a fever, become extremely weak or tired, or feel very ill.

Check with your doctor if you experience confusion, dizziness, vision changes, sleeplessness, or slurred speech. Also report uncontrolled movements, nausea, vomiting, and bleeding gums.

Make sure you know how you react to Dilantin before you drive or perform other activities requiring alertness.

What you must know about alcohol and other drugs

Check with your doctor before drinking alcoholic beverages because alcohol may prevent Dilantin from working well.

Tell your doctor about other medications you're taking. Some of the many medications you need to avoid or use only with your doctor's supervision are blood thinners, antihistamines (found in cold and allergy medications), the ulcer drug Tagamet (cimetidine), and aspirin.

Special directions

• Tell your doctor if you have other medical problems, especially a heart condition, porphyria, and liver or kidney disease.
• See your dentist regularly, and inform him or her that you're taking Dilantin.

Important reminders

If you're pregnant or breast-feeding, check with your doctor before taking this medication.

If you have diabetes, be aware that Dilantin may affect the results of blood and urine glucose tests.

If you're an athlete, you should know that the U.S. Olympic Committee bans and sometimes tests for phenytoin in biathlon and modern pentathlon events.

Dilaudid

Dilaudid is prescribed to relieve pain or cough. This drug's generic name is hydromorphone.

How to take Dilaudid Dilaudid comes in tablet, suppository, and injection forms. Take it only as prescribed. Overuse could lead to dependency and risk of overdose.

To insert a *suppository,* follow these steps: If the suppository is too soft to insert, run cold water over it or chill it in the refrigerator for about 30 minutes before removing the foil wrapper. Then remove the wrapper and moisten the suppository with cold water. Lie down on your side. Using your index finger, gently push the suppository into your rectum as far as possible.

If you're using the *injectable* form, follow your doctor's instructions for performing injections. Alternate among several injection sites to help prevent complications.

What to do if you miss a dose Take the missed dose as soon as you remember. However, if it's almost time for your next regular dose, skip the missed dose and take the next one at the regular time. Don't take a double dose.

What to do about side effects If you think you've taken an overdose or develop symptoms of an overdose, get emergency medical care *immediately.* Symptoms of overdose include seizures, cold and clammy skin, confusion, severe drowsiness or dizziness, slow or troubled breathing, slow heartbeat, extreme nervousness or restlessness, severe weakness, and very small pupils.

Dilaudid may cause drowsiness, dizziness, difficulty thinking clearly, nausea, vomiting, constipation, difficulty urinating, or a false sense of well-being. These problems may go away as your body adjusts to the medication; if they continue, tell your doctor.

Don't drive or perform other activities requiring alertness until you know how you respond to this medication.

To help prevent or relieve constipation, drink plenty of fluids and eat high-fiber foods.

What you must know about alcohol and other drugs

Don't drink alcoholic beverages while taking Dilaudid because the combination can cause an overdose. Check with your doctor before taking other prescription or nonprescription medications. Some can add to Dilaudid's effects.

Special directions

• Let your doctor know if you have other medical problems. They may affect the use of this medication.

• If you've taken Dilaudid regularly for several weeks or more, don't stop taking it without first checking with your doctor, who will want to decrease your dosage gradually to minimize side effects from withdrawal.

Important reminders

If you're pregnant or think you may be, check with your doctor before taking this medication.

Children and older adults are especially sensitive to this medication.

Dimetapp

This medication relieves a stuffy or runny nose and sneezing from colds and allergies. Dimetapp's generic name is brompheniramine with phenylpropanolamine.

How to take Dimetapp

This medication comes in tablet, extended-release tablet, and elixir forms. Carefully follow the label directions. Take Dimetapp with food, milk, or water to reduce stomach upset.

Swallow an *extended-release tablet* whole; don't break, crush, or chew it. If you can't swallow it, consult the doctor, nurse, or pharmacist.

What to do if you miss a dose

Take the missed dose as soon as you remember. But if it's almost time for your next dose, skip the dose you missed and resume your normal dosing schedule. Never take a double dose.

What to do about side effects

Call the doctor *immediately* if you have a rapid or irregular heartbeat, a tight chest, sore throat, fever, unusual tiredness or weakness, or unusual bleeding or bruising.

Common side effects include a dry mouth, thick phlegm, drowsiness and, possibly, nervousness, restlessness, and insomnia. If these effects persist, call your doctor.

Know how you respond to this medication before you drive or perform other activities requiring alertness.

If you have trouble sleeping, take the day's last dose a few hours before bedtime.

Relieve dry mouth with ice chips or sugarless gum or hard candy.

What you must know about alcohol and other drugs

Tell your doctor about other medications you're taking. Taking this drug with alcoholic beverages and other medications that depress the central nervous system (such as antihistamines and pain and seizure medications) increases the side effects of all. And taking this drug with appetite suppressants increases the risk of overdose. Signs of overdose include difficulty breathing, severe drowsiness, persistent headache, and seizures.

Special directions

• Inform the doctor if you have asthma, heart or blood vessel disease, high blood pressure, glaucoma, diabetes, an overactive thyroid, or urinary problems.

• Also report any allergic or unusual reactions to antihistamines.

Important reminders

If you're pregnant or breast-feeding, consult your doctor about using this medication.

This medication should be used cautiously in young children and older adults.

If you're an athlete, you should know that the National Collegiate Athletic Association and the U.S. Olympic Committee disqualify athletes from competitions if urine samples contain excess phenylpropanolamine (an ingredient in Dimetapp).

Diuril

Diuril helps control high blood pressure. Also, by increasing urination, Diuril relieves the body of excess water. This drug's generic name is chlorothiazide.

How to take Diuril Carefully follow the label directions. Take a single daily dose in the morning after breakfast. If you're taking more than one dose a day, schedule the last dose no later than 6 p.m., unless your doctor directs otherwise.

If you're taking the *liquid* form, remember to shake the bottle well before pouring a dose.

What to do if you miss a dose Take the missed dose as soon as you remember. If it's almost time for your next dose, skip the dose you missed, and take your next dose at the regular time. Don't take a double dose.

What to do about side effects If you develop a persistent fever, sore throat, joint pain, unusual bruising or bleeding, or extreme listlessness or fatigue, stop taking Diuril and call the doctor *immediately.*

More common side effects include jitteriness, muscle cramps, numbness and tingling, weakness, fatigue, increased urination and thirst, and sensitivity to sunlight. If these symptoms persist or worsen, call your doctor.

What you must know about other drugs Tell your doctor about other medications (prescription and nonprescription) you're taking because some may reduce Diuril's effectiveness.

Special directions • Tell the doctor if you have other medical problems, particularly diabetes, gout, lupus, pancreatitis, and kidney or liver disease. Also report any allergies you have.

• If the doctor prescribes a special low-salt diet (to help reduce your blood pressure), follow it closely.

• When you take this medication, your body will lose water and potassium. To prevent complications, your doctor may recommend potassium-rich foods (such as citrus fruits and bananas), a potassium supplement, or another medication.

• Notify your doctor if you have severe or continuing vomiting or diarrhea. These conditions can lead to increased potassium and water loss.

Important reminders

Don't take this medication if you're pregnant or breast-feeding.

If you have diabetes, monitor your blood sugar levels carefully.

Older adults are especially sensitive to the effects of this medication.

If you're an athlete, you should know that the National Collegiate Athletic Association and the U.S. Olympic Committee ban the use of chlorothiazide.

Dolobid

Your doctor has prescribed Dolobid to relieve your pain. This medication, which is similar to aspirin, is often used to treat osteoarthritis symptoms, such as joint swelling, stiffness, and pain. The drug's generic name is diflunisal.

How to take Dolobid

Dolobid comes in tablet form. Take Dolobid with food or an antacid and a full glass (8 ounces) of water. Don't crush or break the tablet — swallow it whole.

Also, don't lie down for about 15 to 30 minutes after taking your dose. This helps to prevent irritation of your esophagus.

What to do if you miss a dose

Take the missed dose as soon as you remember. However, if it's almost time for your next dose, skip the missed dose and take your next dose on schedule. Never take a double dose.

What to do about side effects

Check with your doctor if this medication makes you dizzy or if you develop a headache or rash. Also notify the doctor if you have ringing in your ears or changes in your vision.

Because Dolobid can irritate your digestive tract, call your doctor if you experience nausea, heartburn, stomach or abdominal pain, or diarrhea.

Call your doctor *at once* if you have any of the following warning signs of gastrointestinal bleeding or ulcers: severe stomach or abdominal pain; black, tarry stools; and vomiting of blood or material that looks like coffee grounds.

What you must know about alcohol and other drugs

Don't drink alcoholic beverages while taking Dolobid because the combination increases the risk of stomach problems.

Tell the doctor about other medications you're taking. Don't take aspirin, Tylenol (acetaminophen), or other aspirin-related drugs together with Dolobid for more than a few days, unless your doctor gives you other directions, because doing so may cause unwanted side effects.

If you take blood thinners, be aware that Dolobid may increase your risk of bleeding. Antacids may decrease Dolobid's effectiveness.

Special directions

• Tell your doctor if you have other medical problems, especially ulcers, a heart condition, or kidney disease. Also inform the doctor if you're allergic to Dolobid, aspirin, or other medications.

• Before having any kind of surgery (including dental surgery), tell the doctor or dentist that you're taking Dolobid.

• Because this medication may make you dizzy, make sure you know how you react to it before you drive, use machines, or perform other activities that could be dangerous if you're not fully alert.

Important reminders

If you're pregnant or breast-feeding, don't take this medication unless you have your doctor's approval.

If you're an older adult, be aware that you may be especially sensitive to side effects from Dolobid.

Donnatal

This drug is a combination of belladonna and phenobarbital. Donnatal relieves cramping from stomach and intestinal spasms and also decreases stomach acid.

How to take Donnatal

This medication comes in tablet form. Carefully follow the label directions. Unless your doctor gives you other instructions, take the medication 30 to 60 minutes before meals.

What to do if you miss a dose

Take the missed dose as soon as you remember. But if it's almost time for your next dose, skip the missed dose and resume your normal dosage schedule. Never take a double dose.

What to do about side effects

If you experience itching or a rash, unusual bleeding or bruising, a sore throat and fever, eye pain, or yellowish eyes or skin, stop taking the medication and call your doctor *immediately*.

Other side effects include constipation; mouth, nose, throat, or skin dryness; decreased sweating; dizziness; and drowsiness. Call your doctor if these symptoms persist or become worse.

Make sure you know how you respond to this medication before you drive or perform other activities requiring alertness.

If you experience increased sensitivity to light, wear sunglasses and avoid bright lights.

Avoid becoming overheated because Donnatal may cause you to sweat less and thus increase your body temperature.

What you must know about alcohol and other drugs

Don't take this medication with alcoholic beverages or medications that can cause drowsiness (for example, medications for hay fever and other allergies or colds), seizure medication, sleeping medication, or muscle relaxants.

Avoid taking this medication within 1 hour of taking an antacid or diarrhea medication. Taking these medications too close together decreases the effectiveness of Donnatal.

Special directions

• Tell your doctor if you have other medical problems; they may affect the use of this medication.

• Check with your doctor before taking any new medications, either prescription or nonprescription, while taking Donnatal.

Important reminders   If you're pregnant or breast-feeding, check with your doctor before taking this medication.

Children and older adults are especially sensitive to the effects of this medication.

Dramamine

Dramamine is used to relieve nausea and vomiting and to prevent or treat motion sickness. This drug's generic name is dimenhydrinate.

How to take Dramamine   Dramamine comes in the form of tablets, chewable tablets, capsules, and syrup.

Carefully follow the label directions. If you're taking Dramamine to prevent motion sickness, take it at least 1 to 2 hours before traveling. If this isn't possible, take it at least 30 minutes before traveling.

Take this medication with food or a glass of milk or water to lessen stomach irritation, if necessary.

What to do about side effects   Dramamine may make you feel drowsy. Occasionally, this medication causes headache, palpitations, blurred vision, and mouth dryness. If these side effects persist or become severe, call your doctor.

If this medication makes your mouth feel dry, you may get temporary relief by using sugarless hard candy or gum, melting bits of ice in your mouth, or using a saliva substitute.

Because this medication may make you drowsy, make sure you know how you react to it before you drive, use machines, or perform other activities that could be dangerous if you're not fully alert.

What you must know about alcohol and other drugs   Check with your doctor before drinking alcoholic beverages or taking other drugs because the combined effects may make you overly drowsy.

Special directions   • Check with your doctor before you take this medication if you have glaucoma, asthma, an enlarged prostate, or a seizure disorder.

• Don't take Dramamine if you're allergic to Theo-Dur (theophylline), an asthma medication.

• Tell your doctor that you're taking Dramamine before you have any skin tests for allergies because it may affect the test results.

• If you're taking Dramamine to control nausea and vomiting, make sure your doctor knows that you're taking this medication if you should suddenly develop symptoms of appendicitis, such as stomach or lower abdominal pain, cramping, and soreness.

Important reminders   If you're pregnant or breast-feeding, check with your doctor before using Dramamine.

Be aware that children and older adults are especially sensitive to side effects from this medication.

Dulcolax

Dulcolax is used to relieve constipation. This drug's generic name is bisacodyl. Another brand name is Fleet Bisacodyl.

How to take
Dulcolax   Dulcolax is available in tablet, enema, powder for rectal solution, and suppository forms.

Follow your doctor's instructions. If you're using the enema, powder for rectal solution, or suppository form, also follow the manufacturer's package directions exactly.

Whichever Dulcolax form you use, drink six to eight 8-ounce glasses of liquid daily to help soften your stools.

Take the *tablet* on an empty stomach for rapid effect. Because the tablets are specially coated to prevent stomach irritation, don't chew, crush, or take them within an hour of drinking milk or taking antacids. You may want to take tablets at bedtime to produce results the next morning.

If you're using a *suppository* and it's too soft to insert, chill it for 30 minutes or run cold water over it before removing the foil wrapper. To insert it, first wash your hands; then remove the wrapper and moisten the suppository with cold water. Lie on your side and use your finger to gently push the suppository into your rectum.

To use the *enema,* first lubricate your anus with Vaseline (petroleum jelly). Then lie on your side and gently insert the rectal tip of the enema applicator. Squeeze all the solution from the enema bottle.

What to do about side effects Common side effects include nausea, vomiting, abdominal cramps and, with the suppository, a burning sensation in the rectum. If these symptoms persist or worsen, contact your doctor. Also notify the doctor if you notice rectal bleeding, blistering, pain, burning, itching, or other irritation you didn't have before using this medication.

Special directions
• If you have other medical problems, check with your doctor before using Dulcolax.
• Don't use Dulcolax or other laxatives if you have stomach or lower abdominal pain, cramping, bloating, soreness, nausea, or vomiting. Instead, notify your doctor as soon as possible.
• Don't use Dulcolax within 2 hours of taking other medications; doing so can reduce other medications' effects.
• Never use Dulcolax for more than 1 week unless your doctor prescribes it.
• If a change in bowel function persists longer than 2 weeks or keeps returning, check with your doctor before using Dulcolax.
• Don't use Dulcolax unless you need it. Overusing laxatives may damage bowel structures, foster dependence, and cause weakness, poor coordination, dizziness, and light-headedness.

Important reminder Don't use Dulcolax in children under age 6 unless prescribed by a doctor.

Duragesic

Your doctor has prescribed the Duragesic transdermal patch to help relieve your pain. This drug's generic name is fentanyl.

How to apply a Duragesic patch

Apply a new patch to a new site every 72 hours or as ordered by your doctor. First, clip excess hair at the patch site. Don't use a razor because shaving may irritate or scratch your skin.

Wash your skin with clear water if necessary, but don't use soap, oil, lotion, alcohol, or any other substance that may irritate your skin or interfere with the patch's stickiness.

Make sure your skin is completely dry. Then put the patch on your skin and hold it in place for 10 to 20 seconds to make sure it stays on.

What to do if you miss a dose

If you don't apply a new patch when scheduled, do so as soon as you can. Don't apply more than one patch at a time. Doing so may cause serious side effects.

What to do about side effects

Seek medical care *at once* if you have trouble breathing.

Duragesic also may make you feel drowsy and lethargic. It may lower your blood pressure, causing you to feel dizzy or light-headed. You may also experience constipation and problems with urination. If these side effects persist or become severe, contact your doctor.

Don't drive or perform activities requiring alertness until you know how Duragesic affects you.

What you must know about alcohol and other drugs

Don't drink alcoholic beverages or take medications that affect your nervous system (such as many allergy or cold medications, narcotics, muscle relaxants, sleeping pills, and seizure medications). Combined with Duragesic, these medications may produce serious side effects.

Special directions

• Before using Duragesic, inform your doctor of other medical problems you may have. They may affect the use of this medication.

• Don't stop using Duragesic suddenly. Doing so may cause undesirable withdrawal effects. Consult your doctor, who may reduce your dosage gradually before stopping the medication completely.

Important reminders

If you're breast-feeding, consult your doctor before taking Duragesic.

Young children and older adults are especially sensitive to Duragesic.

If you're an athlete, be aware that the U.S. Olympic Committee bans and tests for the use of fentanyl.

Dyazide

Your doctor has prescribed this medication to control your blood pressure. This drug's generic name is hydrochlorothiazide with triamterene. Another brand name is Maxzide.

How to take Dyazide

Take this drug exactly as prescribed. If you're taking one dose a day, take it in the morning after breakfast. If you're taking more than one dose a day, take your last dose before 6 p.m. so the need to urinate won't disturb your sleep. To prevent stomach upset, take this medication with milk or meals.

What to do if you miss a dose

Take the missed dose as soon as you remember unless it's almost time for your next dose. If so, skip the missed dose and take your next dose as scheduled. Never take a double dose.

What to do about side effects

If you feel like your throat is closing and you have trouble breathing, stop taking this medication and get emergency care *at once.* Also stop taking this medication and call your doctor if you experience persistent fever, sore throat, joint pain, or easy bleeding or bruising.

Common side effects include dehydration, low blood sugar level, chronic fatigue, anxiety, irritability, muscle cramps, numbness, pain, "pins and needles" sensation, weakness, increased urination and thirst, and weak, irregular pulse. If these symptoms persist, tell your doctor.

This medication may make you sensitive to sunlight, so limit sun exposure.

What you must know about other drugs

Tell your doctor if you're taking other prescription or nonprescription drugs. For example, taking this medication with angiotensin-converting enzyme inhibitors (such as Capoten) or potassium supplements can raise blood potassium levels, possibly leading to kidney and heart problems.

Special directions
• Because this medication may decrease your body's potassium level, your doctor may instruct you to eat foods high in potassium, such as uncooked dried fruits and fresh orange juice, take a potassium supplement, and cut down on salt.

• Contact your doctor if you develop persistent or severe diarrhea or vomiting, which can cause excessive potassium and water loss and decrease blood pressure too much.

Important reminders
If you're pregnant or breast-feeding, check with your doctor before taking this medication.

Older adults are especially sensitive to this medication.

If you're an athlete, be aware that the National Collegiate Athletic Association and the U.S. Olympic Committee ban the use of hydrochlorothiazide with triamterene.

Dymelor

Dymelor lowers blood sugar levels. This drug's generic name is acetohexamide.

How to take Dymelor
This medication comes in tablet form. Carefully follow the label directions. Take it at the same time each day, and don't take more or less than your doctor has ordered.

What to do if you miss a dose
Take the missed dose as soon as you remember. If it's almost time for your next dose, skip the missed dose. Take your next dose at the regularly scheduled time. Don't take a double dose.

What to do about side effects
This medication may cause unsatisfactorily low blood sugar levels, especially if you delay or miss a meal or snack, exercise more than usual, or drink a significant amount of alcohol. Symptoms of low blood sugar include

cool pale skin, difficulty concentrating, shakiness, headache, cold sweats, and anxiety.

Learn to recognize your reaction to a low blood sugar level so you can take corrective steps quickly.

Check your blood sugar level with a test strip to confirm that it's low. (Be sure to ask your doctor for information if you don't know how to test yourself.) To correct a low blood sugar level, eat or drink something containing sugar, such as glucose tablets or gel, fruit juice, or raisins.

If the symptoms don't subside in 10 or 15 minutes or if you feel worse, eat or drink some more food or liquid that contains a lot of sugar. Also seek medical attention immediately.

Be sure to notify your doctor if your blood sugar levels drop and you have symptoms. That's because the blood sugar–lowering effects of Dymelor may last for days and your symptoms may recur.

Other possible side effects include nausea, vomiting, mild drowsiness, headache, heartburn, dizziness, diarrhea, constipation, appetite changes, and stomach pain, fullness, or discomfort. These side effects may subside as your body adjusts to the medication. If these effects persist, consult your doctor.

Because this medication may make your skin more sensitive to the sun, wear a sunblock with a skin protection factor (SPF) of at least 15. Also wear protective clothing and sunglasses when you're outside. If you develop a severe reaction from sun exposure, contact your doctor and stay out of the sun.

What you must know about alcohol and other drugs Avoid alcoholic beverages until you have discussed their use with your doctor. Combining Dymelor and alcohol can make you ill or cause your blood sugar level to drop.

Tell the doctor what other medications you're taking, including nonprescription drugs. Many contain ingredients that interact with Dymelor to increase or decrease your blood sugar level beyond a safe amount. For example, antidepressants, Chloromycetin (chloramphenicol), sulfa drugs, or oral anticoagulants (blood thinners) may increase your risk of having a low blood sugar level. On the other hand, steroids, glucagon, or thiazide diuretics (water pills) may increase your chances for a high blood sugar level.

Some heart medications (called beta blockers) may make a low blood sugar episode last longer or hide the symptoms of a low sugar level.

What's more, some nonprescription medications (such as aspirin or similar products containing salicylates, appetite control medications, or cold or cough medicines) may affect your sugar level.

Special directions
• Make sure your doctor knows your medical history, especially if you have a heart problem or kidney, liver, or thyroid disease.

• Follow your special meal plan carefully. Diet is the most important part of controlling your diabetes and is necessary for your medication to work.

• Test the amount of sugar in your blood and urine as directed by your doctor. Self-testing helps you keep your diabetes under control and warns you when it's not.

• Don't take any other medication unless it's prescribed or approved by your doctor. This precaution applies especially to nonprescription medications used to treat colds, coughs, asthma, or hay fever. It also applies to appetite control preparations.

• Tell the doctor if you develop an infection because you may need insulin temporarily to control your blood sugar level. Severe infection can cause your glucose level to change rapidly.

• Because this medication may make your skin more sensitive to the sun, wear a sunblock with a skin protection factor (SPF) of at least 15. Also wear protective clothing and sunglasses when you're outside. If you develop a severe reaction from sun exposure, contact your doctor and stay out of the sun.

• Keep follow-up medical appointments so your doctor can check your progress regularly, especially during the first few weeks that you take Dymelor.

• Before any kind of surgery, dental work, or emergency treatment, tell the doctor or dentist that you're taking Dymelor.

• Wear a medical identification tag or bracelet or carry an identification card at all times. Your identification should state that you have diabetes. It should also name your medications.

Important reminders If you're breast-feeding or you become pregnant, check with your doctor before taking this medication.

If you're an older adult, be aware that you may be more sensitive than younger adults to the effects of Dymelor.

Dynapen

Dynapen is prescribed to treat bacterial infections. This drug's generic name is dicloxacillin. Another brand name is Dycill.

How to take Dynapen This antibiotic medication comes in capsule and oral suspension forms.

If you're taking the *capsule* form of Dynapen, don't break, chew, or crush the capsule — swallow it whole.

If you're taking the *oral suspension,* use a dropper or specially marked measuring spoon to measure each dose accurately.

Take your medication with a full glass (8 ounces) of water on an empty stomach, either 1 hour before or 2 hours after meals unless otherwise directed by your doctor.

Continue to take your medication, even after you start to feel better. Stopping too soon may allow your infection to return.

What to do if you miss a dose Take the missed dose as soon as possible. But if it's almost time for your next dose, adjust your dosage schedule as follows.

If you take two doses a day, space the missed dose and the next dose 5 to 6 hours apart.

If you take three or more doses a day, space the missed dose and the next dose 2 to 4 hours apart. Then resume your regular dosing schedule.

What to do about side effects

Call your doctor *at once* if you develop any of the following signs of an allergic reaction: difficulty breathing, a rash, hives, itching, or wheezing.

Check with your doctor if you experience nausea, heartburn, or diarrhea, especially if these symptoms persist or become severe.

What you must know about other drugs

Tell the doctor about other medications you're taking. Probalan (probenecid), a gout medication, may increase the effects of Dynapen. This effect may or may not be beneficial; check with your doctor.

Special directions

• Tell your doctor if you have a history of kidney problems or if you're allergic to other antibiotics.

• If you become allergic to this medication, you should carry a medical identification card or wear a medical identification bracelet stating this.

• If you develop severe diarrhea, don't take any diarrhea medication without first checking with your doctor. Diarrhea medications may make your diarrhea worse or last longer. For mild diarrhea, you may take a diarrhea medication containing kaolin or attapulgite.

• Tell the doctor that you're taking Dynapen before you have medical tests because this medication may alter test results.

Important reminder

If you're pregnant or breast-feeding, check with your doctor before taking this medication.

Dyrenium

This medication is a diuretic, a drug that helps reduce the amount of water in your body. This drug's generic name is triamterene.

How to take Dyrenium

If you're taking one dose a day, take it in the morning after breakfast. Because the medication will increase your urine output, taking it in the morning will help prevent the increase in urine from disturbing your sleep. If you take more than one dose a day, take the last dose no later than 6 p.m. If the medication upsets your stomach, take it with food or milk.

What to do if you miss a dose

Take the missed dose as soon as possible. But if it's almost time for your next dose, skip the missed dose and take your next dose as scheduled.

What to do about side effects

When you first start taking Dyrenium, you may feel unusually tired or dizzy. If this becomes particularly bothersome, call your doctor.

Dyrenium may cause the amount of potassium in your body to increase. Call your doctor *right away* if you develop any of the following signs and symptoms of too much potassium: confusion or nervousness; irregular heartbeat; numbness or tingling in hands, feet, or lips; difficulty breathing; unusual tiredness or weakness; weakness or heaviness in legs.

Also call your doctor right away if you develop a rash or itching.

To keep from becoming dizzy or fainting, change positions slowly. Also get up slowly after sitting or lying down.

What you must know about other drugs

Dyrenium may interfere with the way some medications work. Tell your doctor if you're taking Indocin (indomethacin), Lanoxin (digoxin), Eskalith (lithium), or a medication for high blood pressure.

Also, because Dyrenium may interfere with tests to measure the amount of a heart medication called Cardioquin (quinidine) in your blood, tell your doctor if you're taking Cardioquin.

Because Dyrenium doesn't cause you to lose potassium the way some diuretics do, don't take a potassium supplement. Also avoid drinking low-salt milk or using salt substitutes (which contain potassium), unless your doctor instructs you otherwise.

Special directions

• Tell your doctor if you have diabetes, kidney or liver disease, gout, menstrual problems, breast enlargement, or a history of kidney stones.

• Your doctor may tell you to weigh yourself every day, measure your urine output, and monitor the amount of fluid you drink. Keep a written record of the results and take it with you when you visit the doctor.

Important reminders   If you have diabetes, be especially careful in testing your urine for glucose. That's because Dyrenium may raise your blood sugar level.

If you're an athlete, you should know that the U.S. Olympic Committee and National Collegiate Athletic Association bans and tests for the use of triamterene.

E

Elavil

Your doctor has prescribed Elavil to relieve your depression. The drug's generic name is amitriptyline. Other brand names include Endep and Enovil.

How to take Elavil
Elavil comes as a syrup or tablet. Carefully follow the directions on the bottle.

Take Elavil with food, even for a daily bedtime dose, unless your doctor has told you otherwise.

What to do if you miss a dose
If you take one dose daily at bedtime and you miss a dose, don't take the missed dose in the morning — it may cause disturbing side effects during waking hours. Instead, call your doctor for directions.

If you take more than one dose daily, take the missed dose as soon as possible. But if it's almost time for your next dose, skip the missed dose and go back to your regular schedule. Don't take a double dose.

What to do about side effects
Elavil may make you feel drowsy or dizzy. You may experience an irregular or fast pulse, blurred vision, dry mouth, constipation, sweating, or problems with urinating.

You may also feel light-headed or faint if you get up suddenly from a lying or sitting position. Getting up slowly may help. Notify your doctor if any of these effects persist or become troublesome.

To help combat constipation, increase your fluid and fiber intake. If these steps don't help, your doctor may prescribe a stool softener.

Until you know how Elavil affects you, don't drive, use machinery, or do anything else that requires alertness. The drowsiness and dizziness usually go away after a few weeks of taking this medication.

If Elivil causes mouth dryness, use sugarless gum or hard candy, ice chips, or a saliva substitute. However, if your mouth continues to feel dry for more than 2 weeks, check with your doctor or dentist. Continuing mouth dryness may increase the chance of dental disease, including tooth decay, gum disease, and fungus infections.

Elavil may make your skin more sensitive to sunlight. Sun exposure may cause a rash, itching, redness, other discoloration, or a severe sunburn. Avoid direct sunlight, wear protective clothing including a hat and sunglasses, and use a sunblock with a skin protection factor (SPF) of 15 or higher on your skin and lips. If you have a severe sun reaction, check with your doctor.

What you must know about alcohol and other drugs

When taking Elavil, ask your doctor before drinking alcoholic beverages or taking nonprescription medications, such as allergy, cold, or other medications that make you sleepy.

Tell your doctor if you're taking other medications. Barbiturates (anxiety medication) may decrease Elavil's effectiveness.

Ritalin (methylphenidate) and the ulcer drug Tagamet (cimetidine) may increase Elavil's effect beyond a safe level.

When taken with Elavil, Adrenalin (epinephrine) and Levophed (norepinephrine) may increase your blood pressure. Monoamine oxidase (MAO) inhibitors such as Marplan (isocarboxazid) may cause severe agitation, high fever, or seizures.

Special directions

• Be sure to tell your doctor if you have other medical problems. They may affect the use of Elavil.

• You may need to take this medication for several weeks before you begin to feel better. See your doctor at regular intervals so he or she can check your progress and perhaps adjust the dosage.

• Make sure you tell other doctors and your dentist that you're taking this medication before you have medical tests, surgery, dental work, or emergency treatment.

• Don't stop taking this medication without checking with your doctor, who may reduce the dosage gradually to prevent your condition from becoming worse and to lessen the possibility of withdrawal symptoms, such as headache, nausea, and an overall feeling of discomfort.

• Keep in mind that the effects of this medication may last for 3 to 7 days after you stop taking it.

Important reminders   If you have diabetes and you notice a change in your blood or urine glucose test results, contact your doctor. This medication may affect your sugar levels.

Notify your doctor if you're pregnant or breast-feeding while taking this medication.

Children and older adults may be especially sensitive to Elavil's effects.

Emcyt

This estrogen-like medication is used to treat menopausal symptoms, vaginal dryness, and certain cancers. The drug's generic name is estradiol. Other brand names are Estrace and Estraderm.

How to take Emcyt   Emcyt comes in tablet, vaginal cream, and skin patch forms. Follow your doctor's instructions exactly. If the tablets cause nausea, you may take them with food.

Before applying a *patch,* read the accompanying instructions. Wash and dry your hands. Apply the patch to a clean, dry, nonoily skin area, such as your abdomen or buttocks.

If you're using the *vaginal cream,* your doctor may want you to use it at bedtime so it will be absorbed better. If you don't use it at bedtime, lie down for 30 minutes after use.

What to do if you miss a dose   If you forget to take a *tablet* or change a *skin patch,* do it as soon as possible. But if it's almost time for your next dose, skip the missed dose. Take your next tablet or apply a new patch on schedule. Don't take a double dose of tablets or use more than one patch at a time.

If you forget to apply a dose of *vaginal cream* and don't remember until the next day, skip the missed dose. Resume your regular dosing schedule.

What to do about side effects   Blood clots are a rare but serious complication. Call for emergency help *immediately* if you have sudden or severe headache; sudden loss of coordination; blurred vision or other vision changes; numbness or stiffness in your legs; pain in your chest, groin, or legs; or shortness of breath.

Call your doctor *right away* if you notice rapid weight gain; swelling in your feet and lower legs; breast enlargement, pain, or lumps; or unusual vaginal bleeding. Also call if you become nauseated, lose your appetite, or have stomach bloating or cramps.

If you're using the vaginal cream, call your doctor if you develop swelling, redness, or itching in the vaginal area.

What you must know about other drugs Because many medications can interfere with Emcyt, tell your doctor about other medications (nonprescription and prescription) that you're taking.

Special directions • Because Emcyt can aggravate many medical conditions, tell your doctor about other medical problems you have. Also tell the doctor if any female relatives have had cancer of the breast or female organs.
• Keep all appointments for follow-up visits so your doctor can check your progress and detect side effects early.
• Perform breast self-examinations regularly and report unusual changes.

Important reminders Don't take Emcyt if you're pregnant or breast-feeding. If you have diabetes, be aware that Emcyt may affect your sugar levels.

Emperin with Codeine

This medication is used to treat moderate to severe pain. Generically, the drug is known as aspirin with codeine.

How to take Emperin with Codeine Take Emperin with codeine exactly as your doctor has prescribed. To reduce stomach irritation, take this medication with food or an 8-ounce glass of milk or water.

What to do if you miss a dose If you take this medication regularly and you miss a dose, take the missed dose as soon as you remember. However, if it's almost time for your next dose, skip the missed dose and go back to your regular schedule. Don't take a double dose.

What to do about side effects

If you have trouble breathing or experience itching, a rash, or other signs of an allergic reaction, stop taking this medication and notify your doctor *immediately.*

Side effects may include abdominal pain caused by gas, heartburn, indigestion, and nausea. If these symptoms persist or become severe, contact your doctor.

This medication also may cause dizziness and lightheadedness. Move slowly when you get up from a lying or sitting position.

What you must know about alcohol and other drugs

Don't take alcoholic beverages with this medication because the codeine in it can slow down your nervous system, making you extremely drowsy. Also, the mixture of alcohol and aspirin may irritate your stomach.

Tell your doctor about other medications you're taking, especially antacids, because they may make the Emperin with codeine less effective.

Check with the doctor before taking other medications that slow the nervous system, such as medications for colds or hay fever and other allergies, prescription pain and seizure medications, muscle relaxants, and other medications that make you feel relaxed or sleepy.

Taking this medication with anticoagulants (blood thinners) may increase your risk of bleeding.

If you have diabetes, keep in mind that Emperin with codeine (and other aspirin products) taken regularly may increase the effects of oral diabetes medications. Check with your doctor to see whether the dosage of your diabetes medication needs adjustment.

Check with the doctor before taking Tylenol (acetaminophen).

Special directions

• Tell your doctor if you've ever had an unusual or allergic reaction to aspirin or codeine.
• Inform your doctor if you have other medical problems, especially gout or gallbladder disease.
• Check the labels of all nonprescription and prescription medications to see if they contain aspirin, other salicylates, or salicylic acid. Pepto-Bismol (bismuth subsalicylate) is an example of a commonly used nonpre-

scription medication that contains salicylates. Contact your doctor if you're taking a product that contains a narcotic, aspirin, or other salicylates because combining these medications can lead to overdose.

• Don't take this medication if it smells like vinegar. This odor means that the aspirin is losing its effectiveness.

• Make sure you know how you respond to this medication before you perform activities that require alertness, such as driving or operating machinery.

• Make sure you tell other doctors and your dentist that you're taking this medication before surgery (including dental surgery) or emergency treatment. Because this medication may cause bleeding problems, your doctor may instruct you to stop taking it 5 days before surgery.

• Don't suddenly stop taking this medication if you've been taking it regularly. Your doctor may want to reduce your dosage gradually to avoid withdrawal effects.

Important reminders

If you become pregnant while taking this medication, notify the doctor as soon as possible. Don't take aspirin in the last 3 months of your pregnancy unless directed by your doctor.

If you're breast-feeding, tell the doctor before you take this medication.

Never give a medication containing aspirin to a child or teenager with a fever or other signs of a viral infection, such as chickenpox or flu. The aspirin may cause Reye's syndrome, a serious illness.

Keep in mind that children are especially sensitive to the effects of this medication, particularly if they have a fever or have lost large amounts of body fluids from vomiting, diarrhea, or sweating. Also, the codeine in this medication may make children unusually excited or restless.

Older adults are especially susceptible to the side effects of this medication, particularly breathing problems.

If you're an athlete, you should know that the National Collegiate Athletic Association and the U.S. Olympic Committee ban the use of codeine.

E-Mycin

Your doctor has prescribed E-Mycin to treat your infection. The drug is known generically as oral erythromycin. Other brand names include Erytab and PCE.

How to take E-Mycin
This medication comes in tablet, capsule, and oral liquid forms. Carefully check the label on your prescription bottle, and follow the directions exactly as written.

Take your medication with a full glass (8 ounces) of water 1 hour before meals or 2 hours after. If the tablets are coated or the medication upsets your stomach, you may take it with food. But don't take your medication with fruit juice.

If you're taking the *chewable tablets,* chew or crush them before swallowing. If you're taking the *delayed-release capsules,* swallow them whole.

If you're taking the *oral liquid* form, measure your dose with a special dropper or measuring spoon made especially for medications.

Continue to take your medication for the full treatment time, even if you feel better after a few days. Stopping too soon may allow your infection to return.

What to do if you miss a dose
Take the missed dose as soon as possible. But if it's almost time for your next dose, change your schedule as follows:

If you take two doses a day, space the missed dose and the next one 5 to 6 hours apart.

If you take three or more doses a day, space the missed dose and the next one 2 to 4 hours apart.

Then resume your regular dosage schedule.

What to do about side effects
If you develop a rash or itchy skin, stop taking the medication and call your doctor *immediately.* Sometimes, these symptoms are warning signs of a serious allergic reaction. If you feel unusually restless or have trouble breathing, get medical care *right away.*

Tell your doctor if you have stomach pain, diarrhea, nausea, or vomiting. These symptoms may go away as your body adjusts to E-Mycin, but let your doctor know if they bother you.

What you must know about other drugs Tell your doctor if you're taking other medications. E-Mycin may not work well if taken with certain other antibiotics. Taking E-Mycin with blood thinners may increase your risk of bleeding. Your doctor also may caution you against taking E-Mycin with the asthma drug Theo-Dur (theophylline) because of possible unwanted side effects.

Special directions • Tell your doctor if you have other medical problems, especially liver disease, and if you're allergic to E-Mycin, another medication, or any food.
• Tell other doctors that you're taking E-Mycin before you have medical tests because the drug may interfere with some test results.

Ergostat

Your doctor has prescribed Ergostat to relieve your headaches. This drug's generic name is ergotamine.

How to take Ergostat This medication comes in three forms: tablets to melt under your tongue, an inhaler, and suppositories.

If you're taking the *under-the-tongue tablets,* place the tablet under your tongue so it dissolves. Don't chew or swallow it because it works faster when absorbed into the lining of your mouth.

If you're using the *inhaler,* read the directions that come with it before using the medication. The inhaler gives about 300 measured sprays.

If you're using a *suppository* and it's too soft to insert, keep it in the foil wrapper and run cold water over it or chill it in the refrigerator for about 30 minutes. To insert it, remove the foil wrapper and moisten the suppository with cold water. Then lie on your side and use your index finger to gently push the suppository into your rectum as far as you can.

Don't take more than the prescribed amount of Ergostat without checking with your doctor.

For best results, take Ergostat at the first sign of a headache. Also, lie down in a quiet, dark room for at least 2 hours after taking your medication.

What to do about side effects Call your doctor *right away* if you experience confusion; rapid or slow heartbeat; numbness and tingling of your fingers, toes, or face; red blisters on, or coldness of, your hands and feet; shortness of breath; chest or stomach pains; bloating; or weakness.

If you develop swelling in your legs or feet or you start having headaches more often or more severely than before, check with your doctor as soon as possible.

You may experience diarrhea, dizziness, nausea, or vomiting, but these symptoms usually stop when your body adjusts to the medication. If they continue or become bothersome, check with your doctor. If you're using the inhaler and you get a cold or a sore throat or mouth, call your doctor.

Special directions • Tell your doctor if you're taking other medications, especially if you're taking a beta blocker such as Inderal (propranolol) for high blood pressure or a heart condition.

• Tell your doctor if you have other medical problems, especially diseases of the heart, blood vessels, kidney, liver, or thyroid, and if you have high blood pressure or a skin condition that causes severe itching.

• Your doctor also needs to know if you've recently had a procedure called an angioplasty (to open a blocked blood vessel) or surgery on a blood vessel.

• Avoid alcoholic beverages because they can make your headaches worse.

Important reminders If you're pregnant or breast-feeding, check with your doctor before taking this medication. If you're an older adult, you may be especially prone to side effects from Ergostat.

Ergotrate

Ergotrate is used after delivery or miscarriage to prevent or treat excessive bleeding from your uterus. The drug's generic name is ergonovine.

How to take Ergotrate

Ergotrate comes in tablet form. Carefully check the label on your prescription bottle and follow these directions exactly.

Don't take more Ergotrate, don't take it more often, and don't take it for a longer time than prescribed.

What to do if you miss a dose

If you miss a dose, skip it. Take your next dose on schedule. Don't take a double dose.

What to do about side effects

If you develop a rash or itchy skin, start to wheeze, or feel short of breath, stop the medication and call your doctor *immediately.* These symptoms may be warning signs of an allergic reaction, which could be serious. If you have difficulty breathing, get emergency medical care *immediately.*

Check with your doctor if you experience dizziness, headaches, chest pain, ringing in your ears, or nausea and vomiting. Also be aware that this medication can increase your blood pressure.

You may experience menstrual-like cramps. That's because this medication causes the muscles of your uterus to tighten; this is how it controls bleeding. If your cramping becomes too uncomfortable, call your doctor.

What you must know about other drugs

You may need to avoid certain medications, such as some anesthetics, because they can cause unwanted effects. Tell your doctor if you're taking other prescription or nonprescription medications.

Special directions

• Tell your doctor if you have other medical problems, especially chest pain or other heart problems, blood vessel disease (such as Raynaud's phenomenon), high blood pressure (now or in the past), toxemia, and kidney or liver disease. Also report any new medical problems if they occur while taking this medication.

• Let your doctor know if you're allergic to this medication or you have other drug or food allergies.

• If you have an infection, check with your doctor because Ergotrate may have stronger effects in this case.

• Don't smoke while taking Ergotrate because smoking may increase the risk of harmful side effects.

• Make sure your doctor knows if you're on any special diet, such as a low-salt or low-sugar diet.

• If your bleeding doesn't slow down or if it becomes heavier, call your doctor as soon as possible.

Important reminder If you're breast-feeding, check with your doctor before taking this medication.

Erycette

Your doctor has prescribed Erycette for your skin problem. The drug is known generically as topical erythromycin. Another brand name is EryDerm.

How to apply Erycette This medication is available as an ointment, a gel, a pledget (swab), and a solution. Before applying it, wash the area gently with warm water and soap, rinse well, and pat dry. After shaving, wait about 30 minutes before applying the swab, gel, or solution. Otherwise, the alcohol in your medication may sting.

Keep the medication away from your eyes, nose, and mouth. If you do get some in your eyes, immediately wash them out carefully with cool tap water.

If you're using the *ointment* or *gel*, apply a thin film of medication to cover the area lightly. If you're using the *solution*, dab the medication on with an applicator tip or a moistened pad.

What to do if you miss an application Apply the missed dose as soon as possible. But if it's almost time for your next application, skip the missed one and go back to your regular schedule.

What to do about side effects Expect some mild stinging of your skin for a few minutes after you apply Erycette. This is normal. However, call your doctor if your skin continues to itch or burn. Also call if your skin breaks out in a rash or becomes dry or scaly. These symptoms may go away as your body adjusts to Erycette, but let your doctor know about them, especially if they become bothersome or severe.

What you must know about other drugs

If you're using another medication on your skin along with Erycette, wait at least 1 hour before you apply the second medication to prevent skin irritation.

Special directions

• Tell your doctor if you're allergic to any medication or food.

• If you have acne, don't wash the affected area too often. Doing so could dry your skin and make your acne worse. Wash the area with a mild, bland soap two or three times a day, unless you have oily skin. Check with your doctor for specific instructions.

• If you're using Erycette for acne, you may wear cosmetics, but use only water-based products. Also, don't apply cosmetics heavily or too frequently because your acne could worsen.

Eskalith

This medication acts on the central nervous system to help you control your emotions and cope better with everyday problems. The drug's generic name is lithium. Another brand name is Lithobid.

How to take Eskalith

Carefully follow the label directions on your prescription bottle. Take only the amount prescribed by your doctor.

Take doses of Eskalith every day at regularly spaced intervals to keep a constant amount of the drug in your blood.

Eskalith comes in three forms: regular and sustained-release tablets, regular capsules, and a syrup. If you're taking the *sustained-release tablets,* swallow the tablet whole. Don't crush, chew, or break it before swallowing. If you're taking the *syrup,* dilute it in fruit juice or another flavored beverage.

What to do if you miss a dose

Take the missed dose as soon as you remember. However, if your next scheduled dose is within 2 hours (or 6 hours for sustained-release tablets), skip the missed dose and resume your regular schedule. Never take a double dose.

What to do about side effects

If you have diarrhea, nausea, vomiting, drowsiness, muscle weakness, or clumsiness, stop taking Eskalith and contact your doctor *immediately*.

Contact your doctor *at once* if you feel faint or have a rapid or slow heartbeat, seizures, an irregular pulse rate, troubled breathing, unusual weakness or fatigue, or weight gain.

Inform your doctor if you start to lose hair, become hoarse, experience depression or unusual excitement, notice your skin getting dry, or become more sensitive to cold temperatures. Also report any swelling of the neck, feet, or lower legs.

You may become thirstier, urinate more often, lose bladder control, and have mild nausea and slight hand trembling while taking Eskalith. These side effects usually go away as your body adjusts to the medication. Consult with your doctor if they persist or become bothersome.

What you must know about other drugs

Check with your doctor or pharmacist before taking diuretics (water pills) or nonnarcotic medications for pain or inflammation such as Indocin (indomethacin). These medications can increase the level of Eskalith in your blood and cause serious side effects.

Tell your doctor or pharmacist if you're taking other medications for mental illness. These medications can increase your chance for side effects from Eskalith and may cause lethargy, tremor, and other symptoms.

Check with your doctor or pharmacist before taking Aminophyllin (aminophylline), an asthma medication, or products containing sodium bicarbonate (baking soda) to treat indigestion or sodium chloride. These medications may make Eskalith less effective in treating your condition.

Special directions

• Make sure your doctor knows about your medical history, especially any schizophrenia, brain or kidney disease, diabetes, difficult urination, severe infection, seizures, heart problems, psoriasis, Parkinson's disease, thyroid disease, or leukemia.

• Avoid hazardous activities, such as driving a car or using dangerous tools, until you know how the drug affects you. Eskalith can make you drowsy or less alert.

• To reduce stomach upset, take Eskalith after meals with plenty of water.

• You probably won't get the full benefits of Eskalith for several weeks. However, don't stop taking it if you think you're not getting better. Instead, call your doctor.

• Drink 2 to 3 quarts (2 to 3 liters) of water or other fluids daily and salt your food as you normally do unless your doctor tells you otherwise.

• If you usually drink large amounts of caffeine-containing beverages (such as coffee, tea, or colas), ask your doctor about cutting down on these beverages to get the full benefits of Eskalith.

• During hot weather and activities that make you sweat heavily, drink more fluids and increase your salt intake.

• Check with your doctor if you get an illness that causes vomiting, diarrhea, or heavy sweating. These conditions can make you lose too much water and salt.

• Call your doctor before going on a weight-loss diet or making major changes in your diet. If you lose too much water and salt while dieting, serious side effects could occur.

• Make sure to have your Eskalith blood levels checked regularly because even a slightly increased level can be dangerous.

• Have regular medical checkups so your doctor can make sure the Eskalith is working properly and detect any side effects.

• Carry an identification card (available at drugstores) that tells others how to respond in case you experience serious Eskalith side effects.

• Don't switch to another brand of lithium without your doctor's approval.

• Don't stop taking Eskalith, even if you start to feel better, unless your doctor approves.

Important reminders   If you become pregnant while taking Eskalith, check with your doctor.

If you're breast-feeding, don't take Eskalith without your doctor's approval. Eskalith may be harmful to your baby.

If you're an older adult, you may be especially sensitive to the side effects of this medication.

Eulexin

Your doctor has prescribed Eulexin to treat prostate cancer. The drug's generic name is flutamide.

How to take Eulexin

Take this medication exactly as directed. Continue taking it for the full course of treatment, even after you begin to feel better. Don't stop taking the drug without first talking to your doctor.

When you take Eulexin, you usually take other medications also. If you do, follow your doctor's instructions on their use.

What to do if you miss a dose

Take the missed dose as soon as possible. But if it's almost time for your next dose, skip the missed dose and take your next dose as scheduled. Don't take a double dose.

What to do about side effects

Eulexin may diminish your sexual desire and ability. It can also cause diarrhea, nausea, vomiting, and hot flashes. If these symptoms persist or become severe, call your doctor.

Special directions

• If you vomit shortly after taking a dose of this medication, check with your doctor, who may tell you to take the dose again or to wait until the next scheduled dose.
• Schedule regular medical checkups so your doctor can monitor your progress.

Important reminder

If you want to have children, talk to your doctor about it because Eulexin lowers your sperm count. And the medication it's used with causes sterility, which may be permanent.

F

Feldene

Feldene is used to relieve the joint swelling, pain, and stiffness of arthritis. The drug's generic name is piroxicam.

How to take Feldene

Feldene comes in capsules. Follow your doctor's instructions for taking this medication. To lessen stomach upset, take your dose with food or an antacid. Also, avoid lying down for 15 to 30 minutes after taking your dose to prevent irritation of your esophagus.

Take your medication faithfully every day as directed. Realize that it may take several weeks before you start to feel better.

What to do if you miss a dose

If you remember the missed dose within 1 to 2 hours, take it as soon as possible. Otherwise, skip the missed dose and take your next dose on schedule. Don't take a double dose.

What to do about side effects

Occasionally, Feldene can cause serious bleeding from the digestive tract. Call your doctor *at once* if you have warning signs of internal bleeding, such as black, tarry stools; severe abdominal or stomach pain; severe, continuing nausea or heartburn; or vomiting of blood or material that looks like coffee grounds.

Feldene also can cause nausea, heartburn, drowsiness, dizziness, and increased sensitivity to light. Let your doctor know if these symptoms continue or become bothersome.

Because Feldene may make you more sensitive to sunlight, limit your exposure to bright sun.

What you must know about other drugs

Tell your doctor if you're taking other medications. Don't use aspirin without your doctor's okay because the Feldene may not work as well. If you take Eskalith (lithium), a drug for bipolar disorder, your doctor may need to adjust your Eskalith dosage.

Tell your doctor if you take blood thinners or diabetes medications because these drugs may cause harmful effects when used with Feldene.

Special directions
• Tell your doctor if you have other medical problems, especially stomach ulcers or other digestive disorders, diabetes, and heart or liver disease. Also reveal if you've ever had an unusual or allergic reaction to aspirin or another medication.
• If this medication makes you drowsy or dizzy, don't drive or perform other activities that require alertness.

Important reminders
If you're pregnant or breast-feeding, check with your doctor before using this medication.

If you're an older adult, you may be especially prone to side effects from Feldene.

If you have diabetes, Feldene may mask the signs of infection, so check carefully.

Fioricet

Fioricet is usually prescribed to treat moderately severe tension headaches. The drug's generic name is acetaminophen with butalbital and caffeine.

How to take Fioricet
This medication comes in tablet and capsule forms. Carefully read the medication label and follow the directions exactly. Don't take more than six tablets or capsules in a day. If you don't feel better, call your doctor. Don't increase the dose on your own.

To minimize stomach upset, you may take Fioricet with milk or meals.

What to do if you miss a dose
Take the missed dose as soon as you remember. But if it's almost time for your next dose, skip the missed dose and take the next regular dose. Don't take a double dose.

What to do about side effects
If you experience allergy symptoms (itching, a rash, difficulty breathing or swallowing), stop taking Fioricet and notify your doctor *immediately*.

Fioricet may cause confusion, dizziness, drowsiness, light-headedness, nausea, stomach pain, and vomiting. If these symptoms persist or increase, contact your doctor.

What you must know about alcohol and other drugs

Don't take Fioricet with alcoholic beverages, drugs that relax you or make you feel sleepy, antihistamines, or other drugs that may decrease your activity level.

Check with the doctor or pharmacist before taking any nonprescription medications. Many contain Tylenol (acetaminophen) and should be counted as part of your total daily dosage. In normal amounts, Tylenol safely and effectively relieves pain. But in high doses, it can damage the liver.

Tell your doctor if you're taking Dolobid (diflunisal) because it may increase the effects of the Tylenol.

Special directions

• Inform the doctor about your medical history, particularly if you have diabetes, kidney or liver disease, or blood disorders.
• Be aware of your response to Fioricet before driving or performing other activities requiring alertness.
• Don't stop taking Fioricet suddenly. Your doctor may recommend reducing the dosage before stopping completely. Don't take more than the prescribed amount, and don't take the medication longer than your doctor directs.

Important reminders

If you're pregnant or breast-feeding, check with your doctor before taking Fioricet.

If you're an athlete, you should know that the National Collegiate Athletic Association and the U.S. Olympic Committee have banned the use of butalbital and limit the amount of caffeine that can be present in urine.

Fiorinal

Fiorinal helps to relieve pain and to slow down the nervous system. The drug's generic name is aspirin with butalbital and caffeine.

How to take Fiorinal

This medication is available as tablets and capsules. Take it exactly as ordered. Don't increase your dose or take it longer than ordered by the doctor. If you take too much of this medication, it may cause stomach problems, become habit-forming, or lead to medical problems due to an overdose.

To reduce stomach irritation, take this medication with meals or an 8-ounce glass of milk or water.

What to do if you miss a dose

If you take this medication regularly and you miss a dose, take the missed dose as soon as you remember. However, if it's almost time for your next dose, skip the missed dose and resume your regular schedule. Never take a double dose.

What to do about side effects

If you have breathing difficulty, itching, a rash, or other signs of an allergic reaction, stop taking this medication and notify the doctor *immediately.*

If you think you may have taken an overdose, get emergency help *immediately.* Symptoms of overdose include hearing loss, confusion, ringing or buzzing in the ears, severe excitement or dizziness, seizures, and difficulty breathing.

Side effects may include abdominal pain caused by gas, heartburn, indigestion, and nausea. If these persist or become severe, contact the doctor.

What you must know about alcohol and other drugs

Don't drink alcoholic beverages while taking this medication because the mixture may irritate your stomach and increases nervous system effects, such as drowsiness, dizziness, or light-headedness.

Check with the doctor before taking other medications that slow down the nervous system — medications for colds or hay fever and other allergies; prescription pain and seizure medications; muscle relaxants; and other medications that make you feel relaxed or sleepy.

Special directions

• If you're taking this medication regularly or in large amounts, don't stop taking it without checking with your doctor. Abruptly stopping this medication may cause withdrawal symptoms.

• Other medical problems may affect the use of Fiorinal. Tell your doctor if you have anemia, gout, peptic ulcer or other stomach problems, or heart, kidney, or liver disease because using this medication may make these conditions worse. Also tell the doctor if you have a vitamin K deficiency.

• Don't take this medication if it has a strong, vinegar-like odor. This odor means the aspirin in the medication is breaking down and is no longer effective.

• Before surgery (including dental surgery) or emergency treatment, tell your doctor or dentist that you're taking this medication. Your doctor may tell you to stop taking it for 5 days before surgery to prevent bleeding problems.

• Because this medication may make you dizzy, drowsy, or light-headed, wait until you know how it affects you before you drive, operate machinery, or perform other activities that require alertness.

Important reminders   If you have diabetes and take this medication regularly, it may cause false urine glucose test results. Check with your doctor if you notice any unusual changes in the test results.

If you become pregnant or you're breast-feeding while taking this medication, notify your doctor.

Because Fiorinal contains aspirin, never give it to a child or a teenager who has a fever or other signs of a viral infection, such as flu or chickenpox. Any aspirin may cause Reye's syndrome, a serious illness. Contact your doctor for an alternative product.

Children are especially sensitive to side effects of this medication, particularly if they have a fever or have lost large amounts of body fluids from vomiting, diarrhea, or sweating.

Older adults are also especially sensitive to side effects of this medication and may develop more severe effects than younger adults. They may show signs of confusion, depression, or overexcitement.

If you're an athlete, you should know that the National Collegiate Athletic Association and the U.S. Olympic Committee ban the use of butalbital and limit the amount of caffeine that can be present in the urine.

Flagyl

This medication is usually prescribed to treat an infection of the sex organs (trichomoniasis) or of the intestine (amebiasis). This drug's generic name is metronidazole.

How to take Flagyl
This medication is available in tablets and as an oral suspension. Carefully check the prescription label. Take only the amount prescribed.

To keep a constant amount of this medication in your blood, space doses evenly.

You may crush the tablets before swallowing, if necessary.

If this medication upsets your stomach, take it with meals.

What to do if you miss a dose
Take the missed dose as soon as you remember. However, if it's almost time for your next dose, skip the missed dose and resume your regular schedule. Don't take a double dose.

What to do about side effects
Call your doctor *immediately* if you have seizures or if you experience pain, tingling, numbness, or weakness in your hands or feet.

Headache, dizziness, light-headedness, diarrhea, nausea, vomiting, stomach pain, and appetite loss may occur. Call your doctor if these side effects persist or become bothersome.

Flagyl may make you dizzy. Avoid hazardous activities, such as driving a car or using dangerous tools, until you know how this medication affects you.

Flagyl may cause a metallic taste and may turn your urine reddish brown. These effects are to be expected.

What you must know about alcohol and other drugs
Avoid drinking alcoholic beverages or taking drugs that contain alcohol (such as cough syrup) during treatment with Flagyl and for at least 48 hours afterward.

Check with your doctor before taking a blood thinner (anticoagulant). Combining Flagyl with a blood thinner may increase your chance for bleeding.

Special directions
• Make sure your doctor knows about your medical history, especially if you have heart or liver disease, blood problems, central nervous system problems (such as seizures), or swelling (edema).

• If you're taking this medication to treat an intestinal infection, see your doctor for follow-up visits. You may need to provide stool specimens for 3 months after treatment ends to make sure your infection is gone. To prevent reinfection, wash your hands after bowel movements and before handling and eating food. Avoid eating raw foods.

• If you're taking this medication to treat a sexual infection, avoid intercourse or use a condom. The doctor may want to treat your sexual partner while you're being treated.

Important reminder
If you're in the first 3 months of pregnancy or if you're breast-feeding, check with your doctor before taking this medication.

Flexeril

This medication is a muscle relaxant. It's given to relieve muscle pain, stiffness, and discomfort caused by strains, sprains, or injuries. This drug's generic name is cyclobenzaprine.

How to take Flexeril
Flexeril comes in tablet form. Carefully check the label on your prescription bottle, which tells you how much medication to take. Follow the directions exactly as ordered.

What to do if you miss a dose
If you remember within an hour or so of the missed dose, take it right away. Then go back to your regular schedule. But if you don't remember until later, skip the missed dose and take your next dose on schedule. Don't take a double dose.

What to do about side effects
Drowsiness is the most common side effect of Flexeril. If it persists or becomes severe, call your doctor. Also

check with your doctor if you develop constipation, heartburn, or abdominal pain, or if your mouth feels dry.

What you must know about alcohol and other drugs

Avoid drinking alcohol while you're taking Flexeril because the combination may cause oversedation. For the same reason, avoid using other medications that slow down your nervous system (central nervous system depressants), such as tranquilizers, sedatives, sleeping aids, and many medications·for hay fever, colds, and flu.

Check with your doctor before you take other prescription or nonprescription medications.

Special directions

• Tell your doctor if you have other medical problems, especially heart, kidney, or liver disease; an overactive thyroid gland; glaucoma; or difficulty urinating.

• Because Flexeril can cause drowsiness, make sure you know how you react to it before you drive, use machines, or perform other activities that require alertness.

• If your mouth feels dry, try using sugarless hard candy or gum, ice chips, or a saliva substitute. If your dry mouth lasts for more than 2 weeks, check with your doctor or dentist. Continuing dryness of the mouth may increase the chance of tooth decay, gum disease, and fungal infections.

• If you're constipated from using Flexeril, drink several extra glasses of water daily. If that doesn't help, check with your doctor about using a stool softener.

Important reminder

If you're an athlete, be aware that the U.S. Olympic Committee has banned the use of cyclobenzaprine in biathlon and modern pentathlon events.

Floxin

Your doctor has prescribed Floxin to treat your bacterial infection. This antibiotic is used to kill the bacteria that cause gonorrhea, urinary tract infections, and other infections. The drug's generic name is ofloxacin.

How to take Floxin This medication comes in tablets. Take them exactly as ordered. For best results, take each dose with a full glass (8 ounces) of water. Drink several extra glasses of water daily unless your doctor tells you otherwise.

Continue to take Floxin, even after you begin to feel better. Stopping too soon may allow your infection to return.

What to do if you miss a dose Take the missed dose as soon as possible. However, if it's almost time for your next dose, skip the missed dose and take your next dose as scheduled. Don't take a double dose.

What to do about side effects Call your doctor *right away* if you start to wheeze, feel short of breath, have difficulty breathing, or break out in a rash or hives.

Check with your doctor if you have abdominal pain, diarrhea, dizziness, drowsiness, headache, light-headedness, nausea, vomiting, nervousness, or trouble sleeping.

This medication may make you unusually sensitive to sunlight, so limit your exposure to direct sun.

What you must know about other drugs Tell your doctor about other medications you're taking because many drugs can interfere with absorption of Floxin. These include antacids that contain aluminum or magnesium, iron supplements, Carafate (sucralfate, an ulcer drug), and products that contain zinc.

If you take blood thinners, you should know that combined use with Floxin may increase the risk of bleeding.

If you take Theo-Dur (theophylline), a drug for asthma or bronchitis, Floxin may worsen the side effects from this medication.

Special directions • Make sure your doctor knows about your medical history, especially if you have brain or spinal cord disease or a kidney problem.

• Because Floxin may make you drowsy, make sure you know how you react to it before you drive or perform other activities that might be dangerous if you're not fully alert.

Important reminder If you're pregnant or breast-feeding, don't use Floxin unless you and your doctor have discussed the possible risks.

Folvite

Folvite is a B vitamin (B9) that helps prevent or treat anemia. The drug's generic name is folic acid.

How to take Folvite Follow your doctor's instructions exactly. Don't take more than prescribed.

What to do if you miss a dose Although you should try to remember to take Folvite every day, don't worry if you forget to take it, even for a few days. Don't make up missed doses, and never increase your dosage.

What to do about side effects If you experience wheezing and difficulty breathing, stop taking Folvite and call your doctor *immediately.*

What you must know about other drugs Avoid the antibiotic Chloromycetin (chloramphenicol) while you're taking Folvite. Chloromycetin may decrease the effects of Folvite.

Special directions • Because certain medical problems may affect the use of Folvite, be sure to tell your doctor about other medical problems you have, especially a blood disorder known as pernicious anemia. Taking Folvite while you have pernicious anemia may cause serious side effects.
• Eat plenty of foods high in folic acid content. Such foods include green vegetables, potatoes, fruits, grains, and organ meats. Eat fresh foods when possible; cooking may reduce a food's folic acid content.

Important reminder If you're pregnant or breast-feeding, ask your doctor whether you should continue taking Folvite.

Fulvicin

Your doctor has prescribed Fulvicin to treat your fungal infection. This drug's generic name is griseofulvin. Another brand name is Grisactin.

How to take Fulvicin

Take Fulvicin tablets, capsules, or liquid exactly as prescribed. To help clear up your infection completely, take the medication for the full length of time ordered by your doctor, even if you begin to feel better after a few days.

Take Fulvicin with or after meals, preferably with fatty foods (for example, whole milk or ice cream). This reduces stomach upset and helps your body absorb the medication.

What to do if you miss a dose

Take the missed dose as soon as possible unless it's almost time for your next dose. If so, skip the missed dose and take the next dose as scheduled. Don't take a double dose.

What to do about side effects

If you develop a rash or itchy skin, stop taking Fulvicin and call your doctor *immediately*. Sometimes an allergic reaction such as this can be serious. If you become restless or have difficulty breathing, get emergency care *immediately*.

Fulvicin may cause a blood problem that can increase your risk of infection. This side effect can become serious, especially when you take the medication for a long period. Promptly report fever, weakness, sore throat, or mouth sores to your doctor.

Fulvicin may cause a headache, which usually goes away as your body adjusts to the medication. If it persists or worsens, call your doctor.

Because this drug increases your skin's sensitivity to sunlight, wear sunglasses and a wide-brimmed hat and use a sunblock when in the sun.

What you must know about alcohol and other drugs

Avoid alcoholic beverages. Drinking them while you're taking Fulvicin may cause a rapid heartbeat, sweating, and flushed skin.

Because Fulvicin may interfere with the action of birth control pills, consider using another birth control method while you're taking Fulvicin and for 1 month after stopping it.

Avoid barbiturates; they may decrease Fulvicin's effects. Also, oral blood thinners may not work as well when taken with Fulvicin.

Special directions

• Tell the doctor about other medical conditions you have, particularly liver disease, lupus or lupuslike disease, or porphyria.

• Because Fulvicin may make you dizzy or less alert than usual, don't drive or perform other activities requiring alertness until you know how you respond to this medication.

Important reminder

If you think you're pregnant, stop the medication and check with your doctor.

G

Gantanol

Your doctor has prescribed Gantanol to treat your infection. The drug's generic name is sulfamethoxazole.

How to take Gantanol

Take the medication exactly as prescribed by your doctor. Take it at the same times every day so that the amount of drug in your bloodstream remains constant. Keep taking your medication even if you feel better after a few days.

With each dose, drink a full glass (8 ounces) of water. Also make a point of drinking several more glasses of water throughout the day to help prevent unwanted side effects.

What to do if you miss a dose

Take the missed dose as soon as you can. But if it's almost time for your next dose, don't take a double dose. Instead, adjust your schedule as follows:

• If your doctor has prescribed two doses a day, wait 5 to 6 hours after taking the missed dose and then take your next dose. After that, resume your regular dosage schedule.

• If your doctor has prescribed three or more doses a day, wait 2 to 4 hours after taking the missed dose and then take the next dose. After that, resume your regular dosage schedule.

What to do about side effects

Call your doctor *right away* if your skin itches, develops a rash, blisters, turns red, or starts to peel. Tell your doctor if you experience increased sensitivity to the sun, or if you develop a sore throat, fever, or pallor while taking this medication.

Right after you start taking the medication, you may experience diarrhea, headaches, dizziness, loss of appetite, nausea or vomiting, and fatigue. If these symptoms continue for more than a day, tell your doctor.

Gantanol may make your skin more sensitive to the sun, so limit your exposure while you're taking the medication.

What you must know about other drugs

Before you take any other drug, check with your doctor or pharmacist because Gantanol can interfere with the way some other drugs work.

In particular, tell your doctor if you're taking any oral drug to control diabetes. Gantanol may increase the effects of this oral drug, making it necessary to adjust your dose.

Special directions

• Tell your doctor if you've ever had a reaction to any type of sulfa drug or any drug containing sulfur, a diuretic (water pill) such as Lasix (furosemide), or an oral drug for diabetes.

• Also tell your doctor if you have a history of anemia, a glucose-6-phosphate dehydrogenase (G6PD) deficiency, urinary obstruction, kidney or liver disease, severe allergies, asthma, blood disorders, or porphyria.

• Because this medication makes some people dizzy, wait until you know how you respond to it before driving or operating any machinery.

Important reminder

Don't take this drug if you're pregnant or breast-feeding.

Gantrisin (oral)

This oral medication is prescribed to help treat infections. The drug's generic name is sulfisoxazole.

How to take oral Gantrisin

Oral Gantrisin comes in tablet and liquid forms. Take or use the medication exactly as prescribed, at the same times every day. Continue it even after you start to feel better.

Drink a full glass (8 ounces) of water with each dose. Also drink several more glasses of water throughout the day to help prevent unwanted side effects.

What to do if you miss a dose

Take the missed dose as soon as you can. But if it's almost time for your next dose, don't take a double dose. Instead, adjust your dosing schedule as follows:

• If your doctor has prescribed two doses a day, wait 5 to 6 hours after taking the missed dose before taking the next dose. Then resume your regular dosage schedule.

• If your doctor has prescribed three or more doses a day, wait 2 to 4 hours after taking the missed dose before taking the next dose. Then resume your regular dosing schedule.

What to do about side effects

Call your doctor *right away* if you notice any of these side effects: itching or rash; red, blistering, or peeling skin; decreased urine output; or difficulty swallowing.

Right after you start taking oral Gantrisin, you may experience diarrhea, headaches, dizziness, loss of appetite, nausea or vomiting, and fatigue. If these symptoms continue for more than a day, tell your doctor.

Oral Gantrisin may make your skin more sensitive to sunlight, so limit your exposure to the sun.

What you must know about other drugs

Oral Gantrisin may change how your body responds to certain drugs. Don't take it with drugs containing ammonium chloride (such as some cough medicines), para-aminobenzoic acid (also known as PABA, found in some multivitamins), or vitamin C.

Oral Gantrisin may also change the effects of birth control pills, oral drugs for diabetes, blood thinners, and Folvite (folic acid). If you're taking any of these medications, let your doctor or pharmacist know.

Special directions

• Tell your doctor if you've ever had a reaction to any type of sulfa drug or any drug containing sulfur, a diuretic (water pill) such as Lasix (furosemide), or an oral drug for diabetes.

• Also tell your doctor if you have a history of anemia, a glucose-6-phosphate dehydrogenase (G6PD) deficiency, urinary obstruction, kidney or liver disease, severe allergies, asthma, blood disorders, or porphyria.

Important reminder

Don't take this drug if you're pregnant or breast-feeding.

Gantrisin (for eyes)

Ophthalmic Gantrisin is prescribed to treat eye infections. Its generic name is sulfisoxazole.

How to use ophthalmic Gantrisin

If you're using the *eyedrops*, follow these steps. First wash your hands. Then tilt your head back and pull your lower eyelid away from your eye to form a pouch. Without touching your eye with the applicator, squeeze the prescribed number of drops into the pouch. Then gently close your eye and don't blink. Keep your eye closed for 1 to 2 minutes to allow the drops to cover the eye.

If you're using the *ointment*, follow these steps. First wash your hands. Then pull your lower eyelid away from your eye to form a pouch. Without touching your eye with the applicator tip, squeeze a thin strip of ointment, about ½ to 1 inch long, into the pouch. Gently close your eye. Keep your eye closed for 1 to 2 minutes to give the medication time to cover the eye. After applying the medication, wash your hands again.

Use all of the medication as prescribed by your doctor even if your symptoms go away after a few days. Otherwise, your infection may return.

What to do if you miss a dose

Apply the missed dose as soon as possible. However, if it's almost time for your next dose, skip the missed dose and apply the next dose on schedule.

What to do about side effects

You may notice that your eyes sting or burn for a few minutes after you use the drops or ointment. This is to be expected. Also expect your vision to blur briefly after you apply the eye ointment.

If you're sensitive to the medication, your eyelids may swell, itch, and burn constantly. If this happens, notify your doctor.

What you must know about other drugs

Ophthalmic Gantrisin isn't compatible with any type of silver eye preparation. If you're using silver nitrate or a mild silver protein for the eye, tell your doctor or pharmacist.

Special directions • Tell your doctor if you've ever had an allergic reaction to any type of sulfa medication.

• Don't share your medication with anyone. If someone in your family develops the same symptoms that you have, call your doctor.

Garamycin

Garamycin is used to treat eye infections. This drug's generic name is gentamicin.

How to use Garamycin is available as eyedrops and as an ointment.
Garamycin Carefully read the instructions on the medication label, which tell you how much to use for each dose.

If you're using the *eyedrops*, follow these steps: Wash your hands. Tilt your head back and pull your lower eyelid away from your eye to form a pouch. Squeeze the correct number of drops into the pouch and gently close your eye. Don't blink. Keep your eye closed for 1 to 2 minutes to allow the medication to cover the eye. If you think you didn't get a drop into your eye, use another drop. Repeat on the other eye, if directed.

If you're applying the *ointment*, follow these steps: Wash your hands. Pull your lower eyelid away from your eye to form a pouch. Squeeze a thin strip of ointment into the pouch, and gently close your eye. Keep your eye closed for 1 to 2 minutes to allow the medication to cover the eye. Repeat on the other eye, if directed.

What to do if you Use the eyedrops or apply the ointment as soon as possi-
miss a dose ble. But if it's almost time for the next dose, skip the missed dose and take your next dose on schedule.

What to do about Your eyes may temporarily feel irritated if you're using
side effects the eyedrops.

If you're applying the ointment, expect your eyes to burn or sting; you may also have blurred vision.

If these side effects persist or become bothersome, tell your doctor.

Special directions Tell your doctor if you're allergic to this medication or to related antibiotics, such as Amikin (amikacin), Kantrex (kanamycin), Mycifradin (neomycin), streptomycin, or Tobrex (tobramycin).

Glucotrol

Your doctor has prescribed this medication, in combination with a special diet and exercise program, to control your blood sugar level. This drug's generic name is glipizide.

How to take Glucotrol Take Glucotrol exactly as prescribed. Take it at the same time each day, about 30 minutes before a meal, to ensure the best blood sugar control. If you take one dose a day, take it in the morning.

What to do if you miss a dose Take the missed dose as soon as possible. But if it's almost time for your next dose, skip the missed dose and take the next dose as scheduled.

What to do about side effects Glucotrol may cause nervousness, increased sweating, fast heartbeat, headache, and yellowing of your skin and the whites of your eyes. If these symptoms persist or worsen, tell your doctor.

If Glucotrol increases your sensitivity to sunlight, limit your exposure, wear protective clothing, and use a sunblock.

What you must know about alcohol and other drugs Avoid alcoholic beverages. They can lower your blood sugar level and also cause stomach pain, nausea, vomiting, dizziness, and excessive sweating.

Glucotrol can change the effects of many drugs, and other drugs can reduce Glucotrol's effectiveness. Check with your doctor before taking other medications, either prescription or nonprescription.

Special directions • Tell your doctor about other medical conditions you have, especially heart, kidney, liver, or thyroid disease.
• If you develop new medical problems, especially infections, tell your doctor.

- Follow your prescribed diet and exercise plan carefully.
- Test your blood sugar level as your doctor instructs.
- Wear a medical identification bracelet at all times and carry an identification card indicating your medical problems and medications.
- Tell family members how to treat the symptoms of high and low blood sugar (hyperglycemia and hypoglycemia) so they're prepared if you have a reaction and can't direct them.

Important reminders   If you're pregnant or think you may be, tell your doctor, who will change your medication to insulin. If you plan to breast-feed, check with your doctor first.

If you're an older adult, you may be especially sensitive to Glucotrol.

Gyne-Lotrimin

This drug is prescribed to treat fungal infections of the vagina. Its generic name is clotrimazole.

**How to use
Gyne-Lotrimin**   Gyne-Lotrimin comes as a vaginal cream or vaginal tablet. Fill the applicator with cream to the level indicated or unwrap a tablet, wet it with lukewarm water, and place it on the applicator. Lie down with your knees apart, insert the applicator in your vagina, and deposit the cream or tablet.

Continue to use Gyne-Lotrimin even if your symptoms clear up in a few days. Otherwise your infection may return. Because fungal infections may be slow to clear up, you may need to use Gyne-Lotrimin every day for several weeks or more.

**What to do if you
miss a dose**   Apply the missed dose as soon as possible. However, if it's almost time for your next dose, skip the missed dose and take your next dose on schedule.

**What to do about
side effects**   Check with your doctor if you feel burning or irritation in your vagina.

Special directions Tell your doctor if you have other medical problems, especially liver disease.

Important reminder If you're pregnant, don't use Gyne-Lotrimin without first checking with your doctor.

H

Halcion

Your doctor has prescribed Halcion to help you sleep. This drug's generic name is triazolam.

How to take Halcion

Follow your doctor's instructions exactly. Don't increase your dose, even if you think your current dose isn't working. Instead, call your doctor.

Because Halcion can be habit-forming, don't take it for a longer time than your doctor prescribed.

What to do about side effects

This medication may make you feel tired, drowsy, or dizzy. If the symptoms are severe, or if you feel excessively tired or "hungover" the day after you've taken the medication, your dose may be too high. Call your doctor so he or she can adjust your dosage.

What you must know about alcohol and other drugs

Avoid drinking alcoholic beverages while you're taking Halcion because alcohol increases depressant effects of Halcion on the central nervous system. At the same time, Halcion increases the depressant effects of alcohol. As a result, you could overdose. For this same reason, avoid taking narcotic drugs unless told otherwise by your doctor.

Inform your doctor if you're taking the drug Tagamet (cimetidine) for an ulcer or E-Mycin (erythromycin) for an infection. Either of these medications could cause Halcion to stay in your bloodstream for a prolonged period of time.

Also tell your doctor if you're taking Retrovir (zidovudine [the AIDS drug that's also called AZT]). Halcion could cause your body to absorb a greater amount of Retrovir. Therefore, the doctor may need to decrease your dosage.

Special directions

• Halcion may aggravate certain medical problems. For this reason, be sure to tell your doctor if you have glaucoma, a history of alcohol or drug abuse, a mental disorder, myasthenia gravis, Parkinson's disease, or kidney or liver disease.

• Because Halcion may make you drowsy or light-headed, don't drive or operate any machinery until you know how you respond to the medication.

• After you stop taking Halcion, you may have difficulty sleeping for the next few nights. This is not unusual and should stop on its own.

Important reminders Don't take this medication if you think you might be pregnant, or if you're breast-feeding. If you're an older adult, be aware that this medication could make you drowsy during the day, which could lead to falls.

If you're an athlete, you should know that the U.S. Olympic Committee and the National Collegiate Athletic Association have banned triazolam and sometimes test for it.

Haldol

Your doctor has prescribed Haldol to treat your psychiatric condition. This drug's generic name is haloperidol.

How to take Haldol Take this medication exactly as prescribed. To prevent stomach upset, take it with food or milk.

If you're using the *liquid* form, take it by mouth even if it comes with a dropper. If it doesn't come in a dropper bottle, use a specially marked measuring spoon.

What to do if you miss a dose Take the missed dose as soon as possible, and space any doses remaining for that day at regular intervals. The next day, resume your regular dosage schedule. Don't take a double dose.

What to do about side effects If you develop a fever, a fast heartbeat, difficult or rapid breathing, profuse sweating, or seizures, stop taking Haldol and get emergency care *immediately.*

Haldol may cause blurred vision and a dry mouth, which usually disappear as your body adjusts to the drug. If they persist or are bothersome, tell your doctor. Also call if you notice fine, shaky movements of your tongue or any uncontrollable movements of your mouth, face, arms, or legs.

Haldol may cause you to perspire less and to be more sensitive to sunlight.

After you stop taking Haldol, side effects such as trembling or uncontrolled movements, nausea, or vomiting may occur. If they do, call your doctor promptly.

What you must know about alcohol and other drugs

Don't drink alcoholic beverages while taking Haldol because the combination could cause an overdose. Also, check with your doctor before taking any prescription or nonprescription medications.

Special directions

• Tell your doctor about other medical problems you have because they may affect the use of this medication.
• Don't drive or perform other activities requiring alertness until you know how you react to this medication.
• Don't stop taking this medication without first consulting your doctor.
• Decreased perspiration can cause your body temperature to rise, increasing your chance of heatstroke. Be careful not to become overheated.
• Relieve mouth dryness with sugarless hard candy or gum, ice chips, mouthwash, or a saliva substitute. If this dryness continues for more than 2 weeks, tell your doctor or dentist.
• Because Haldol may make your skin more sensitive to light, wear protective clothing and sunglasses and use a sunblock when outdoors.

Important reminders

If you're pregnant or think you may be, check with your doctor before taking Haldol. And don't breast-feed while taking this medication.

Children and older adults are especially sensitive to Haldol's side effects.

If you're an athlete, be aware that the U.S. Olympic Committee and the National Collegiate Athletic Association have banned haloperidol.

Herplex Liquifilm

Your doctor has prescribed this brand of eyedrops or eye ointment to treat your viral eye infection. This drug's generic name is idoxuridine. Another brand name is Stoxil.

How to use Herplex Liquifilm

Use the medication exactly as prescribed. Follow these steps:

First wash your hands; then gently clean away any crusting around the affected eye. If it's dried, moisten it with warm water.

Next, gently pull down the lower lid to create a pocket.

If you're using the *eyedrops*, tilt your head back and carefully squeeze the prescribed number of drops into the pocket.

If you're using the *ointment*, squeeze a thin strip — ½ to 1 inch (1.3 to 2.5 centimeters) long — into the pocket.

Close your eyes gently. Don't blink. Hold your fingers lightly on the innermost corner of the affected eye (near the bridge of your nose) for 1 minute to keep the medication from being lost down your tear duct. Keep your eyes closed for 1 to 2 minutes so the medicine can reach the infection.

To keep the medication as germfree as possible, don't touch the dropper, don't lay it down, and don't let it touch anything else, including your eye. After using the ointment, wipe the tip of the tube with a clean tissue. Keep the container tightly closed.

Use Herplex Liquifilm for the entire time prescribed, even if your symptoms disappear. But don't use it more often or for a longer time than prescribed; overuse could cause other eye problems.

What to do if you miss a dose

Apply the missed dose as soon as possible unless it's almost time for your next regular dose. If so, skip the missed dose and take your next dose as scheduled.

What to do about side effects

Stop taking Herplex Liquifilm and call your doctor if you develop itching, swelling, redness, pain, or persistent burning in your eyes. Also tell the doctor if you experience blurred or dimmed vision.

Herplex Liquifilm may make your eyes more sensitive to light, so wear sunglasses and avoid bright lights.

What you must know about other drugs

Don't use other eye medications, especially those that contain boric acid, along with Herplex Liquifilm. Boric acid can interfere with Herplex Liquifilm or cause side effects.

Special directions

• Before using this medication, tell your doctor if you have other medical conditions or if you've ever had an unusual reaction to this medication, any iodine-containing preparation, or another medication or food.

• Don't share your medication with family members; also, use separate washcloths and towels to help prevent the spread of infection.

• Never use old medication because it can cause your eyes to burn. Also, old medication may have lost its ability to fight infection.

• If your symptoms don't get better within 1 week or if they worsen, tell your doctor.

Important reminder

If you're pregnant or think you may be, check with your doctor before using Herplex Liquifilm.

Hiprex

This medication is usually prescribed to prevent and treat infections of the urinary tract. This drug's generic name is methenamine. Another brand name is Mandelamine.

How to take Hiprex

This drug is available in regular and enteric-coated tablets, an oral suspension, and granules (for oral solution).

Carefully follow the directions on the label of your prescription bottle. Take only the amount prescribed by your doctor.

If you're taking the *enteric-coated tablets,* swallow them whole. Don't crush or break them.

If you're taking the *oral suspension*, use the proper device, such as a specially marked medication spoon, to measure doses accurately. Don't use a household teaspoon.

If you're taking the *granules,* dissolve the packet contents in 2 to 4 ounces of cold water, stir well, and then take the dose immediately.

Continue to take this medication for the full time prescribed by the doctor, even if you feel better. Stopping too soon can allow your infection to return.

What to do if you miss a dose

Take the missed dose right away. However, if it's almost time for your next regular dose, don't take a double dose. Instead, follow these directions:

• If the doctor has prescribed two daily doses, space the missed dose and the next dose 5 to 6 hours apart.

• If the doctor has prescribed three or more daily doses, space them 2 to 4 hours apart.

Then resume your regular dosage schedule.

What to do about side effects

Contact your doctor *right away* if you develop a rash or lower back pain, if you feel pain or burning when you urinate, or if you see blood in your urine.

What you must know about other drugs

If you're taking water pills (diuretics) or drugs that make your urine less acidic (urinary alkalizers), check with your doctor or pharmacist. These medications may prevent Hiprex from working properly. Urinary alkalizers include Diamox (acetazolamide), Neptazane (methazolamide), sodium bicarbonate (baking soda), and antacids that contain calcium or magnesium.

Special directions

• You shouldn't take Hiprex if you're severely dehydrated or if you have severe liver or kidney disease.

• For Hiprex to work well, your urine must be acidic (pH 5.5 or below). Before you start taking this medication, test your urine pH with Nitrazine paper. If you don't know how to test your urine, ask your doctor, nurse, or pharmacist.

• To help make your urine acidic, eat more acidic foods, such as cranberries, cranberry juice with vitamin C added, prunes, and plums. Also, eat fewer alkaline foods, such as milk, other dairy products, and most fruits. Avoid taking antacids.

• Drink plenty of fluids during treatment.

Hismanal

Hismanal is used to relieve or prevent the symptoms of hay fever and other allergies. The drug's generic name is astemizole.

How to take Hismanal
This medication is available as a tablet. Take it on an empty stomach 1 hour before or 2 hours after meals.

What to do if you miss a dose
If you take this medication regularly and you miss a dose, take it as soon as possible. However, if it's almost time for your next dose, skip the missed dose and go back to your regular schedule. Don't take a double dose.

What to do about side effects
You may experience headaches, drowsiness, nervousness, dry mouth, dizziness, nausea, or diarrhea. Contact your doctor if these symptoms persist or become severe.

What you must know about alcohol and other drugs
Check with your doctor before drinking alcoholic beverages because the combined effects of alcohol and this medication may increase the risk of drowsiness.

If you're taking this medication regularly and also taking large amounts of aspirin (perhaps for arthritis), be sure to tell your doctor. Hismanal may mask warning signs — such as ringing in the ears — that you're taking too much aspirin.

Special directions
• Tell your doctor if you have other medical problems, especially asthma, an enlarged prostate, urinary tract blockage or difficulty urinating, or glaucoma. They may affect the use of Hismanal.
• Make sure you know how you react to this medication before you drive, use machinery, or perform other activities that require alertness.
• Inform the doctor that you're taking this medication before you have skin tests for allergies because this medication may affect the test results.

Important reminders
Tell your doctor if you're breast-feeding or you become pregnant while taking this medication.

Be aware that children and older adults are especially sensitive to the effects of Hismanal.

HydroDIURIL

This thiazide diuretic lowers your blood pressure by reducing the amount of water in your body. This drug's generic name is hydrochlorothiazide. Another brand name is Oretic.

How to take HydroDIURIL

This medication comes in tablet and liquid forms. If you're taking one dose a day, take it in the morning after breakfast. If you're taking more than one dose a day, take the last dose before 6 p.m. so you won't have to wake up to urinate.

If you're taking the *liquid* form, use a specially marked dropper or medicine spoon. Don't use a household teaspoon.

What to do if you miss a dose

Take the missed dose as soon as you remember, unless it's almost time for your next regular dose. If so, skip the missed dose and take your next dose as scheduled. Never take a double dose.

What to do about side effects

If you experience persistent fever, sore throat, joint pain, or easy bruising and bleeding, stop taking this medication and call your doctor *immediately.*

This medication may cause dehydration, low blood sugar level, fatigue, muscle cramps, numbness, "pins and needles" sensation, and weakness. If these side effects persist, tell your doctor.

What you must know about other drugs

Questran (cholestyramine), Colestid (colestipol), and nonsteroidal anti-inflammatory drugs (NSAIDs) decrease HydroDIURIL's effects. If you're taking any of these medications along with HydroDIURIL, follow your dosage schedule exactly to minimize drug interactions. Avoid taking Proglycem (diazoxide), which may worsen HydroDIURIL's side effects.

Special directions

• Before taking HydroDIURIL, tell your doctor if you're allergic to sulfa drugs or other medications.

• Because this medication may decrease your body's potassium level, the doctor may instruct you to eat foods high in potassium, such as uncooked dried fruits and fresh orange juice, take a potassium supplement, and decrease your salt intake.

• Inform your doctor if you're already on a special diet such as one for diabetes.

• Contact your doctor if you experience persistent or severe diarrhea or vomiting.

• Because HydroDIURIL may increase your sensitivity to sunlight, limit sun exposure, wear protective clothing and sunglasses, and use a sunblock.

Important reminders If you're pregnant or breast-feeding, check with your doctor before taking this medication.

If you have diabetes, you should know that HydroDIURIL may interfere with blood or urine glucose tests.

If you're an older adult, you may be especially sensitive to side effects.

If you're an athlete, be aware that the National Collegiate Athletic Association and the U.S. Olympic Committee have banned diuretics and test for them.

Hytrin

This medication relaxes your blood vessels so that the blood passes through them more easily, helping to lower your blood pressure. This drug's generic name is terazosin.

How to take Hytrin Follow your doctor's instructions exactly. Hytrin won't cure your high blood pressure; it will only help control it. That's why you need to continue to take this medication even if you feel well. You may even need to take it for the rest of your life.

What to do if you miss a dose Take the missed dose as soon as you remember, as long as you remember on the same day as the missed dose. If you don't remember until the next day, skip the missed dose and take the next dose as scheduled. If you miss several doses, call your doctor before resuming your medication.

What to do about side effects

Hytrin may make you feel dizzy or light-headed, especially when getting up after sitting or lying down. Other possible side effects include an irregular heartbeat, swelling in the feet and lower legs, stuffy nose, and nausea. Call your doctor if any of these symptoms becomes bothersome.

What you must know about other drugs

Don't take any other drugs — even nonprescription ones — without first talking with your doctor. This is especially true for diet, asthma, cold, cough, hay fever, and sinus medications — all of which may increase your blood pressure.

Special directions

• Because your first dose of Hytrin will most likely make you drowsy or dizzy, take it at bedtime. For this same reason, be careful if you need to get up during the night.
• To reduce the chance of dizziness, get up slowly. If you begin to feel light-headed once you're standing, lie down so you don't faint. Then sit up for a few moments before standing.
• You're more likely to feel dizzy if you drink alcoholic beverages, stand for a long period of time, or exercise — especially when the weather is hot. So, be careful about drinking alcoholic beverages. And pay attention to standing or exercising, particularly in hot weather.
• Also, don't drive or operate any machinery until you know how you're going to respond to the medication.
• Remember to keep your appointments with your doctor, even if you feel well, and to check your blood pressure frequently.

Important reminder

Let your doctor know if you think you're pregnant or if you're breast-feeding.

I J

Imodium

Imodium is used to treat diarrhea. This drug's generic name is loperamide.

How to take Imodium

This medication is available in tablet, capsule, and liquid forms.

If you buy Imodium without a prescription and are treating yourself, follow the instructions on the package carefully. Don't take more than the recommended amount.

If you're taking Imodium by prescription, follow your doctor's instructions carefully.

What to do if you miss a dose

If you're taking Imodium on a regular schedule, skip the missed dose and resume your regular dosage schedule. Never take a double dose.

What to do about side effects

Constipation may occur. If it's severe and occurs suddenly, check with your doctor *immediately.*

What you must know about other drugs

Check with your doctor or pharmacist if you're taking an antibiotic to treat infection. Some antibiotics cause diarrhea. Taking Imodium at the same time may worsen or prolong the diarrhea.

Before taking a narcotic pain reliever, check with your doctor or pharmacist. Combining a narcotic with Imodium may increase your chance for severe constipation.

Special directions

• Don't take Imodium if you have colitis.
• Make sure your doctor knows about your medical history. Especially mention any liver disease, a severely enlarged prostate, or dependence on narcotics; Imodium can make these conditions worse.
• After the initial dose, take the medication after each passage of unformed stool until your diarrhea goes away (unless the doctor tells you otherwise).

- If your diarrhea doesn't go away after 2 days or if you develop a fever, stop taking Imodium and contact your doctor.
- If you lose a great deal of fluid from diarrhea, you may suffer dehydration, a serious condition. Call your doctor *right away* if you have any of the following symptoms: dry mouth, increased thirst, decreased urination, dizziness, light-headedness, or wrinkled skin.
- Until you achieve a solid stool, replace the fluid your body has lost from diarrhea. Drink plenty of clear liquids that don't contain caffeine (such as caffeine-free cola and tea, ginger ale, gelatin, and broth). As your condition improves, you may eat bread, crackers, hot cereal, and other bland foods. Avoid caffeine, spicy or fried foods, vegetables, fruits, bran, candy, and alcoholic beverages because these could make your diarrhea worse.

Important reminders   If you're pregnant or breast-feeding, check with the doctor before using Imodium.

Check with the doctor before giving Imodium to children.

If you're an older adult, losing fluid from diarrhea can be especially dangerous. Call your doctor or pharmacist for special instructions on how to replace lost fluid.

Imuran

Imuran decreases the body's natural immunity, which helps to prevent a rejection reaction after organ transplant. This drug is also used to treat rheumatoid arthritis. Its generic name is azathioprine.

How to take Imuran   Check the label on your prescription bottle and follow the directions exactly.

What to do if you miss a dose   If your dosing schedule is once a day, don't take the dose you missed and don't double the next dose. Instead, resume your normal dosage schedule and check with your doctor.

If you're taking more than one dose a day, take the missed dose as soon as you remember it. If it's time for your next dose, take both doses together, then resume your usual schedule. If you miss more than one dose, notify your doctor.

If you vomit after taking a dose, notify your doctor, who will instruct you either to take the dose again or to wait until your next scheduled dose.

What to do about side effects

Notify your doctor *immediately* if you have a fever, chills, wet cough, or other symptoms of infection; black, tarry stools; bloody urine; unusual bruising or bleeding; or increased fatigue or weakness.

What you must know about other drugs

Tell your doctor about other medications you're taking. If you're taking Zyloprim (allopurinol), you'll need a lower Imuran dose.

Special directions

• Tell your doctor if you have other medical problems. They may affect the use of Imuran.

• Schedule regular checkups so that your doctor can monitor Imuran therapy and check for side effects.

• Don't stop taking Imuran without first consulting your doctor.

• During and after Imuran therapy, don't receive any vaccinations unless your doctor approves. Imuran increases your risk of getting the infection that the vaccine prevents.

• Caution close associates who just received the oral polio vaccine that they could pass the polio virus to you. If you can't avoid these people, wear a protective mask over your nose and mouth.

• Because Imuran increases your risks of infection and bleeding, take these precautions:

— Avoid people with known infections.

— Call your doctor immediately if you think you're getting sick.

— Be careful not to cut yourself using a toothbrush, dental floss, or a razor.

— Avoid touching your eyes or nose.

— Avoid contact sports or other activities in which bruising or injury can occur.

Important reminders If you become pregnant, stop taking Imuran and notify your doctor. Also, don't breast-feed while taking this medication.

Inderal

Prescribed to relieve angina (chest pain) and to treat certain heart conditions, Inderal may also be used to prevent some kinds of severe headaches. This drug's generic name is propranolol.

How to take Inderal Inderal comes in tablets, extended-release capsules, and an oral solution. Take this medication exactly as the doctor has ordered. Take it with meals, preferably at the same time each day, so you're less likely to forget.

Once a day, preferably before the first dose, take your pulse (if instructed by your doctor). If your pulse rate is less than 50 beats per minute, don't take the next dose. Instead, call your doctor as soon as possible.

Don't stop taking Inderal suddenly; doing so may increase your angina.

What to do if you miss a dose Take the missed dose right away if you remember within 1 hour or so. However, if it's within 8 hours of your next regular dose, skip the missed dose and resume your regular dosage schedule. Never take a double dose.

What to do about side effects Call your doctor *right away* if you have a persistent cough, shortness of breath, difficulty breathing, unusual tiredness, lethargy, restlessness, and anxiety.

Check with your doctor if you feel depressed or dizzy or can't sleep at night. Also call if you start wheezing, develop a rash, or have a very slow heart rate, especially less than 50 beats per minute. To minimize dizziness, rise slowly from a sitting or lying position and avoid sudden changes in position. To avoid insomnia, take your last dose no later than 2 hours before bedtime.

What you must know about other drugs

To avoid harmful interactions, tell your doctor if you're taking other medications. Also, check with the doctor before you take new medications.

In particular, your doctor needs to know if you're taking insulin or other drugs for diabetes, the ulcer drug Tagamet (cimetidine), asthma medications, or medications for heart conditions.

Special directions

• Tell your doctor if you have other medical problems, especially other heart problems, asthma, lung disease, diabetes, low blood sugar, an overactive thyroid, or liver disease.

• Because Inderal may make you dizzy, make sure you know how you're reacting to it before you drive or perform other activities that might be dangerous if you're not fully alert.

• Before you have surgery, tell the doctor that you're taking Inderal.

Important reminders

If you're pregnant or breast-feeding, check with your doctor before taking this medication.

If you're an athlete, you should know that the U.S. Olympic Committee and the National Collegiate Athletic Association have banned propranolol and conduct tests for it.

Indocin

Indocin is prescribed to relieve fever, pain, swelling, or joint stiffness. This drug's generic name is indomethacin.

How to take Indocin

Indocin comes in regular and sustained-release capsules, liquid, and suppositories. Take the *capsules* or *liquid* on a full stomach or with an antacid unless your doctor instructs otherwise. Don't mix the liquid with the antacid or any other liquid before taking it; take the antacid first. Take capsules with a full glass (8 ounces) of water, and don't lie down for 15 to 30 minutes afterward.

If you're taking a *sustained-release capsule,* swallow it whole. Don't crush, break, or chew it.

To use a *suppository,* follow these steps. If the suppository is too soft to insert, run cold water over it or chill it in the refrigerator for about 30 minutes. Remove the foil wrapper and moisten the suppository with cold water. Lie on your side and use your index finger to gently push the suppository into your rectum as far as possible. Keep the suppository in place for at least 1 hour.

What to do if you miss a dose

If you're using the *regular capsules, liquid,* or *suppositories,* take a missed dose when you remember it. But if it's almost time for your next dose, skip the missed dose and take the next one as scheduled.

If you're taking *sustained-release capsules* once or twice a day, take the missed dose if it's no more than 2 hours after the scheduled time for that dose. But if it's later, skip the missed dose and take the next dose at its scheduled time.

What to do about side effects

If you develop a hivelike rash or itching, stop taking Indocin and call your doctor *immediately.* If you become restless, start wheezing, and have difficulty breathing or develop puffiness around your eyes, seek emergency care *immediately.*

Stop taking the medication and call your doctor *at once* if you have stomach pain; pass black, tarry stools; have severe nausea, heartburn, or indigestion; or vomit that looks like coffee grounds.

Also tell your doctor about other side effects, including weakness, sore throat, or swelling of your face, feet, or lower legs.

What you must know about alcohol and other drugs

Don't drink alcoholic beverages while taking Indocin. Tell your doctor if you're taking other medications because many drugs can interact with Indocin. In particular, mention blood pressure medications, Dolobid (diflunisal), Benemid (probenecid), and Eskalith (lithium).

Special directions

• Tell the doctor if you have other medical problems. They may affect the use of this medication.
• Don't drive or perform other activities requiring alertness until you know how you react to this medication.

Important reminders If you're pregnant or think you may be, check with your doctor before taking this medication. Don't breast-feed while taking Indocin. If you're an older adult, you may be especially sensitive to side effects.

Insulin

Your doctor has prescribed insulin injections to control your blood sugar level.

How to use insulin You've been given instructions on the kind of insulin to use, the correct dose, the number of injections you need each day, and the times to perform them. Follow these instructions exactly — they're tailored especially for you.

Use the guidelines below to help you prepare and administer your insulin injection.

Drawing up insulin into the syringe To draw up insulin into the syringe correctly, follow these steps.

1 Before you do anything else, wash your hands.

2 If your insulin is the intermediate- or long-acting kind (cloudy), mix it by slowly rolling the bottle between your hands (as shown) or gently tipping it over a few times. Never shake the bottle vigorously.

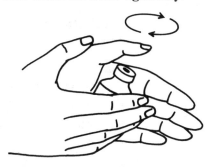

3 Inspect the insulin solution. Don't use the insulin if it looks lumpy or grainy, seems unusually thick, sticks to the bottle, or appears even a little discolored or if the bottle looks frosty. Use regular insulin (short-acting) only if it's clear and colorless.

4 Remove the colored protective cap on the bottle. Don't remove the rubber stopper.

5 Wipe the top of the bottle with an alcohol swab.

6 Remove the needle cover of the insulin syringe.

7 Draw air into the syringe by pulling back on the plunger. The amount of air that you draw into the syringe should be equal to your insulin dose.

8 Gently push the needle through the top of the rubber stopper.

9 Push the plunger in all the way to inject the air from the syringe into the bottle.

10 Turn the bottle with syringe upside down in one hand. Make sure the tip of the needle is covered by the insulin.

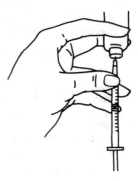

With your other hand, pull the plunger back slowly to draw the correct dose of insulin into the syringe.

11 Check the insulin in the syringe for air bubbles. To remove air bubbles, push the insulin slowly back into the bottle and draw up your dose again.

12 Check your dose again; then remove the needle from the bottle and recover the needle.

Mixing two types of insulin If you're mixing more than one type of insulin in the same syringe, you also need to know the following:
• When mixing two types of insulin, first draw into the syringe the same amount of air as the amount of insulin you'll be withdrawing from each bottle.

• If you're mixing regular insulin with another type of insulin, *always* draw up the regular insulin into the syringe first. When mixing two types of insulin other than regular insulin, you can draw them in any order, but use the same order each time.

• Some insulin mixtures must be injected immediately. Others may be stable for a while, meaning you can fill the syringe ahead of time. Ask your doctor, nurse, or pharmacist which type you have.

• If your mixture is stable and you mixed it in advance, gently turn the filled syringe back and forth to remix the insulins before injecting. Don't shake the syringe.

Giving the injection   Inject the insulin into fatty tissue on the thighs, abdomen, upper arms, or buttocks. The abdomen is preferred because insulin is absorbed into the bloodstream most evenly from the abdomen. Rotate among sites within the same anatomic area as you've been instructed, such as moving from left to right in rows, from the top to the bottom of the area. Remember, inject each new dose at least 1 inch from the previously used site.

After you've prepared your syringe, inject the insulin, following these steps.

1 Use an alcohol pad to clean the site for the injection, and let the area dry.

2 Remove the needle's protective covering. Pinch a large area of skin and hold it firmly. With your other hand, push the needle straight into the pinched skin at a 90-degree angle. Make sure the needle is all the way in.

Note: If you're thin or greatly overweight, you may be given special instructions for giving yourself insulin injections.

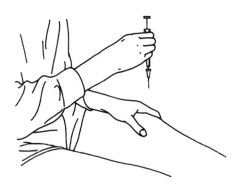

3 Push the plunger all the way down to inject the dose quickly (in less than 5 seconds).

4 Then hold an alcohol pad near the needle, and pull the needle straight out of the skin.

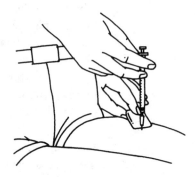

5 Press the pad against the injection site for several seconds. Don't rub.

If you're using an insulin pump for continuous insulin infusion, follow your doctor's and the pump manufacturer's instructions exactly.

What to do if you miss a dose

Follow your doctor's instructions. What you must do depends on the type and amount of insulin you're taking as well as how much time has elapsed since your last insulin injection.

What to do about side effects

Contact your doctor *immediately* if you develop itching, hives, a rash, difficulty breathing, or wheezing after your insulin injection. You may be having an allergic reaction; your doctor will need to change your type of insulin.

Insulin may cause low blood sugar, especially if you delay or miss a meal or snack, exercise much more than usual, or drink alcoholic beverages. Watch for cool, pale skin; difficulty concentrating; shakiness; headache; cold sweats; or anxiety — but keep in mind that everyone has different symptoms. Be sure to learn your own early symptoms so you can take quick action.

If you have symptoms of low blood sugar, eat or drink something containing sugar, such as glucose tablets or Jello or fruit juice. If possible, check your blood sugar level to confirm that it's low. If symptoms don't go away in 15 minutes, again eat or drink something containing sugar and wait another 15 minutes. If symptoms still don't go away, seek emergency medical care *immediately.*

Notify your doctor if you have frequent or severe low blood sugar reactions — your insulin dosage or type may need to be changed.

Also tell your doctor if you note skin changes at injection sites, such as pitting or thickening.

What you must know about alcohol and other drugs

Because alcohol can cause severely low blood sugar, ask your doctor whether you can safely drink alcoholic beverages and, if so, how much.

Beta blockers such as Inderal (propranolol), Atromid-S (clofibrate), Pondimin (fenfluramine), monoamine oxidase (MAO) inhibitors (drugs for depression), salicylates (aspirin), or Achromycin (tetracycline) can prolong a low blood sugar reaction when taken with insulin. Corticosteroids such as Orasone (prednisone) and thiazide diuretics (water pills) can decrease insulin's ability to lower your blood sugar level. Check with your doctor before taking any of these drugs.

Special directions

• Tell your doctor if you have other medical problems, especially infections or kidney, liver, or thyroid disease. Other medical problems may affect the use of insulin.

• Although disposable syringes are usually used only once, you may wish to reuse a syringe until its needle becomes dull. If you reuse the syringe, check with your nurse, doctor, or pharmacist for cleaning instructions. Make sure you recap the needle after each use. Throw away the syringe when the needle becomes dull or bent or comes into contact with any surface other than the cleaned and swabbed area of skin.

• Don't use insulin after the expiration date on the package, even if the bottle has never been opened. Instead, check with your pharmacist about the possibility of exchanging bottles.

• Keep unopened bottles of insulin refrigerated until needed. Never freeze insulin. Remove the insulin from the refrigerator and allow it to reach room temperature before injecting it.

• You may keep an insulin bottle in use at room temperature for up to 1 month. Throw away any insulin that has been kept at room temperature for longer than 1 month.

• Don't expose insulin to extremely hot temperatures or to sunlight. Extreme heat will reduce its effectiveness.

• See your doctor regularly so he or she can check your condition and adjust your insulin therapy as needed.

• If you've been smoking for a long time and suddenly stop, tell your doctor, who will probably reduce your insulin dosage.

• Follow your prescribed diet and exercise plan strictly. Don't miss or delay any meals.

• When you become sick with a cold, fever, or the flu, make sure you take your insulin, but check with the doctor to determine the dose. Take your insulin even if you feel too sick to eat. This is especially true if you have nausea, vomiting, or diarrhea.

• Learn how to check your own blood sugar level and urine for ketones (an acid that may be released from your bloodstream into your urine when your blood sugar level is too high).

• You'll develop high blood sugar if you're not getting enough insulin. Contact your doctor if you experience excessive thirst, hunger, and urination or if your blood sugar levels are high even without symptoms. If left untreated, high blood sugar can cause diabetic coma, an emergency condition.

• Wear a medical identification bracelet or necklace and carry an identification card indicating that you have diabetes and listing your insulin type and dosage.

• Keep a glucagon kit and a syringe and needle available, and teach your family how to prepare and use it if you develop severe low blood sugar. Keep some kind of quick-acting, sugary food handy to treat low blood sugar symptoms.

• Discuss any travel plans with your doctor, especially if you're changing time zones. You may need to make some temporary adjustments to your insulin dosage.

Important reminder If you become pregnant, tell your doctor, who will adjust your insulin therapy.

Iron supplements (oral)

Iron supplements are used to help correct iron deficiency. Your body needs enough iron to produce the number of red blood cells that you need to stay healthy. Brand names for iron supplements include Feosol, Feostat, and Fumerin.

How to take oral iron supplements

Iron supplements come in many forms — for example, tablets, capsules, and elixir. Carefully follow your doctor's instructions. For best results, take the supplement on an empty stomach either 1 hour before or 2 hours after meals. Take the supplement with water or, even better, orange juice because the vitamin C in the juice increases iron absorption into your blood.

If necessary to reduce stomach upset, take iron supplements with food or immediately after meals.

If you're taking the *elixir*, sip it through a narrow straw to keep it from staining your teeth.

What to do if you miss a dose

Skip the missed dose and take your next dose as scheduled. Don't take a double dose.

What to do about side effects

Constipation, nausea, and black, tarry stools are common. If these problems become bothersome or severe, tell your doctor.

What you must know about other drugs

Don't take iron supplements at the same time as antacids (such as Maalox), Questran (cholestyramine), Chloromycetin (chloramphenicol), or vitamin E. Ask a nurse, pharmacist, or doctor to help you schedule these medications to minimize interactions.

Special directions

• Tell your doctor if you're allergic to any iron medication or to another drug, food, or chemical.

• Don't take high doses of iron for longer than 6 months without consulting your doctor. Prolonged overuse could lead to lead poisoning. Also, unabsorbed iron could hide blood in your stools, possibly delaying discovery of a serious disorder.

• To help prevent constipation, drink plenty of fluids, exercise regularly, and eat foods high in fiber, such as fresh fruits and vegetables and foods containing bran and oats.

• Remove tooth stains caused by liquid iron supplements with baking soda or hydrogen peroxide solution (3%).

Important reminders If you're pregnant or breast-feeding, check with your doctor before taking an iron supplement.

Carefully follow the directions for giving an iron supplement to a child. Overdose and iron poisoning are especially dangerous in children.

If you're an older adult, check with your doctor before taking an iron supplement.

ISMO

Your doctor has prescribed ISMO to help prevent your angina attacks. This drug's generic name is isosorbide mononitrate.

How to take ISMO ISMO is available in regular and extended-release tablet form. You will probably be taking two doses daily, 7 hours apart. Follow the label directions exactly. Be careful not to crush or chew the extended-release tablets.

What to do if you miss a dose Take the missed dose as soon as possible. But if it's within 2 hours of your next scheduled dose (or within 6 hours if you're taking an extended-release form), skip the missed dose and take the next one as scheduled. Never take two doses at once.

What to do about side effects ISMO may make you feel tired or dizzy and may give you a headache. Try taking aspirin or Tylenol (acetaminophen) to relieve your headache. Daily headaches are a common side effect and may just indicate that your medication is working. If you suddenly stop getting headaches, check with your doctor — your medication may not be working as well anymore. Because ISMO can make you light-headed or dizzy when you get up from a lying or sitting position, try getting up slowly.

You may also experience emotional ups and downs. If you experience heart problems, such as an irregular heartbeat or chest pain, contact your doctor for advice. ISMO may cause abdominal pain or diarrhea as well as upper respiratory infection, coughing, flushing, and rash. If any of these effects persists or becomes severe, notify your doctor.

What you must know about alcohol and other drugs

Don't drink alcohol while you're taking ISMO. Also be sure to let your doctor know if you're taking other heart medications, such as Cardizem (diltiazem) or Nitrostat or Nitro-Dur (nitroglycerin), for acute angina attacks because your dosage may need adjustment.

Special directions

• Tell your doctor about other medical conditions you have. They may affect the use of ISMO.

• Don't suddenly stop using this medication if you've been taking it regularly. Doing so could trigger an angina attack. Call your doctor first.

• Also call your doctor if you find any partially dissolved tablets in your stools.

Important reminders

Be sure to tell your doctor if you're breast-feeding.

Isopto Hyoscine

Your doctor has prescribed Isopto Hyoscine eyedrops to dilate your pupils. This medication is used before eye exams, before and after eye surgery, and to treat certain eye conditions. This drug's generic name is scopolamine.

How to use Isopto Hyoscine eyedrops

First, wash your hands. Then follow these steps: Tilt your head back. With your middle finger, apply pressure to the inside corner of the affected eye. (And continue to apply pressure for 2 to 3 minutes after you've put the drops in your eye.) Using your index finger, pull the lower eyelid away from the eye to form a pouch. Squeeze the prescribed number of drops into the pouch. Gently close your eyes. Don't blink. To help the eyedrops become absorbed, keep your eyes closed for 1 to 2 minutes. Wash your hands again.

If required, repeat the procedure with the other eye.

To help keep your medication as germfree as possible, take care not to touch the applicator tip to any surface, including your eye. Close the bottle tightly between uses.

What to do if you miss a dose

Apply the missed dose as soon as possible. However, if it's almost time for your next dose, adjust your dosing schedule as follows:

• If you apply one dose daily, skip the missed dose. Apply the next day's dose on schedule.

• If you apply more than one dose daily, skip the missed dose and apply the next dose on schedule. Don't take a double dose.

What to do about side effects

If you begin to have blurred vision or irritated eyes, check with your doctor, especially if these symptoms continue or become bothersome. You may also notice that your eyes are unusually sensitive to bright light. Wear sunglasses to protect your eyes when you're outdoors or in a brightly lighted room.

Special directions

• Tell your doctor if you have other medical problems, especially glaucoma or other eye problems, Down syndrome, or spastic paralysis.

• Because Isopto Hyoscine eyedrops may blur your vision, make sure you can see clearly before you drive or perform other activities that might be dangerous if you're not seeing well.

Important reminders

If you're an older adult, you may be especially prone to side effects from Isopto Hyoscine eyedrops. If your vision becomes blurred, take extra care to prevent slips and falls.

Isordil

This medication is used to treat angina attacks and certain other heart conditions. This drug's generic name is isosorbide dinitrate. Another brand name is Sorbitrate.

How to take Isordil

For best results, take this medication exactly as your doctor has instructed.

Regular or extended-release tablets or capsules are used to prevent angina attacks. Take the medication with a full glass (8 ounces) of water and on an empty stomach (30 minutes before or 1 to 2 hours after meals). Swallow the extended-release tablet or capsule whole. Don't crush, break or chew it.

Sublingual (under-the-tongue) or chewable tablets are used to relieve the pain of an attack that's occurring. Place a sublingual tablet under your tongue and let it dissolve. Don't chew or swallow it, and don't swallow saliva until the tablet dissolves completely. Chew a chewable tablet well and hold it in your mouth for about 2 minutes before swallowing.

If you still have chest pain after taking three sublingual or chewable tablets in 15 minutes, get emergency medical care.

What to do if you miss a dose

Take the missed dose as soon as possible. But if it's within 2 hours of your next scheduled dose (or within 6 hours if you're taking an extended-release form), skip the missed dose and take the next one as scheduled. Never take two doses at once.

What to do about side effects

Seek emergency medical care *immediately* if you think you may have taken an overdose or if you develop signs and symptoms of an overdose — bluish lips, nails, or palms; extreme dizziness or fainting; extreme head pressure; shortness of breath; severe tiredness or weakness; weak and rapid heartbeat; fever; or seizures.

More common side effects — dizziness, rapid or pounding heartbeat, skin redness, headache, nausea, or vomiting — should go away after you've been taking the medication for a while. If they don't, consult your doctor.

To minimize dizziness or fainting, get up slowly from a lying or sitting position.

What you must know about other drugs

If you're also taking a blood pressure medication or another heart medication, your blood pressure may decrease even more. Check with your doctor.

Special directions
• Tell your doctor about other medical conditions you have. They may affect the use of Isordil.
• Don't suddenly stop using this medication if you've been taking it regularly. Doing so could trigger an angina attack.
• If you're taking extended-release tablets or capsules, call your doctor if you find any partially dissolved tablets in your stools.

Important reminders
If you're pregnant or think you may be, check with your doctor before taking this medication. If you're an older adult, you may be especially susceptible to Isordil's side effects.

Isuprel

This medication is prescribed to relieve the wheezing and shortness of breath caused by asthma, bronchitis, or emphysema or to treat heart rhythm problems. This drug's generic name is isoproterenol.

How to take Isuprel
Isuprel comes as an aerosol inhaler, a solution used with a nebulizer inhaler, and a sublingual (under-the-tongue) tablet. Follow your doctor's instructions closely.

To use the *aerosol inhaler* or *nebulizer solution,* first clear your nose and throat. Then breathe out, exhaling as much air as you can. Put the mouthpiece in your mouth, release the spray, and inhale deeply. Hold your breath for a few seconds, and then remove the mouthpiece and exhale slowly.

Wait 1 to 2 minutes before using it again. You may not need another spray.

If you're also taking another inhaled medication, take Isuprel first and wait 5 minutes before taking the other medication.

To take a *sublingual tablet,* place the tablet under your tongue and let it dissolve. Don't chew or swallow it, and don't swallow saliva until it dissolves completely.

Avoid taking Isuprel at bedtime, if possible. It may disturb your sleep.

What to do if you miss a dose

Take the missed dose as soon as you can. Then evenly space your remaining doses for the day. Never take a double dose.

What to do about side effects

Seek emergency care *immediately* if you think you may have taken an overdose or if you develop symptoms of an overdose — chest pain, seizures, chills, fever, severe muscle cramps, nausea, vomiting, shortness of breath, severe trembling or weakness, and rapid, slow, or fluttering heartbeat.

Also seek emergency care if your skin develops a bluish color and you experience severe dizziness, facial flushing, increased difficulty breathing, a rash, or swelling of your face or eyelids.

Isuprel may cause a headache and rapid or pounding heartbeat. These side effects should go away after you use the medication for a while. If they persist, call your doctor.

What you must know about other drugs

Tell your doctor about other prescription or nonprescription medications you're taking, especially Inderal (propranolol) or another beta blocker, Adrenalin (epinephrine), or a digitalis glycoside (heart medication).

Special directions

• Tell your doctor about other medical problems you have. They may affect the use of this medication.
• If you don't breathe easier after taking this medication, call your doctor right away.
• Avoid caffeine-containing food and drink — coffee, tea, cola, and chocolate.

Important reminders

If you're pregnant or think you may be, or if you're breast-feeding, check with your doctor before taking this medication.

If you're an athlete, be aware that the U.S. Olympic Committee has banned isoproterenol and conducts tests for it.

K

Kaopectate

Used to treat diarrhea, this medication actually combines two generic drugs: kaolin and pectin.

How to take Kaopectate

Carefully read and follow all the instructions and precautions on the medication bottle. Also follow any special directions your doctor may have given you. Shake the bottle vigorously before pouring your dose.

Special directions

• If you still have diarrhea after taking this medication for more than 48 hours, don't take any more; contact your doctor *promptly*.

• Besides using Kaopectate to treat your diarrhea, you also need to replace lost body fluids and modify your diet. During the first 24 hours, drink plenty of clear liquids, such as apple juice, broth, plain gelatin, and decaffeinated tea. Eat bland foods, such as applesauce, bread, cooked cereals, and crackers. Avoid bran, alcoholic beverages, caffeine, candy, fried or spicy foods, fruits, and vegetables. These foods can worsen your diarrhea.

• If your body loses too much fluid from diarrhea, you will become severely dehydrated. Call your doctor if you have the following symptoms: dizziness, dry mouth, increased thirst, decreased urination, and wrinkled skin.

Important reminders

Don't give this medication to a child age 3 or younger. Because the fluid loss caused by diarrhea may lead to severe health problems, call the doctor instead.

If you give this medication to a child over age 3, make sure the child drinks at least 3 to 4 quarts (3 to 4 liters) of liquid each day until the diarrhea is gone.

If you're an older adult, you may develop severe health problems from the fluid loss caused by diarrhea. Drink extra fluids to offset this loss.

Keflet

This antibiotic is used to treat various infections, but not colds or flu. The drug's generic name is cephalexin. Other brand names include Keflex and Keftab.

How to take Keflet

Keflet comes in tablets, capsules, and a liquid (oral suspension). Carefully check your medication label. This tells you how much to take at each dose and when to take it. Follow the directions exactly.

If you're taking *tablets or capsules*, take them with food or milk to decrease possible stomach upset.

If you're taking the *liquid*, store it in the refrigerator. Keep the bottle closed tightly and shake it well before using. Discard unused liquid after 14 days.

To make sure that your infection clears up completely, take your medication for the entire time your doctor prescribed, even if your symptoms subside.

What to do if you miss a dose

Take the missed dose as soon as you remember. But if it's almost time for your next dose and your dosing schedule is three or more times a day, space the dose you missed and the next scheduled dose 2 to 4 hours apart. Then resume your normal dosing schedule.

What to do about side effects

Occasionally, this medication produces serious side effects, including allergic reaction, anemia, and colitis. If you experience a fever, rash, itching, restlessness, or difficulty breathing, stop taking the medication and seek emergency medical care *immediately.*

If you experience fatigue, weakness, pale skin, nausea, vomiting, loss of appetite, or diarrhea, report these effects to your doctor *promptly.*

What you must know about other drugs

To ensure that you benefit from treatment, tell your doctor about other medications you're taking. Probalan (probenecid) may increase the effects of Keflet.

Special directions

• Tell your doctor if you're allergic to any medications, especially other antibiotics.

• Inform your doctor if you have other medical problems, particularly kidney disease.

• Check with your doctor before taking new medications (prescription or nonprescription) or if new medical problems develop.

• Avoid taking diarrhea medication without consulting your doctor. Interactions with many diarrhea medications can increase or prolong diarrhea.

• If symptoms don't subside in a few days or if they worsen, call your doctor.

Important reminder   If you're pregnant or breast-feeding, check with your doctor before taking this medication.

Klonopin

This medication helps to prevent seizures. The drug's generic name is clonazepam.

How to take   Klonopin is available in tablet form. Carefully check the
Klonopin   prescription label, and follow the directions exactly. Don't take more than the prescribed amount.

Take this medication faithfully every day in regularly spaced doses.

What to do if you   If you're taking this medication regularly and you miss a
miss a dose   dose, take the missed dose as soon as possible. However, if it's almost time for your next dose, skip the missed dose and take your next dose on schedule. Don't take a double dose.

What to do about   Get emergency help *at once* if you have the following
side effects   signs of overdose: slurred speech, confusion, severe drowsiness, and staggering.

Also call your doctor at once if this medication starts to slow your breathing or makes breathing difficult. Check with your doctor if you become drowsy, your mouth starts to water, or you notice odd changes in your behavior.

What you must   Don't drink alcoholic beverages while taking Klonopin
know about alcohol   because the combination may cause oversedation. For
and other drugs   the same reason, avoid other central nervous system depressants (drugs that slow down your nervous system)

while using Klonopin. Examples of depressants include sleeping pills, tranquilizers, narcotic painkillers, and many cold and flu medications.

Special directions

• Tell your doctor about your medical history, especially if you have liver or lung disease, kidney problems, or glaucoma.

• Tell your doctor about other medications you're taking.

• See your doctor regularly to determine if you need to continue taking this medication because it may become habit-forming.

• Your doctor may want you to carry medical identification stating that you're taking this medication.

• Before any medical tests, tell the doctor that you're taking Klonopin because it may alter the test results.

• Because this medication can cause drowsiness, make sure you know how you react to it before you drive, use machines, or perform other activities that require alertness.

Important reminders

If you're pregnant or breast-feeding, check with your doctor before taking this medication.

If you're an athlete, you should know that the National Collegiate Athletic Association and the U.S. Olympic Committee have banned the use of clonazepam.

Kwell

This medication is prescribed to treat scabies and lice infestations. Its generic name is lindane.

How to apply Kwell

This medication comes as a cream, lotion, or shampoo. The cream and lotion forms are used to treat scabies. The shampoo form is used to treat lice.

Don't exceed the amount your doctor has ordered, and don't use Kwell more often or for a longer time than ordered because this could cause poisoning.

To use the cream or lotion, apply a thin layer to your freshly washed and dried skin. Use enough medication to cover the entire skin surface from the neck down, including the soles of your feet. Rub in the cream or lotion well; then leave it on. After the prescribed number of hours (usually 8 to 12 hours), wash yourself thoroughly. If you need a second application, wait 1 week before repeating.

To use the *shampoo,* apply it undiluted to freshly washed and dried hair. Apply enough to your dry hair to thoroughly wet both the affected areas and surrounding hair-covered areas. Rub the shampoo into your hair and scalp. If you're applying it while taking a bath, make sure the shampoo doesn't drip onto other parts of your body or into the bath water. Leave it on for 4 to 5 minutes, then add enough water to create a lather. Rinse your hair thoroughly; then dry it with a clean towel. When your hair is dry, comb it with a fine-toothed comb dipped in white vinegar to remove any remaining lice eggs.

What to do about side effects

Call your doctor *right away* if you have symptoms of Kwell poisoning, such as seizures, dizziness, nervousness, restlessness, clumsiness, a fast heartbeat, muscle cramps, or vomiting.

If you use Kwell repeatedly, your skin may become irritated and you may have symptoms of Kwell poisoning. Report skin irritation to your doctor.

Special directions

• Don't swallow Kwell. This medication is poisonous and can be fatal.

• Keep the medication away from your eyes, nose, mouth, and lips. If any gets in your eyes, *immediately* flush your eyes with water and notify the doctor.

• Don't use Kwell on open cuts, sores, or inflamed areas of your skin.

• Don't inhale vapors from this medication.

• Your sexual partner and members of your household may need to be treated with Kwell because scabies and lice spread through close contact.

• After you wash the medication off your body, change and sterilize (dry-clean or wash in very hot water) all your clothing and bed linens.

• After using Kwell shampoo, clean your combs and brushes with it; then wash them thoroughly. Don't use Kwell as a regular shampoo.

Important reminder

If you're pregnant or breast-feeding, tell your doctor before using Kwell.

L

Laniazid

This medication is prescribed to treat tuberculosis. Its generic name is isoniazid. Another brand name is Tubizid.

How to take Laniazid

Take Laniazid exactly as your doctor has prescribed. Take it at the same time each day to help you avoid missed doses. If the medication upsets your stomach, take it with food or an antacid.

Keep taking Laniazid as your doctor directs, even after you feel better. Otherwise, your tuberculosis may not clear up completely. You may need to take this medication for 1 or more years.

What to do if you miss a dose

Take the missed dose as soon as you remember. However, if it's almost time for your next dose, skip the missed dose and go back to your regular dosage schedule. Don't take a double dose.

What to do about side effects

Call your doctor *right away* if you experience any of the following side effects:
- nausea, vomiting, diarrhea, or loss of appetite
- blurred vision, loss of vision, or eye pain
- clumsiness or unsteadiness
- burning, numbness, tingling, or weakness in your hands or feet
- fever, hives, itching, or a rash
- abdominal pain, yellowing of the skin or whites of the eyes, dark urine, or light-colored stools
- behavioral changes, hallucinations, or seizures.

What you must know about alcohol and other drugs

Avoid drinking alcoholic beverages while taking Laniazid; combining them increases the risk of liver problems.

Tell your doctor about prescription and nonprescription drugs you're taking because some drugs interact with Laniazid. For example, you should avoid taking any antacid that contains aluminum within 1 hour of the time you take Laniazid because the antacid will decrease Laniazid's effectiveness. Also, Laniazid increases the blood levels and potential side effects of Dilantin (phenytoin).

Special directions

• Don't drive or perform other activities requiring alertness and clear vision until you know how your body responds to this medication.
• Avoid eating Swiss cheese and tuna. Coupled with Laniazid, these foods can cause chills, headache, lightheadedness, red and itchy skin, increased sweating, and a rapid or pounding heartbeat. If these symptoms occur, call your doctor.

Important reminders

If you're pregnant or breast-feeding, check with your doctor before taking Laniazid.

If you're an older adult, you may be especially sensitive to Laniazid's side effects.

Lanoxin

Prescribed to treat heart conditions, Lanoxin helps to improve the strength and efficiency of the heart and to control an irregular heartbeat. This drug's generic name is digoxin. Another brand name for the drug is Lanoxicaps.

How to take Lanoxin

This medication is available as capsules, elixir, and tablets. Carefully check the label on your prescription bottle and follow the directions exactly as ordered.

If you're taking the *elixir,* measure your dose only with the specially marked dropper.

Ask your doctor about checking your pulse rate. If he or she wants you to, you should check your pulse rate before each dose. If it's much slower or faster than your usual rate (or less than 50 beats per minute) or if it changes rhythm or force, check with your doctor. Such changes may mean side effects are occurring.

Don't stop taking Lanoxin without first checking with your doctor. Stopping suddenly may cause a serious change in your heart's function.

What to do if you miss a dose
If you remember within 12 hours, take the missed dose as soon as you remember. However, if you don't remember until later, skip the missed dose and take your next dose on schedule. Don't take a double dose.

What to do abut side effects
Call your doctor *right away* if you develop any of the following symptoms:
• increased shortness of breath
• sudden weight gain (3 pounds [1.36 kilograms] or more in 1 week)
• swelling of your ankles or fingers
• visual changes: blurred vision, double vision, light flashes, or the appearance of yellow-green halos around images
• digestive problems: loss of appetite, nausea, vomiting, or diarrhea
• changes in your pulse rate
• hallucinations.
Check with your doctor if this medication makes you feel tired, weak, or agitated.

What you must know about other drugs
Tell your doctor about other medications you're taking because many prescription and nonprescription drugs can interact with Lanoxin. For example, Lanoxin may become toxic if taken with many medications, including certain antibiotics, heart medications, steroids, and water pills.

Other medications can decrease the absorption of Lanoxin, including cholesterol-lowering drugs, antacids, and some diarrhea medications.

Special directions
• Tell your doctor if you have other medical problems, especially kidney, liver, or lung disease or a history of rheumatic fever.
• Before having any kind of surgery (including dental surgery) or emergency treatment, tell the doctor or dentist that you're taking Lanoxin.

Important reminders If you're pregnant or breast-feeding, check with your doctor before using this medication.

If you're an older adult, be aware that you may be especially prone to unwanted effects from Lanoxin.

Larodopa

This medication is usually given to treat Parkinson's disease. Its generic name is levodopa. Another brand name is Dopar.

How to take Larodopa Carefully check the label on your prescription bottle, which tells you how much to take at each dose. Take only the amount prescribed by your doctor.

What to do if you miss a dose Take the missed dose as soon as possible. However, if your next scheduled dose is within 2 hours, skip the missed one and resume your regular dosage schedule. Never take a double dose.

What to do about side effects Call your doctor if you have fatigue, headache, shortness of breath, insomnia, depression, mood or behavior changes, or unusual and uncontrolled body movements. Also tell the doctor if you feel faint, dizzy, or light-headed when rising from a lying or sitting position.

Anxiety, confusion, or nervousness may occur. If these symptoms persist or are bothersome, call your doctor.

Larodopa may make you drowsy or less alert. Your urine and sweat may turn red or black. This is normal and doesn't require medical attention.

What you must know about other drugs Check with your doctor or pharmacist before taking other prescription or nonprescription drugs. Other drugs can change the way Larodopa works.

Monoamine oxidase (MAO) inhibitors (drugs for depression) can cause very high blood pressure when taken within 14 days of Larodopa. Check with your doctor about stopping treatment.

Special directions • Make sure your doctor knows your medical history before you take Larodopa.

• Avoid potentially hazardous activities, such as driving a car, until you know how the drug affects you.

• If Larodopa upsets your stomach, take it with food. Don't take it with high-protein foods, such as poultry and eggs; they can make the drug less effective.

• When getting out of bed, change positions slowly and dangle your legs for a few moments to reduce dizziness.

• If your diet usually includes avocados, bacon, beans, liver, oatmeal, peas, pork, sweet potatoes, or tuna, check with your doctor to find out if you should cut down on these foods. They contain large amounts of vitamin B_6 (pyridoxine), which can make Larodopa less effective. Also, don't take supplements containing vitamin B_6 unless your doctor approves them.

• Contact your doctor if you believe your behavior or mental status is changing.

• You may not notice Larodopa's effects for several weeks. If you don't think the drug is working, don't stop taking it; call your doctor. Also, if your symptoms persist or get worse, check with the doctor.

Important reminders If you're breast-feeding, check with your doctor before taking Larodopa.

If you have diabetes, the doctor may need to adjust your dosage of insulin or other diabetes medication. Also, you may need to switch to another type of urine glucose test.

Lasix

Your doctor has prescribed Lasix to help reduce the amount of water in your body. This drug's generic name is furosemide.

How to take Lasix Lasix comes in tablet and liquid forms. Take a single dose in the morning after breakfast; if you're taking more than one dose a day, take the last dose no later than 6 p.m., unless your doctor instructs otherwise. This schedule will reduce the chances of your sleep being interrupted by the need to urinate.

If you're taking the *liquid* form, use a special measuring spoon (not a household teaspoon) to measure each dose accurately.

To reduce stomach upset, take Lasix with food or milk.

What to do if you miss a dose

Take the missed dose as soon as possible. But if it's almost time for your next dose, skip the one you missed and take the next dose at its scheduled time. Don't take a double dose.

What to do about side effects

Contact your doctor *immediately* if you develop an infection or a fever.

Lasix may cause dehydration and lower your body's levels of potassium, chloride, sodium, calcium, or magnesium. As a result, your doctor may tell you to have your blood tested regularly.

Lasix commonly causes dizziness, fatigue, and increased urination, particularly when you first start taking it. If any of these effects persists or becomes severe, tell your doctor.

Because Lasix increases your sensitivity to light, wear a hat and sunglasses and use a sunblock outdoors.

What you must know about alcohol and other drugs

Limit your intake of alcoholic beverages. Taking an aminoglycoside antibiotic, such as Amikin (amikacin), with Lasix increases the risk of developing hearing problems. Indocin (indomethacin) can decrease Lasix's effects, and Atromid-S (clofibrate) can enhance its effects.

Special directions

• Tell your doctor about other medical problems you have. They may affect the use of this medication.
• Because Lasix may lower your body's potassium level, eat plenty of foods with high potassium content (for example, oranges or other citrus fruits).
• To prevent excessive water and potassium loss, call your doctor if you become ill and experience continuing vomiting or diarrhea.
• Minimize dizziness by getting up slowly after lying down or sitting. Also, avoid overexertion and standing for long periods.

Important reminders   If you're pregnant or breast-feeding, check with your doctor before taking Lasix.

If you're an older adult, you may be especially prone to the side effects of Lasix.

If you have diabetes, Lasix may affect your blood sugar levels. Report any consistent change in your home test results.

If you're an athlete, be aware that the National Collegiate Athletic Association and the U.S. Olympic Committee ban the use of furosemide.

Lescol

Lescol is prescribed to help lower cholesterol levels in the blood. This drug's generic name is fluvastatin.

How to take Lescol   This medication comes in capsule form. You may take Lescol with or between meals but it works the best if you take it at bedtime. Carefully follow the label directions.

What to do if you miss a dose   Take the missed dose as soon as you remember. If it's almost time for your next dose, skip the missed dose, and return to your regular schedule. Don't take a double dose.

If you normally take your dose at bedtime but don't remember it until morning, don't take the missed dose in the morning. Skip the missed dose and take the next dose on schedule.

What to do about side effects   Lescol may make you feel dizzy, wakeful, or tired. You may also experience diarrhea, constipation, abdominal pain, gassiness, or stomach upset as well as headaches or rash.

Lescol can also cause back pain; cold- and flulike symptoms, such as runny nose, coughing, sinus infection or pain, or bronchitis; and blood problems such as leukopenia (low white blood cell count). Be sure to notify your doctor if you experience muscle aches or pain. Also contact your doctor if any of these effects persists or becomes severe.

What you must know about alcohol and other drugs

Don't drink alcohol while taking Lescol.

Several drugs interact with Lescol, so inform your doctor if you take any of the following drugs: Lanoxin (digoxin), Rifadin (rifampin), Questran (cholestyramine), Colestid (colestipol), Tagamet (cimetidine), Prilosec (omeprazole), Zantac (ranitidine), Sandimune (cyclosporine) or other immunosuppressants, E-Mycin (erythromycin), Lopid (gemfibrozil), or Niacor (niacin).

Special directions

• Be sure to tell your doctor if you have liver or kidney disease.

• Stay on a standard low-cholesterol diet while you're taking Lescol. Exercise and weight control are very important in controlling your condition.

• Your liver function will be regularly tested while you take Lescol. Keep in mind that Lescol can affect certain liver and thyroid tests.

Important reminder

Don't take Lescol if you're pregnant, breast-feeding, or of childbearing age.

Levatol

Your doctor has prescribed Levatol to treat your high blood pressure. The drug's generic name is penbutolol.

How to take Levatol

Levatol comes in tablets. Follow your doctor's instructions exactly. Try not to miss any doses because your condition may worsen if you don't take this medication regularly.

What to do if you miss a dose

Take the missed dose as soon as possible. However, if it's within 8 hours of your next dose, skip the dose you missed and resume your regular schedule. Don't take a double dose.

What to do about side effects

Call your doctor *right away* if breathing becomes difficult or you experience cold hands and feet, confusion, hallucinations, irregular heartbeat, depression, nightmares, a rash, or swelling of your feet or ankles.

Check with your doctor if you feel dizzy, drowsy, or unusually tired or weak. Also tell the doctor if you have trouble sleeping or with your sexual functioning.

What you must know about other drugs

Tell the doctor about other prescription or nonprescription medications you're taking. In particular, your doctor needs to know if you take other medications for high blood pressure, such as Catapres (clonidine). Also tell the doctor if you use nonsteroidal anti-inflammatory drugs, such as aspirin or Motrin (ibuprofen), or if you're taking drugs for diabetes or asthma.

Special directions

• Tell the doctor if you have other medical problems, especially asthma, bronchitis, emphysema, a slow heart rate, depression, diabetes, or diseases of the heart, kidneys, liver, or thyroid.

• Because Levatol may cause dizziness, make sure you know how it affects you before you drive or perform other activities that require full alertness.

• Tell your doctor or dentist that you're taking this medication before you have surgery.

• Don't stop taking Levatol suddenly. Check with your doctor first.

Important reminders

If you're pregnant or breast-feeding, check with your doctor before using Levatol.

If you're an older adult, you may be especially prone to Levatol's side effects.

If you have diabetes, this medication may cause your blood sugar level to fall or may mask signs of low blood sugar.

If you're an athlete, be aware that the U.S. Olympic Committee and the National Collegiate Athletic Association have banned penbutolol and conduct tests for it.

Levo-Dromoran

This medication is usually prescribed to treat moderate to severe pain. Its generic name is levorphanol.

How to take Levo-Dromoran

This drug is available in tablet and injection forms. Carefully check the label on your prescription bottle, which tells you how much to take at each dose. Take only the amount prescribed by your doctor.

If you're taking the *injection* form of Levo-Dromoran at home, make sure you fully understand your doctor's instructions and follow them carefully.

What to do if you miss a dose

Take the missed dose as soon as you remember. However, if it's almost time for your next dose, skip the missed dose and resume your regular schedule. Don't take a double dose.

What to do about side effects

Get emergency help *immediately* if you think you may have taken an overdose. Symptoms of an overdose include slow or troubled breathing, seizures, confusion, severe drowsiness, weakness, dizziness, restlessness, and nervousness.

You may experience milder forms of dizziness or drowsiness, as well as light-headedness, fainting, an unusual feeling of well-being, nausea, vomiting, or constipation. These side effects usually go away over time as your body adjusts to the medication. But you should check with your doctor if they persist or become bothersome.

What you must know about alcohol and other drugs

Avoid alcoholic beverages, sedatives (drugs that relax you and make you feel sleepy), antihistamines such as Benadryl (diphenhydramine), and other central nervous system depressants while taking Levo-Dromoran because of the risk of oversedation.

Special directions

• Don't take Levo-Dromoran if you're allergic to it or to similar medications, such as codeine and morphine.
• Make sure your doctor knows about your medical history, especially if you've had an abnormal heart rhythm, a head injury, liver or kidney problems, seizures, or a respiratory disorder, because this medication could cause serious problems. Also tell your doctor if you've ever been addicted to any drug.
• Avoid hazardous activities, such as driving a car or using dangerous tools, because Levo-Dromoran may make you drowsy or less alert.

• Don't stop taking this drug suddenly without first checking with your doctor. Levo-Dromoran is a narcotic. If you use it for a long time, you may become dependent on it and have withdrawal symptoms when you stop taking it.

Important reminders If you're pregnant or breast-feeding, be sure to tell your doctor before taking this medication.

If you're an older adult, you may be especially sensitive to side effects, particularly breathing problems, when taking Levo-Dromoran.

Librium

This medication is used to relieve mild to moderate anxiety and tension. Its generic name is chlordiazepoxide. Another brand name is Libritabs.

How to take Librium Librium comes in tablets and capsules. Carefully read the medication label, and follow the directions exactly. Take this medication only as your doctor prescribes. Taking too much may lead to dependency.

What to do if you miss a dose Take the missed dose as soon as you remember. But if it's almost time for the next dose, skip the dose you missed and take your next dose at the regular time. Don't take a double dose.

What to do about side effects You may feel drowsy or have a hangover-like feeling. If these symptoms persist or worsen, tell your doctor.

What you must know about alcohol and other drugs Remember to tell your doctor about other medications you're taking. And avoid alcoholic beverages while you're taking this medication. Librium increases the effects of alcohol and other drugs that depress the central nervous system, including some allergy and cold remedies, seizure medications, and pain relievers.

Special directions • Before starting Librium, tell the doctor if you're allergic to any other medications.

• Also inform the doctor about your medical history because certain disorders may affect Librium therapy. For example, a brain disease increases the risk of side effects, and sleep apnea may worsen with Librium.

• Make sure that you know how you respond to this medication before driving a car or performing other activities requiring alertness.

• If you think that this drug isn't helping you after a few weeks, consult your doctor. Don't increase the dosage on your own.

• If you've been taking Librium for a long time, don't suddenly stop taking it. Unpleasant withdrawal symptoms may occur. Consult your doctor to help you gradually reduce the dosage before completely stopping this medication.

Important reminders

If you're pregnant or breast-feeding, tell your doctor before taking Librium.

Children and older adults who take Librium may experience more side effects.

If you're an athlete, you should know that the U.S. Olympic Committee and the National Collegiate Athletic Association ban the use of chlordiazepoxide. Taking it may disqualify you from amateur athletic competitions.

Lidex

This medication helps relieve redness, swelling, itching, and other skin discomfort. Its generic name is fluocinonide.

How to apply Lidex

Lidex comes in cream, ointment, gel, and solution forms. Apply it exactly as your doctor directs. Wash your hands after using your finger to apply it. Don't bandage or wrap the skin being treated unless your doctor directs you to do so.

What to do if you miss an application

Apply the missed dose as soon as possible. But if it's almost time for your next dose, skip the missed dose and apply the next dose on schedule.

What to do about side effects Although side effects are uncommon, Lidex can cause such skin reactions as burning, itching, dryness, changes in color or texture, or a rash and inflammation (dermatitis). Tell your doctor if such effects occur.

Special directions • If you have other medical problems, be sure to let your doctor know. They may affect the use of this medication.

• Don't get Lidex in your eyes. If you do, flush your eyes with water.

• If your doctor instructs you to use an occlusive dressing (an airtight covering, such as plastic wrap or a special patch) over Lidex, make sure you understand how to apply it.

• Don't use leftover medication for other skin problems without first consulting your doctor.

• If you're applying Lidex to a child's diaper area, avoid using tight-fitting diapers or plastic pants. They may cause unwanted side effects.

Important reminders Consult your doctor if you become pregnant while using Lidex.

Don't apply this medication to your breasts before breast-feeding.

Children and adolescents who use Lidex should have frequent medical checkups because this medication can affect growth and cause other unwanted effects.

If you're an older adult, you may be especially susceptible to certain side effects, such as skin tearing and blood blisters.

Lioresal

Lioresal is used to relax certain muscles and relieve the spasms, cramping, and tightness caused by disorders such as multiple sclerosis or some spinal injuries. This drug's generic name is baclofen.

How to take Lioresal This medication comes in tablet form. Read your medication label carefully, and follow the directions exactly. To prevent possible stomach upset, take Lioresal with milk or meals.

What to do if you miss a dose
Take the missed dose as soon as you remember, as long as it's within about an hour of the scheduled time. If you don't remember until later, skip the dose you missed and resume your normal dosing schedule. Don't take a double dose.

What to do about side effects
Common side effects include drowsiness, dizziness, weakness, fatigue, seizures, and nausea. Contact your doctor if seizures develop or if other side effects persist or worsen.

What you must know about alcohol and other drugs
Tell your doctor if you drink alcoholic beverages and take other medications that depress the central nervous system (antidepressants, antihistamines, and barbiturates, for example). These medications increase Lioresal's side effects.

Special directions
• Tell your doctor if you have other medical problems, particularly diabetes, seizure disorder, kidney disease, mental or emotional problems, stroke, and brain disorders.
• Make sure you know how you react to this medication before you drive, operate machinery, or do anything else that could be hazardous if you aren't alert, well coordinated, and able to see well.
• Don't stop taking this medication abruptly because unwanted side effects may occur. Ask your doctor how to gradually reduce your dosage before stopping completely.

Important reminders
If you have diabetes, Lioresal may raise your blood sugar level. Check your blood sugar level carefully. If you notice a change, tell your doctor.

If you're breast-feeding or you become pregnant while taking this medication, contact your doctor.

If you're an older adult, be aware that you may be especially sensitive to Lioresal and may experience more side effects.

If you're an athlete, you should know that the U.S. Olympic Committee and the National Collegiate Athletic Association ban the use of baclofen. Using it may disqualify you from certain amateur athletic events.

Lomotil

Commonly prescribed to treat diarrhea, this medication works by slowing down intestinal movements. It's a combination of the generic products diphenoxylate and atropine.

How to take Lomotil

Lomotil comes in tablet and liquid forms. Carefully read the label on the medication bottle to know how much to take and when.

If you're taking the *liquid* form, make sure to measure the correct amount by using a specially marked measuring spoon or dropper. Using a regular household teaspoon may give you an incorrect dose.

What to do if you miss a dose

If you're taking Lomotil on a regular schedule and you forget to take a dose, take the missed dose when you remember. However, if it's almost time for your next dose, skip the missed dose and take the next one on schedule. Don't take a double dose.

What to do about side effects

Call your doctor if Lomotil causes bloating, constipation, loss of appetite, or stomach pain with nausea and vomiting.

This medication also may make you feel sleepy or dizzy and can cause dry mouth. If these symptoms persist or become bothersome, call your doctor.

Special directions

• Tell your doctor if you have other medical problems, especially liver disease or glaucoma.

• To help replace the fluid lost in your stool, follow these suggestions: drink clear liquids, such as apple juice, broth, ginger ale, or tea. Eat bland foods, such as plain bread or crackers, cooked cereals, and applesauce.

• Avoid citrus fruits, tomatoes, tomato sauce, caffeine, and alcoholic beverages because these foods can make diarrhea worse.

• Call your doctor if your diarrhea continues after 2 days or you develop a fever.

• Because Lomotil may cause drowsiness, make sure you know how you respond to it before you drive a car or perform activities that require mental alertness.

• Don't use this medication for any bout of diarrhea other than the prescribed condition. This medication can make certain forms of diarrhea worse.

Important reminders   If you're pregnant or breast-feeding, check with your doctor before using this medication.

If you're an older adult, you may be especially prone to side effects from Lomotil.

Don't give this medication to a child age 2 or younger because of the high risk of side effects.

Lopid

Your doctor has prescribed Lopid to reduce cholesterol and triglyceride (fat) levels in your blood. This medication's generic name is gemfibrozil.

How to take Lopid   Lopid is available in tablets and capsules. Take the drug exactly as prescribed. Don't take more or less of it, don't take it more or less often, and don't take it for a longer or shorter period than your doctor has ordered.

If your doctor tells you to take two doses a day, take one dose 30 minutes before breakfast and take the second dose 30 minutes before your evening meal.

What to do if you miss a dose   Take the missed dose as soon as you remember. But if it's almost time for your next dose, skip the missed dose and take your next dose as scheduled. Never take a double dose.

What to do about side effects   While taking Lopid, you may have stomach pain, heartburn, nausea, and diarrhea. If these symptoms persist or become severe, tell your doctor.

What you must know about other drugs   Because Lopid may increase the effects of blood thinners such as Coumadin (warfarin), don't take these two medications together.

Special directions   • Carefully follow the special diet your doctor has ordered for you so that Lopid can work properly.

• Don't stop taking Lopid without first asking your doctor. If you stop taking it, your cholesterol and triglyceride levels could rise again.

Important reminder   If you're pregnant or breast-feeding, check with your doctor before taking this medication.

Lopressor

This medication is usually prescribed to treat high blood pressure. It's generic name is metoprolol.

How to take Lopressor   Lopressor is available in regular and sustained-release tablets. Take only the amount prescribed. To help the drug work better, take the tablets with meals.

What to do if you miss a dose   Take the missed dose as soon as possible. However, if it's within 4 hours of your next regular dose, skip the missed dose and resume your regular dosage schedule. Never take a double dose.

What to do about side effects   Call your doctor *right away* if you experience wheezing or difficulty breathing, confusion, hallucinations, slow or irregular heartbeat, cold feet or hands, or swelling of the feet or ankles.

You may experience trouble sleeping, drowsiness, dizziness, light-headedness, reduced sexual ability, or unusual fatigue or weakness. Call your doctor if these effects persist.

What you must know about other drugs   Check with your doctor before taking other drugs, including nonprescription drugs. Some may prevent Lopressor from working properly.

Barbiturates and Rifadin (rifampin) may decrease Lopressor's effects.

Thorazine (chlorpromazine), Tagamet (cimetidine), and Calan (verapamil) may cause your blood pressure to drop too much if you take any of them with Lopressor.

Monoamine oxidase (MAO) inhibitors (drugs for depression) may cause severe high blood pressure if taken within 14 days of taking Lopressor.

Special directions

• Make sure your doctor knows about your medical history, especially if you have heart or blood vessel disease, diabetes, kidney or liver disease, depression, asthma, hay fever, hives, bronchitis, emphysema, an unusually slow heartbeat, or an overactive thyroid.

• Ask your doctor about checking your pulse rate regularly while taking Lopressor. If it's slower than your usual rate (or less than 50 beats per minute), don't take your next dose; call your doctor.

• If Lopressor makes you urinate frequently, take it early in the day to prevent sleep disruption.

• Avoid potentially hazardous activities such as driving a car. Lopressor may make you drowsy or dizzy.

• Follow any diet the doctor prescribes.

• Don't stop taking Lopressor, even if you're feeling well or side effects occur. Check with your doctor.

Important reminders

If you're pregnant or breast-feeding, check with your doctor before taking Lopressor.

If you're an older adult, you may be especially sensitive to the side effects of this medication.

If you have diabetes, check with your doctor. Lopressor may decrease your blood sugar level and may mask signs of low blood sugar (such as a change in your pulse rate). Also, the dosage of your diabetes medication may need to be changed.

If you're an athlete, you should know that the U.S. Olympic Committee and the National Collegiate Athletic Association ban the use of metoprolol.

Lorcet

This medication helps relieve moderately severe pain. Its generic components are acetaminophen and hydrocodone. Another brand name is Vicodin.

How to take Lorcet

Available in tablets, capsules, and oral liquids, this medication can usually be taken every 4 to 6 hours as needed.

Carefully read the medication label and follow the directions exactly. If you don't feel better, call the doctor. Don't increase the dose on your own.

What to do if you miss a dose

Take the missed dose as soon as you remember. But if it's almost time for the next dose, skip the missed dose and resume your regular schedule. Don't take a double dose.

What to do about side effects

If you have a rash, difficulty breathing, or other signs of an allergic reaction, stop taking Lorcet and notify the doctor *immediately*.

Other possible side effects include confusion, dizziness, drowsiness, light-headedness, itching, stomach pain, nausea, vomiting, and constipation. If these symptoms continue or become severe, call the doctor.

What you must know about alcohol and other drugs

Avoid taking Lorcet with alcoholic beverages, medications that relax or sedate you, antihistamines, and other drugs that decrease your activity level.

Check with the doctor or pharmacist before taking any nonprescription medications. Many contain acetaminophen and should be counted toward your daily dosage. In normal doses, acetaminophen is safe and effective; in high doses, it can damage the liver.

Tell your doctor if you're taking Dolobid (diflunisal) because it may increase acetaminophen's effect.

Special directions

• Inform the doctor about your medical history, especially head injury, severe headaches, diabetes, kidney or liver disease, or blood disorders.
• Avoid driving and other activities that require mental alertness until you know how Lorcet affects you.
• To combat possible constipation, consume plenty of fluids and fiber.
• Lorcet may be habit-forming. Take just the amount prescribed and only as long as directed.
• Don't take Lorcet if you're allergic to acetaminophen or to codeine, morphine, or other opiates.

Important reminders

If you're pregnant or breast-feeding, talk to your doctor before taking Lorcet.

Sharing this medication is against federal law.

If you're an athlete, you should know that the U.S. Olympic Committee and the National Collegiate Athletic Association ban the use of this medication.

Lorelco

Prescribed to lower cholesterol levels in the blood, Lorelco may help to prevent the medical problems that can be caused by cholesterol clogging your blood vessels. The drug's generic name is probucol.

How to take Lorelco

Lorelco comes in tablets. Follow your doctor's directions exactly. Take your medication with meals for best results.

Continue to take your medication as directed, even if you feel well. Don't stop taking Lorelco without checking first with your doctor.

What to do if you miss a dose

Take the missed dose as soon as possible. But if it's almost time for your next dose, skip the missed dose and take your next dose on schedule. Don't take a double dose.

What to do about side effects

Let your doctor know if Lorelco causes any digestive distress, such as diarrhea, gas, abdominal pain, bloating, nausea, or vomiting. Also tell the doctor if you begin to sweat heavily for no apparent reason.

What you must know about other drugs

Tell your doctor about other medications you're taking. In particular, your doctor should know if you're taking medications for depression or a heart condition. Use of such medications with Lorelco may cause serious heartbeat irregularities.

Also tell your doctor if you're taking another cholesterol-lowering drug called Atromid-S (clofibrate) because combined use with Lorelco may cause harmful side effects.

Special directions

• Tell your doctor if you have other medical problems, especially gallbladder disease or gallstones, liver disease, or a heart condition. They may affect the use of Lorelco.

• Carefully follow the special diet your doctor gave to you because eating properly is necessary for Lorelco to work well.

• Because Lorelco is less effective if you're very overweight, your doctor may want you to go on a reducing diet. However, check with your doctor first before you start a weight-loss diet.

• Before you have medical tests, tell the doctor that you're taking Lorelco because it may affect test results.

• Keep all appointments for follow-up visits so your doctor can check your progress and make sure your medication is working to lower your cholesterol levels.

Important reminders If you're planning to become pregnant, don't use Lorelco. For 6 months after stopping the medication, use birth control so that your body can be entirely rid of Lorelco before you conceive.

Don't use Lorelco if you're breast-feeding.

Lotrimin

This drug is prescribed to treat fungal infections of the skin. Its generic name is clotrimazole.

How to use Lotrimin Lotrimin comes as a topical lotion, cream, or solution. For any of these forms, apply enough to cover the affected skin area, and rub it in gently. Don't put a bandage over the treated area unless instructed by your doctor. Avoid getting the medication in your eyes.

Continue to use your medication even if your symptoms clear up in a few days. Otherwise your infection may return. Because fungal infections may be slow to clear up, you may need to use Lotrimin every day for several weeks or more.

What to do if you miss a dose Apply the missed dose as soon as possible. However, if it's almost time for your next dose, skip the missed dose and apply your next dose on schedule.

What to do about side effects Call your doctor if redness, blistering, or swelling occurs. Also call if the treated area burns or stings.

Special directions • Tell your doctor if you have other medical problems, especially liver disease.

• Check with your doctor if symptoms of your skin infection haven't gone away within 4 weeks.

M

Maalox

Maalox relieves heartburn, acid indigestion, and symptoms of an ulcer. Another brand name is Di-Gel. This product is made up of the generic compounds aluminum and magnesium hydroxides. Some brands also contain simethicone, an ingredient that relieves the symptoms of excess gas.

How to take Maalox

Maalox is available in tablets, capsules, and liquid. Follow the instructions on the package exactly.

If your doctor gave you special instructions on how to use Maalox and how much to take, follow those instructions.

If you're using Maalox to relieve heartburn or acid indigestion, don't take it for more than 2 weeks unless your doctor tells you to.

If you're using it to relieve symptoms of an ulcer, take it exactly as directed and for the full time of treatment ordered by the doctor. For best results, take it 1 and 3 hours after meals and at bedtime (unless the doctor puts you on a different schedule).

What to do if you miss a dose

If you're taking this medication on a regular schedule, take the missed dose as soon as you remember it. However, if it's almost time for your next regular dose, skip the missed dose and resume your regular schedule. Never take a double dose.

What to do about side effects

Constipation or diarrhea may occur. If these problems persist or become more severe, call your doctor.

What you must know about other drugs

Check with your doctor or pharmacist before taking any other medication. Maalox can change the way other medications work just as other medications can change the way Maalox works.

As a general rule, don't take Maalox within 2 hours of taking any other medication by mouth. If you're taking

Achromycin (tetracycline), Nizoral (ketoconazole), Cipro (ciprofloxacin), or Hiprex (methenamine), stretch that 2-hour wait to 3 hours before taking Maalox.

Special directions

• Make sure your doctor knows about your medical history, particularly of bone fractures, appendicitis, colitis, severe constipation, hemorrhoids, an inflamed bowel, intestinal blockage or bleeding, rectal bleeding, a colostomy or an ileostomy, diarrhea, edema, or heart, kidney, or liver disease. Maalox can make these conditions worse or cause serious problems.

• If your stomach condition doesn't improve or recurs, consult your doctor.

• Have regular checkups, especially if you're taking this medication over a long period of time.

Important reminder

If you're an older adult and have bone problems, check with your doctor before taking this medication.

Macrodantin

This medication is usually prescribed to treat urinary tract infections. Its generic name is nitrofurantoin. Another brand name is Macrobid.

How to take Macrodantin

Macrodantin is available in tablets, capsules, and an oral suspension. Check the prescription label carefully and take only the amount prescribed.

If you're taking the *oral suspension,* shake it hard before each dose. You should use a specially marked measuring spoon (not a household teaspoon) to measure doses accurately.

To reduce stomach upset, take this drug with milk or meals.

What to do if you miss a dose

Take the missed dose as soon as you remember. However, if it's almost time for your next regular dose and the doctor has prescribed three or more doses daily, space the missed dose and the next dose 2 to 4 hours apart; then resume your regular schedule.

What to do about side effects

Contact your doctor *immediately* if you have chest pain, fever, chills, a sore throat, a cough, troubled breathing, dizziness, drowsiness, headache, numbness or tingling of the face or mouth, joint pain, itching, a rash, yellow skin or eyes, or unusual tiredness or weakness.

Macrodantin may cause stomach or abdominal pain or upset, diarrhea, nausea, vomiting, and appetite loss. These side effects usually go away over time as your body adjusts to the drug. Check with your doctor if they persist or become more severe.

Macrodantin can also turn your urine brown or darker than usual.

What you must know about other drugs

Check with your doctor or pharmacist before taking other drugs. Many of them can worsen the side effects of Macrodantin.

Antacids that contain magnesium can make Macrodantin less effective. If you need this kind of antacid, take it at least 1 hour before or after you take the Macrodantin.

Special directions

• Make sure your doctor knows about your medical history, especially if you have glucose-6-phosphate dehydrogenase (G6PD) deficiency, kidney or lung disease, diabetes, asthma, anemia, vitamin B deficiency, electrolyte imbalance, or nerve damage.

• Store Macrodantin in its original container, and keep it away from all metals except aluminum and stainless steel.

Important reminders

If you're pregnant or breast-feeding, check with your doctor before using Macrodantin.

If you have diabetes, don't use the copper sulfate test (Clinitest) to test your urine glucose because Macrodantin may cause a false-positive result. Check with your doctor about which test to use.

Matulane

Prescribed to treat cancer, Matulane stops the growth of cancer cells by destroying them. The generic name for this drug is procarbazine.

How to take Matulane

Matulane capsules must be taken exactly as the doctor prescribes; don't use more or less than indicated and don't take them more often than indicated.

Don't stop taking this medication, even if it makes you feel ill, without first checking with your doctor.

If you vomit soon after taking a dose, check with your doctor to find out whether you should take another dose right away or wait until it's time for your next scheduled dose.

What to do if you miss a dose

If you remember within a few hours, take the missed dose immediately. But if several hours have passed or it's almost time for your next dose, skip the missed dose and take your next dose on schedule. Don't take a double dose.

What to do about side effects

Stop taking Matulane and call your doctor *at once* if you have chest pain, rapid or irregular heartbeat, severe headache, or a stiff neck. Also call your doctor *right away* if you become extremely tired or weak or if you start to bruise or bleed easily.

This medication may cause nausea, vomiting, or loss of appetite. Ask your doctor, nurse, or pharmacist how to reduce the intensity of these side effects. Watch for signs of infection, such as fever and sore throat, and report them to your doctor. Also report hallucinations.

Because Matulane can make you drowsy, make sure you know how you react to it before you drive or perform other activities that require you to be fully alert.

What you must know about alcohol and other drugs

Don't drink alcoholic beverages while taking Matulane; the combination can cause harmful side effects.

Also, tell your doctor about other medications you're taking. In general, you need to avoid medications that slow down the central nervous system, such as tranquilizers, sleeping pills, anesthetics, and cold and flu remedies.

Don't take the pain reliever Demerol (meperidine) with Matulane; this combination can cause low blood pressure that's life-threatening.

Also check with your doctor before you have vaccinations or take new medications — even aspirin.

Special directions

• Tell your doctor if you have other medical problems, especially an infection or liver or kidney disease.
• Avoid foods with a high tyramine content — cheeses, for example, and Chianti wine. Ask your doctor for a complete list of foods to avoid.

Important reminders

Tell your doctor if you're pregnant or intend to have children in the future. Also let the doctor know if you're breast-feeding or plan to do so during treatment.

Older adults may be especially sensitive to side effects from Matulane.

Maxair

Maxair opens the air passages in your lungs and helps you breathe more easily. This medication is used to treat the symptoms of asthma, chronic bronchitis, emphysema, and other lung diseases. Its generic name is pirbuterol.

How to take Maxair

Maxair comes in an aerosol inhaler. Follow your doctor's instructions for using it; don't use more of it or take it more often than prescribed.

Shake the aerosol canister well before each use. Keep the spray away from your eyes because it may cause irritation. Also, don't take more than two inhalations at any one time unless your doctor gives you other instructions. Wait 1 to 2 minutes after the first inhalation to make sure that a second inhalation is necessary.

What to do if you miss a dose

If you're using the inhaler on a regular schedule, take the missed dose as soon as possible. Then take any remaining doses for that day at regularly spaced intervals. Don't take a double dose.

What to do about side effects

Let your doctor know if Maxair makes you feel nervous or dizzy or if you have headaches or trouble sleeping. Also tell the doctor if you develop palpitations or a fast heartbeat and if your throat feels dry or sore.

Occasionally, Maxair causes changes in smell or taste. Don't worry; these effects are temporary and will go away when you stop using the medication.

If Maxair makes your throat and mouth feel dry, try rinsing your mouth with water after each dose.

What you must know about other drugs

Tell your doctor if you're taking beta blockers such as Inderal (propranolol) to treat high blood pressure or a heart condition. Combining these medications with Maxair can reduce the helpful effects of Maxair on your lungs.

Special directions

• Tell your doctor if you have other medical problems, especially heart disease or a seizure disorder. These problems can affect your use of Maxair.

• If the dosage of Maxair you've been using no longer seems to work, check with your doctor. This may mean your condition is getting worse.

Important reminder

If you're pregnant, check with your doctor before using this medication.

Maxidex

This adrenal corticosteroid is used to treat a wide variety of disorders ranging from skin rash to cancer. Its generic name is oral dexamethasone. Another brand name is Decadron.

How to take Maxidex

Maxidex comes in tablet, oral solution, and elixir forms. Read the prescription label carefully before taking it and follow the directions exactly. Don't take Maxidex more often than prescribed.

Take your medication with food to prevent stomach irritation. If you're taking only one dose daily, take it in the morning for best results.

Don't stop taking Maxidex abruptly; check with your doctor.

What to do if you miss a dose

Take the missed dose as soon as possible; then take any remaining doses for that day at regularly spaced intervals. If it's almost time for your next dose, skip the missed dose and take the next one on schedule. Don't take a double dose.

What to do about side effects

Call your doctor *at once* if you have trouble breathing or start to retain water — the medication may be causing a serious heart problem.

Check with your doctor if you experience mood changes or difficulty sleeping. Also call if you feel weak, are unusually thirsty, urinate frequently, or lose weight despite eating regularly.

What you must know about other drugs

Tell your doctor about other medications you're taking, including nonprescription drugs and vaccinations. The doctor may want you to avoid certain pain relievers such as aspirin because they can increase the risk of stomach problems.

If you take barbiturates (found in some sleeping pills and seizure medications) or certain other drugs, your doctor may want to change your dosage levels of Maxidex.

Special directions

• Tell your doctor if you have other medical problems, especially a fungal infection, ulcers, high blood pressure, diabetes, or diseases of the kidney, liver, blood, bones, or other organs.

• Keep all appointments for follow-up visits.

• Your doctor may want you to carry a medical card stating that you're using this medication and that you may need additional medication during an emergency, a severe asthma attack or other illness, or unusual stress.

Important reminder

If you're pregnant or breast-feeding, check with your doctor before using Maxidex.

Maxidex Ophthalmic Suspension

This medication is prescribed to treat eye problems. Its generic name is ophthalmic dexamethasone.

How to use Maxidex Ophthalmic Suspension

This medication is available in eyedrop form. To use the eyedrops, first wash your hands; then shake the bottle of eyedrops.

Tilt your head back and pull your lower eyelid away from the affected eye to form a pouch. Squeeze the correct number of drops into the pouch and gently close your eyes. Don't blink.

Keep your eyes closed for 1 to 2 minutes to allow the medication to be absorbed. If you think you didn't get a drop in your eye, use another drop.

Repeat the procedure on the other eye, if directed.

Try to keep your medication as germfree as possible. Don't touch the applicator tip to any surface, including your eye. Keep the bottle tightly closed between uses.

What to do if you miss a dose

Administer the missed dose as soon as possible. Then administer any remaining doses for that day at regularly spaced intervals. But if it's almost time for your next dose, skip the missed dose and go back to your regular schedule.

What to do about side effects

Stop using Maxidex Ophthalmic Suspension and call your doctor *right away* if you notice any changes in vision. Tell your doctor if you develop further problems with your eyes, such as blurred vision, burning, stinging, redness, or wateriness.

Special directions

• Tell your doctor if you have other medical problems with your eyes, such as a corneal abrasion or glaucoma. Also tell the doctor if you're allergic to any medications.

• Once your eye infection is cured, don't save your medication and use it for a new eye infection. Always check with your doctor first.

• Don't share your medication with family members, even if they have symptoms that resemble yours. If a family member has the same symptoms, call the doctor.

• Don't rub or scratch around your eye while using Max-idex Ophthalmic Suspension. You might accidently hurt your eye.

• Keep all appointments for follow-up visits with your doctor.

Medrol

Medrol is usually given to treat severe inflammation caused by allergies, asthma, skin problems, or arthritis. The generic name for this drug is methylprednisolone.

How to take Medrol   Medrol is available in tablets, as an enema, or as an injection. Read the prescription label carefully and take only the amount prescribed.

If you're taking the *tablets*, take them in the morning unless the doctor tells you otherwise. Taking them with food helps prevent stomach upset.

If you're taking the *enema,* use the entire contents of the bottle unless your doctor gives you other instructions. Insert the rectal applicator tip gently. If the doctor has instructed you to take the enema slowly, shake the bottle every so often during administration.

Don't stop taking Medrol suddenly after long-term use; this action can be fatal. Check with your doctor for instructions on reducing the dosage gradually.

What to do if you miss a dose   If you're taking one dose every other day and you remember your missed dose on the same morning you are scheduled to take it, take the missed dose immediately; then resume your regular schedule. If you don't remember the missed dose until later in the day, take it the next morning; then skip a day and start your regular schedule again.

If you're taking one dose a day, take the missed dose as soon as you remember it; then resume your regular schedule. If you don't remember it until the next day, skip the missed dose. Don't take a double dose.

If you're taking several doses a day, take the missed dose as soon as possible; then resume your regular schedule. If you don't remember it until it's time for your next regular dose, you can take the two doses together.

What to do about side effects

Call your doctor *as soon as possible* if you experience decreased or blurred vision, frequent urination, increased thirst, confusion, excitement, hallucinations, depression, mood swings, a false sense of well-being, unusual feelings of self-importance or of being mistreated, or restlessness.

If you've been taking this medication for a long time, report any of the following side effects to your doctor:
- nausea or vomiting
- stomach pain or burning
- bloody or black, tarry stools
- skin problems, including thin, shiny skin
- reddish purple lines on the arms, legs, face, trunk, or groin
- pitting, scarring, or skin depression (at the place of injection)
- filling out of the face or swelling of the feet or lower legs
- irregular heartbeat
- menstrual problems
- muscle cramps, pain, or weakness
- pain in the back, hips, arms, shoulders, ribs, or legs
- unusual bruising or wounds that won't heal
- unusual weakness or fatigue
- rapid weight gain.

This medication may cause increased appetite, indigestion, nervousness, or trouble sleeping. Call your doctor if any of these side effects persists or becomes too bothersome.

If you're using the *enema,* call your doctor if you experience rectal pain, bleeding, burning, blistering, itching, or any other irritation that wasn't present before you started using Medrol.

If you've been taking Medrol for a long time, you may experience side effects when you stop taking it. For instance, you may experience stomach upset, loss of appetite, fatigue, weakness, joint pain, fever, dizziness, lethargy, depression, fainting, or dizziness or light-headedness when rising from a sitting or lying position. Also, your inflammation (the reason you took the drug in the first place) may recur.

What you must know about alcohol and other drugs

Avoid drinking alcohol while taking this drug. Combining alcohol with Medrol increases the chance for stomach problems.

Check with your doctor or pharmacist if you're taking other drugs. They may change the way Medrol works, Medrol may change the way they work, or serious problems could occur. For instance, barbiturates, Dilantin (phenytoin), and Rifadin (rifampin) may make Medrol less effective, while aspirin and Indocin (indomethacin) may increase the risk of stomach upset and bleeding.

Don't get immunizations when taking this medication unless your doctor approves them, and avoid people who've recently taken oral polio vaccine.

Special directions

• Tell your doctor about other medical problems you have, especially bone, heart, liver, or kidney disease; colitis; diverticulitis; a stomach or an intestinal disorder; diabetes; infection; glaucoma; high blood pressure; kidney stones; high cholesterol levels; an overactive or underactive thyroid; myasthenia gravis; or lupus.

• Also tell the doctor if you've ever had tuberculosis or if you've recently had surgery or a serious injury.

• Follow any special diet your doctor has prescribed (for example, low-salt, high-potassium). The doctor may also want you to add protein to your diet and take potassium supplements.

• Have regular medical exams so the doctor can check your progress.

• If Medrol is injected into one of your joints, don't put too much strain or stress on that joint at first. While the joint is healing, move it only as much as the doctor permits. Call the doctor if you have persistent redness or swelling at the place of injection.

Important reminders

If you're pregnant or breast-feeding, tell your doctor before taking Medrol.

Older adults are especially likely to develop high blood pressure or bone disease when taking this medication.

If you have diabetes, you may need to change the dosage of your diabetes medication. Call your doctor for instructions.

If you're an athlete, you should know that the U.S. Olympic Committee and the National Collegiate Athletic Association restrict athletes' use of methylprednisolone.

Mellaril

This medication is used to treat a variety of conditions, including depression, agitation, and psychotic disorders. The generic name for this drug is thioridazine.

How to take Mellaril

Mellaril comes in tablet, oral solution, and oral suspension forms.

If your medication is in a bottle with a dropper, use the dropper to measure each dose. Dilute the dose in half a glass (4 ounces) of fruit juice, soda, milk, water, or semi-solid food.

If your medication is in *liquid* form, shake the bottle well before using.

To prevent stomach irritation, take Mellaril with food or a glass of water.

Don't let the medication touch your skin; it could cause a rash.

Don't stop taking Mellaril unless your doctor tells you to; sudden withdrawal may cause a severe reaction.

What to do if you miss a dose

If you take one dose a day and you remember the missed dose on the day it's scheduled to be taken, just take it as soon as possible. Otherwise, skip the missed dose and resume your regular schedule.

If you take more than one dose a day and you remember the missed dose within an hour, take it right away. Otherwise, skip the missed dose and take your next dose as scheduled.

What to do about side effects

Call your doctor *right away* if you have uncontrolled movements of your mouth, tongue, cheeks, jaw, or arms and legs. Also call if you have a fever, sore throat, fast heartbeat, rapid breathing, profuse sweating, fainting or dizziness, difficulty urinating, or blurred vision.

Check with your doctor if you become constipated or unusually tired, if you have a dry mouth, or if your skin color changes when you've been in the sun.

Because Mellaril makes your skin more sensitive to sunlight, avoid direct exposure to the sun.

Mellaril can also make you drowsy, so don't drive or perform any potentially hazardous activities while taking it. The drowsiness should become less noticeable after several weeks.

What you must know about alcohol and other drugs

Tell your doctor if you're taking barbiturates, Lithane (lithium), or blood pressure medication.

Don't drink alcoholic beverages while you're taking Mellaril; the combination could cause oversedation.

So that your body can absorb Mellaril completely, avoid taking antacids 2 hours before to 2 hours after your dose.

Special directions

Tell your doctor if you've ever had an allergic reaction to a phenothiazine such as Thorazine or if you have a history of a blood or bone marrow disorder, heart disease, encephalitis, respiratory disease, seizures, glaucoma, an enlarged prostate, urine retention, Parkinson's disease, a low calcium level, or stomach ulcers.

Important reminders

If you're breast-feeding or pregnant, talk with your doctor before taking this medication.

If you're an athlete, you should know that the U.S. Olympic Committee and the National Collegiate Athletic Association ban the use of thioridazine and sometimes test for it.

Metamucil

This medication is prescribed to encourage bowel movements and relieve constipation. The generic name for this product is psyllium. Another brand name is Perdiem.

How to take Metamucil

Metamucil comes in chewable pieces, wafers, and mixable granules and powders. If your doctor prescribed it for you, follow his or her directions for taking it. If you bought it without a prescription, read the package instructions carefully before using it.

If you're using the *dry powder or granule* forms, always mix your dose with liquid first. Never swallow the dry powder or granules without liquid. After mixing, drink your medication immediately or it may congeal.

Drink lots of fluids while taking Metamucil. Begin by taking a full glass (8 ounces) of cold water or fruit juice with each dose. Then drink a second glass of water or juice. Throughout the day, try to drink at least 6 to 8 full glasses of liquid. Don't take this medication before meals; it tends to make you feel full.

You may have to wait 2 to 3 days for this medication to work, although many people have bowel movements within 12 hours of taking it.

What to do about side effects

If you take too much Metamucil or swallow the dry powder or granules without liquid, the medication may block your digestive tract. Call your doctor *right away* if you have severe constipation or difficulty swallowing.

Metamucil can also cause some digestive distress, such as nausea, vomiting, abdominal cramps, or diarrhea. Check with your doctor if these symptoms continue or become severe or if you develop a rash while taking Metamucil.

Special directions

• Tell your doctor if you have other medical problems, especially ulcers or another digestive disease.

• Also tell the doctor if you're on a low-salt diet (because Metamucil is high in sodium) or if you must limit foods that contain phenylalanine, such as breads, cheese, and eggs.

• Don't get into the "laxative habit." If you overuse laxatives, you may become dependent on them. In severe cases, laxative overuse can damage the nerves, muscles, and other tissues of the digestive tract.

• To prevent constipation, eat plenty of whole-grain foods, such as bran and other cereals, as well as vegetables and fresh fruits. Getting regular exercise and drinking lots of fluids will also help keep you regular.

Important reminder If you have diabetes, choose a sugar-free brand of Metamucil.

Mevacor

Prescribed to lower the levels of cholesterol and other fats in the blood, Mevacor works by blocking an enzyme that the body needs to make cholesterol. The generic name for this drug is lovastatin.

How to take Mevacor Mevacor comes in tablets. Check the prescription label carefully and take only the amount prescribed by your doctor.

Mevacor works better when taken with food. If the doctor has prescribed one dose a day, take it with your evening meal. If several doses a day are prescribed, take them with meals or snacks.

Don't stop taking Mevacor unless the doctor approves. When you stop treatment your blood cholesterol level may rise again.

What to do if you miss a dose Take the missed dose as soon as possible. However, if it's almost time for your next dose, skip the missed dose and resume your regular schedule. Never take a double dose.

What to do about side effects Contact the doctor *right away* if you have blurred vision, fever, unusual weakness or fatigue, or muscle aches or cramps.

Because this medication can cause blurred vision, be sure to have regular eye exams.

What you must know about other drugs Check with your doctor or pharmacist if you're taking Niacor (niacin), an immunosuppressive drug such as Sandimmune (cyclosporine), or Lopid (gemfibrozil). These drugs increase the risk of side effects from Mevacor.

Special directions • Don't take this medication if you have liver disease.
• Make sure your doctor knows your medical history, especially if you've had an organ transplant, if you're

about to have major surgery (including dental surgery), or if you have low blood pressure, uncontrolled seizures, or a severe metabolic or endocrine disorder.

• Also tell the doctor if you drink large amounts of alcoholic beverages, which can affect your cholesterol level.

• Follow any special diet the doctor prescribes (a low-fat, low-cholesterol diet, for example).

• Have regular medical checkups so the doctor can make sure the medication is working properly and detect any side effects.

• Be sure to follow through with regular liver function tests if the doctor orders them.

Important reminder   If you're pregnant or breast-feeding, check with your doctor before taking Mevacor. This medication can cause serious problems in a fetus or breast-feeding baby.

Micro-K

Because your body needs additional potassium for good health, your doctor has prescribed Micro-K, a brand name for the generic product potassium chloride. This supplement will help restore the potassium your body has lost during illness or treatment with certain medications. Another brand name for potassium chloride is K-Dur.

How to take Micro-K   Micro-K comes in tablets, extended-release tablets and capsules, an oral liquid, and a soluble powder.

If you're taking the *liquid* or *soluble powder,* dilute your dose in at least a half glass (4 ounces) of cold water or juice to prevent stomach irritation. With the soluble powder, wait for any fizzing to stop before you drink the dissolved medication.

If you're taking the *extended-release tablets* or *capsules,* you should swallow them whole — don't chew, crush, or break them. If you have trouble swallowing, check with your doctor or pharmacist.

Take your medication with food or right after meals to prevent stomach upset.

What to do if you miss a dose

If you remember the missed dose within 2 hours, take it with food or liquids as soon as possible; then go back to your regular dosing schedule. But if you don't remember it until later, skip the missed dose and take your next dose on schedule. Don't take a double dose.

What to do about side effects

Stop taking this medication and call your doctor *right away* if you experience any of the following:

• confusion

• irregular or slow heartbeat

• "pins and needles" feeling in your hands, feet, or lips

• shortness of breath or difficulty breathing

• unusual tiredness or weakness

• unexplained anxiety

• weakness or heaviness of your legs.

Micro-K can also cause nausea, vomiting, abdominal pain, or diarrhea. Call your doctor if these effects persist or become bothersome.

What you must know about other drugs

Tell your doctor if you're taking other medications. You may be told to avoid certain medications that slow intestinal movements (including anticholinergic drugs, such as atropine); combining these drugs with Micro-K can increase the risk of side effects.

Make sure your doctor knows if you're taking an angiotensin-converting enzyme inhibitor such as Vasotec (enalaprilat) or a potassium-sparing diuretic such as Dyrenium (triamterene); combining such products with Micro-K can cause your potassium levels to rise dangerously.

Special directions

• Tell your doctor if you have other medical problems, especially Addison's disease, stomach ulcers, severe diarrhea, and kidney or heart disease. These medical problems can affect your use of Micro-K.

• Don't use salt substitutes or drink low-salt milk unless your doctor tells you to do so. These products may contain potassium and thus could increase your potassium levels too much. Also, check the ingredients of processed foods to avoid added potassium.

Micronase

Micronase is a diabetes medication prescribed in combination with a special diet and exercise program to control your blood sugar level. The generic name for Micronase is glyburide. Another brand name is DiaBeta.

How to take Micronase

Take Micronase exactly as prescribed. To ensure the best blood sugar control, take it at the same time each day. If you take one dose a day, take it in the morning with breakfast. If you're taking more than one dose a day, you may need to take the doses before breakfast and dinner or with meals. Check with your doctor.

What to do if you miss a dose

Take the missed dose as soon as possible. But if it's almost time for your next dose, skip the missed dose and take the next dose as scheduled.

What to do about side effects

Micronase may cause nervousness, increased sweating, fast heartbeat, headache, and yellowing of your skin and the whites of your eyes. If any of these symptoms persists or worsens, tell your doctor.

Micronase can increase your sensitivity to sunlight. If this occurs, wear protective clothing, use a sunblock, and limit sun exposure.

What you must know about alcohol and other drugs

Avoid alcoholic beverages. They can lower blood sugar levels and also can cause stomach pain, nausea, vomiting, dizziness, and excessive sweating.

Micronase can change the effects of many drugs, just as other drugs can reduce its effects. Check with your doctor before taking other medications, either prescription or nonprescription.

Special directions

• Tell your doctor about any other medical conditions you have, especially heart, kidney, liver, or thyroid disease.
• If you develop new medical problems, particularly infections, tell your doctor.
• Follow your prescribed diet and exercise plan carefully.
• Test your blood sugar level as your doctor instructs.

• Wear medical identification at all times and carry a card that indicates you're taking Micronase.

Important reminders   If you're pregnant or think you may be, tell your doctor, who will change your medication to insulin. If you plan to breast-feed, check with your doctor.

If you're an older adult, be aware that you may be especially sensitive to Micronase.

Midamor

This medication helps reduce the amount of water in your body without reducing your potassium level. It can be used to control high blood pressure. The generic name for Midamor is amiloride.

How to take
Midamor   Midamor comes in tablets. Read the label carefully and follow the directions exactly.

If you take a single dose daily, take it in the morning because Midamor increases urination. If you take more than one dose daily, you should take the last dose no later than 6 p.m.

If the medication upsets your stomach, take it with meals or milk.

What to do if you
miss a dose   Take the missed dose as soon as possible. But if it's almost time for your next dose, skip the missed dose and go back to your regular schedule. Don't take a double dose.

What to do about
side effects   Midamor can cause headaches, nausea, vomiting, diarrhea, and loss of appetite. If these effects persist or become severe, contact your doctor.

Because Midamor can increase sun sensitivity, avoid direct sunlight when possible, wear protective clothing, and use a sunblock with a skin protection factor (SPF) of 15 or higher. If you develop a severe sun reaction, contact your doctor.

What you must know about other drugs   Tell your doctor if you're taking another medication for high blood pressure or if you're taking potassium supplements or another potassium-sparing water pill. Combining these medications with Midamor could cause your potassium level to rise dangerously.

Tell your doctor if you're taking Eskalith (lithium); Midamor may increase Eskalith's side effects.

Check with your doctor before using nonprescription pain relievers; they can decrease Midamor's effectiveness.

Special directions   • Check with your doctor before changing your diet. Taking a potassium supplement or eating a high-potassium diet is unnecessary and could be dangerous. Symptoms of too much potassium include confusion, nervousness, fatigue, irregular heartbeat, weakness, shortness of breath, and numbness or tingling in your hands, feet, or lips.

• Tell the doctor or dentist that you're taking Midamor before you undergo surgery (including dental surgery), emergency treatment, or medical tests.

Important reminders   If you become pregnant while taking Midamor, notify your doctor.

Older adults are especially sensitive to Midamor and should be alert for symptoms of potassium overload.

If you're an athlete, you should know that the National Collegiate Athletic Association and the U.S. Olympic Committee ban the use of amiloride.

Miltown

Miltown is usually prescribed to treat anxiety or tension. This drug's generic name is meprobamate. Another brand name is Equanil.

How to take Miltown   Miltown is available in both tablets and sustained-release capsules. Check the prescription label carefully and take only the amount prescribed.

If you've been taking Miltown regularly for several weeks or more, don't stop taking it suddenly. This could cause withdrawal problems. Check with your doctor for instructions on how to discontinue the drug gradually.

What to do if you miss a dose

If you remember within an hour or so, take the missed dose immediately. Otherwise, skip the missed dose and resume your regular schedule. Never take a double dose.

What to do about side effects

If you think you've taken an overdose, get emergency help *immediately.* Overdose symptoms include severe drowsiness, dizziness, light-headedness, shortness of breath, slow or troubled breathing, slow heartbeat, slurred speech, severe weakness, and staggering.

If you experience any of the following symptoms, contact your doctor *as soon as possible:* a fast, pounding, or irregular heartbeat; shortness of breath; troubled breathing; a rash, hives, or itching; confusion; or unusual bleeding or bruising.

Because Miltown can make you drowsy or less alert, avoid potentially hazardous activities, such as driving a car, while you're taking it.

To relieve dry mouth, use sugarless gum or hard candy or suck on ice chips.

What you must know about alcohol and other drugs

Avoid alcoholic beverages, sedatives (drugs that relax you and make you feel sleepy), antihistamines such as Benadryl (diphenhydramine), and other central nervous system depressants while taking Miltown because of the risk of oversedation.

Special directions

• Don't take Miltown if you're allergic to aspirin or if you have porphyria.
• Make sure your doctor knows your medical history, especially if you've had liver or kidney problems, seizures, depression, or drug abuse or addiction problems.
• If you're taking Miltown over a long period of time, see the doctor regularly so your progress can be checked and any unwanted side effects detected.

Important reminders

If you're pregnant, check with your doctor about taking Miltown.

Also check with your doctor if you're breast-feeding. Miltown can make your baby drowsy.

If you're an athlete, you should know that the U.S. Olympic Committee and the National Collegiate Athletic Association ban the use of meprobamate.

Minipress

Your doctor has prescribed Minipress to treat your high blood pressure. This medication works by relaxing blood vessels so that blood can pass through them more easily, reducing pressure. The generic name for Minipress is prazosin.

How to take Minipress

Minipress comes in capsules. Your doctor may direct you to take your first dose at bedtime because the first dose of Minipress sometimes causes dizziness and an irregular heartbeat. If so, take care not to fall if you get out of bed during the night.

Take your doses at the same times every day so that taking your medicine becomes part of your daily routine.

What to do if you miss a dose

Take the missed dose as soon as possible. However, if it's almost time for your next dose, skip the missed dose and take your next dose on schedule. Don't take a double dose.

What to do about side effects

Minipress can make you feel dizzy, faint, or light-headed, especially when you rise suddenly from a lying or sitting position. Getting up slowly may help.

If the medication makes you feel drowsy, nauseated, or tired — or if it gives you a headache — tell your doctor.

What you must know about other drugs

Tell your doctor if you're taking other medications. Combining Minipress with beta blockers such as Tenormin (atenolol) may lower your blood pressure too much.

Special directions

• Tell your doctor if you have other medical problems, especially chest pain, kidney disease, or a heart condition. Other medical problems can affect your use of Minipress.

• Remember, Minipress won't cure your high blood pressure, but it will help control it. You may have to take high blood pressure medication for the rest of your life.

• Along with Minipress, your doctor may prescribe a special low-salt diet. (Too much salt can increase blood pressure.) If so, you'll need to limit your consumption of canned soup, pickles, ketchup, olives, hot dogs, soy sauce, carbonated beverages, and other high-salt foods.

• Keep all appointments for follow-up visits, even if you feel well, so your doctor can check your progress and adjust your medication, if necessary.

Important reminder   If you're an older adult, you may be especially vulnerable to side effects from Minipress, particularly dizziness and light-headedness. Take care to prevent falls.

Moban

Moban is usually prescribed to treat emotional, nervous, or mental disorders. The generic name for this drug is molindone.

How to take Moban   Moban is available in tablets and a solution. Take only the amount prescribed.

If you're taking the *solution,* drink it undiluted or mix it with water, milk, fruit juice, or a carbonated beverage. To reduce stomach irritation, take it with food or a full glass (8 ounces) of water or milk.

Check with your doctor before you discontinue this medication. He or she may want to reduce your dosage gradually.

What to do if you miss a dose   Take the missed dose as soon as possible. However, if it's within 2 hours of your next regular dose, skip the missed dose and resume your regular schedule. Never take a double dose.

What to do about side effects   Before taking Moban, talk to your doctor about the risk of permanent side effects. Moban may cause a movement disorder that doesn't go away — even after you stop taking the drug. Symptoms of this disorder include lip smacking or puckering, cheek puffing, rapid or wormlike tongue movements, and other uncontrolled movements of the mouth, tongue, cheeks, jaw, arms, and legs.

Call your doctor *promptly* if you experience sedation, difficulty talking or swallowing, loss of balance, muscle spasms, restlessness or the need to keep moving, or trembling and shaking of the hands.

You may experience constipation, blurred vision, decreased sweating, difficulty urinating, drowsiness, dry mouth, headache, nausea, stuffy nose, and dizziness or light-headedness when getting up suddenly from a lying or sitting position. Check with your doctor if these side effects persist.

Moban can make you drowsy or less alert, so avoid potentially hazardous activities, such as driving a car, until you know how it affects you.

What you must know about alcohol and other drugs
Avoid alcoholic beverages, barbiturates, sedatives (drugs that relax you and make you feel sleepy), antihistamines such as Benadryl (diphenhydramine), and other central nervous system depressants while taking this medication because of the risk of oversedation.

Antacids and diarrhea medications can decrease the effectiveness of Moban, so avoid taking them 2 hours before or after taking a dose of Moban.

Special directions
Make sure your doctor knows about your medical history, especially if you have or have had brain damage; a head injury; cerebrovascular, heart, respiratory, or liver disease; intestinal blockage; difficulty urinating; enlarged prostate; glaucoma; seizures; or Parkinson's disease.

Important reminders
If you're an older adult, you may be especially prone to side effects from Moban.

If you're an athlete, you should know that the U.S. Olympic Committee and the National Collegiate Athletic Association ban the use of molindone in some athletic events.

Monistat

This medication is usually prescribed to treat fungus infections such as athlete's foot, jock itch, and vaginal yeast infections. The generic name for this drug is miconazole. Another brand name is Micatin.

How to use Monistat

Monistat is available in cream, lotion, powder, spray, and vaginal cream, as well as in vaginal suppositories. Some preparations are available without a prescription. If you're treating yourself, follow the package instructions carefully. If your doctor prescribed Monistat or recommended it to you, follow his instructions for using it.

If you're using the *spray,* shake it well before applying. Spray it on the affected area from a distance of 4 to 6 inches. If you're using the spray on your feet, spray it between your toes, on your feet, and in your socks and shoes. Don't inhale the spray.

If you're using the *powder* on your feet, sprinkle it between your toes, on your feet, and in your socks and shoes.

If you're using the *vaginal cream* or *suppositories,* insert the applicator or suppository high into your vagina at bedtime for the number of days specified on the package or prescribed by your doctor. Wear a sanitary pad to prevent clothing stains. To help clear up your infection, wear only freshly washed cotton underwear and avoid using tampons during treatment.

If you're using the cream, don't apply an airtight cover (such as plastic wrap) over the treated area unless the doctor tells you to; this may irritate your skin.

Take Monistat for the full treatment period prescribed, even if your condition improves. If your condition doesn't improve within 4 weeks or if it gets worse, call the doctor.

What to do if you miss a dose

Administer the missed dose as soon as possible. However, if it's almost time for your next dose, skip the missed dose and resume your regular schedule.

What to do about side effects

Call your doctor *as soon as possible* if you notice a rash, burning, redness, blistering, or another type of skin irritation that wasn't there before you started using Monistat.

Special directions
• If you have liver disease, check with your doctor before using this medication.

• If you plan to use a vaginal form of Monistat and are already using another vaginal medication, check with your doctor or pharmacist before starting treatment.

• If you have sexual intercourse during treatment, don't stop using the medication. Avoid using a latex contraceptive diaphragm because it could interact with Monistat and cause problems. Be aware that your sexual partner may also need to be treated.

Important reminder
If you're pregnant, check with your doctor before using the vaginal form of this medication.

MSIR

MSIR is usually prescribed to relieve pain. The generic name for this drug is morphine. Another brand name is MS Contin.

How to take MSIR
Take only the amount prescribed.

If you're taking the *extended-release tablets,* be sure to swallow them whole. Don't break, crush, or chew them.

If you're taking the *liquid,* use a measuring spoon (not a household teaspoon) to measure your dose. Mix it with juice to improve its taste.

If you're using the *suppositories,* remove the foil wrapper and moisten the suppository with cold water. Lie on your side. Using your finger, push the suppository well up into your rectum.

If you're using the *injection form*, your doctor or nurse will teach you how to administer it.

If you've been taking MSIR regularly, don't suddenly stop taking it. Ask the doctor how to discontinue it gradually.

What to do if you miss a dose
If you're taking MSIR on a regular schedule, take the missed dose as soon as possible. But if it's almost time

for your next regular dose, skip the missed dose and resume your regular schedule. Never take a double dose.

What to do about side effects

Get emergency help *immediately* if your heartbeat seems unusually fast, slow, or pounding; if you start wheezing or have trouble breathing; if your hands and face swell; or if you start sweating a lot.

Call your doctor *right away* if your breathing rate drops to 8 to 10 breaths a minute, if you have hallucinations, or if you feel confused, dizzy, or unusually weak or tired.

If itching or a rash develops, you may be having an allergic reaction. Stop the medication and contact your doctor.

Nausea, vomiting, or constipation may occur, especially at first. If these side effects continue, call your doctor.

If the medication makes you feel nauseated, wait until the nausea subsides before eating your meals. If the nausea is severe or if you vomit, ask the doctor for medication to prevent this side effect.

To help prevent constipation, eat a well-balanced, high-fiber diet, including bran, fruit, and raw, leafy vegetables.

To avoid feeling faint or dizzy, get up slowly from a lying or sitting position.

Because MSIR can make you drowsy and less alert, avoid potentially hazardous activities, such as driving a car, until you know how you react to it.

What you must know about alcohol and other drugs

Don't drink alcoholic beverages while you're taking MSIR.

Also avoid sleeping pills and antihistamines.

Check with your doctor or pharmacist if you're taking other prescription or nonprescription drugs. Some drugs can change the way MSIR works.

Special directions

• Review your medical history with your doctor before you start taking MSIR.

• Take MSIR on a regular schedule; don't wait until your pain is severe.

Important reminders If you're pregnant or breast-feeding, check with your doctor before taking MSIR.

Children and older adults are especially sensitive to this drug.

If you're an athlete, you should know that the U.S. Olympic Committee bans the use of morphine.

Myambutol

Myambutol is used to treat tuberculosis. The generic name for this medication is ethambutol.

How to take Myambutol Take this medication exactly as your doctor directs, preferably at the same time each day so that taking it becomes routine.

If the medication upsets your stomach, you can take it with food.

Keep taking Myambutol as directed, even after you feel better. Otherwise, your tuberculosis may not clear up completely. Keep in mind that you may need to take the medication for 1 year or more.

What to do about side effects Call your doctor *immediately* if you experience blurred vision, blindness, eye pain, or trouble differentiating between red and green. Also call your doctor *at once* if you have chills or fever; pain or swelling in your joints (especially in your feet); burning, numbness, tingling, or weakness in your hands or feet — or if you cough up mucus tinged with blood.

Other possible side effects, such as an upset stomach, diarrhea, loss of appetite, severe fatigue, dizziness, itching, and rashes, may go away as your body adjusts to the medication. However, be sure to discuss any of these side effects with your doctor.

Because Myambutol can affect your level of alertness as well as your vision, don't drive or perform other potentially dangerous activities until you know how you react to it.

Special directions • Before taking this drug, tell your doctor if you have optic neuritis (eye nerve damage), cataracts, recurrent eye infections, or vision problems related to diabetes, gout, or kidney disease. Myambutol can aggravate these conditions.

• Your doctor may order you to have regular blood tests to monitor for certain disorders such as gout.

• Your doctor may also ask you to schedule regular eye exams while you're taking Myambutol.

• Notify the doctor if your symptoms don't disappear or you feel worse after 2 to 3 weeks of Myambutol therapy.

Important reminders If you're breast-feeding, check with your doctor before taking this medication.

Myambutol is not recommended for children under age 13.

Mycelex Troches

This medication comes in the form of throat lozenges and is prescribed to treat fungal infections. Its generic name is clotrimazole.

How to use Mycelex Troches Hold a lozenge in your mouth and allow it to dissolve slowly and completely. This may take 15 to 30 minutes. Try not to swallow your saliva during this time. Don't chew the lozenges or swallow them whole.

Continue to use your medication, even if your symptoms clear up in a few days. Otherwise your infection may return. Because fungal infections may be slow to clear up, you may need to use Lotrimin every day for several weeks or more.

What to do if you miss a dose Apply the missed dose as soon as possible. However, if it's almost time for your next dose, skip the missed dose and apply your next dose on schedule.

What to do about side effects Check with your doctor if you experience nausea and vomiting.

Special directions • Tell your doctor if you have other medical problems, especially liver disease.

• If your symptoms don't go away within 1 week or if they become worse, check with your doctor.
• Tell the doctor before you have liver tests. Mycelex Troches may alter the test results.

Important reminders Don't give Mycelex Troches to children under age 5. Children may be too young to use them without choking.

Myciguent

This medication is usually prescribed to treat skin infections, minor burns, or minor wounds. Its generic name is neomycin.

How to apply Myciguent Myciguent is available in a cream and an ointment. You can buy it without a prescription. If you're treating yourself, follow the package instructions carefully. Don't apply it to a puncture wound, deep wound, serious burn, or raw area unless your doctor approves. If your doctor prescribed the medication or gave you special instructions on how to use it, follow his instructions carefully.

To apply Myciguent, wash the affected area with soap and water; then dry it thoroughly. Apply a generous amount of medication to the affected area and rub it in gently. If you're using the *cream* form of the drug, rub it in until it disappears. If you wish, you can cover the treated area with a gauze dressing.

To eliminate your infection completely, continue to use the medication for the full term of treatment, even if your symptoms go away.

What to do if you miss an application Apply the missed dose as soon as possible. However, if it's almost time for your next regular treatment, skip the one you missed and resume your regular treatment schedule.

What to do about side effects Call your doctor *immediately* if you have breathing problems, dizziness, fainting, or a fever — or if you notice a rash, itching, redness, or other symptoms of skin irritation that weren't there before you started using Myciguent.

The doctor should also be advised of any hearing changes you're experiencing.

What you must know about other drugs

Check with your doctor or pharmacist before applying another medication to the same skin area where you're using Myciguent.

Special directions

• Check with your doctor before using this medication if you have a kidney problem or if you've ever had an allergic or unusual reaction to another antibiotic, including Mycifradin (the oral form of neomycin), Amikin (amikacin), Garamycin (gentamicin), Kantrex (kanamycin), Netromycin (netilmicin), streptomycin, and Nebcin (tobramycin).

• Keep this medication away from your eyes.

• If your skin condition doesn't improve within 1 week or if it gets worse, call your doctor or pharmacist.

• Don't use this medication for a long time without your doctor's approval.

Mycolog II

Your doctor has prescribed Mycolog II to treat your fungal infection and relieve the discomfort it's causing. The generic name for this product is nystatin with triamcinolone.

How to use Mycolog II

This combination medication comes in cream and ointment forms. Follow your doctor's directions for using it. Be exact; don't use it more often than prescribed or for a longer time than recommended.

To apply the cream or ointment, rub a small amount into the affected area gently and thoroughly. Take care to keep it away from your eyes.

Don't put a bandage, wrap, or other tight dressing over the treated skin unless your doctor directs you to do so. Wear loose-fitting clothing when using this medication on your groin area.

Use Mycolog II for the full time of treatment, even if your symptoms go away. If you stop using it too soon, your infection may return.

What to do if you miss a dose
Apply the missed dose as soon as possible. But if it's almost time for your next dose, skip the missed dose and take your next dose on schedule.

What to do about side effects
Call your doctor *right away* if you start to have skin irritation, such as blistering, burning, dryness, itching, or peeling.

If you use this medication for a long time, you may experience other side effects. Let your doctor know if you show any of the following signs: acne or oily skin; increased growth or loss of hair; reddish purple lines on your arms, face, legs, trunk, or groin; or thin skin that bruises easily.

Special directions
• Because certain medical conditions may prevent your using Mycolog II, tell your doctor if you have (or have had in the past) herpes, chickenpox, tuberculosis, or viral infections of the skin.
• Don't use this medication for other skin problems unless you've checked first with your doctor.
• If your skin problem isn't better within 2 to 3 weeks, call your doctor.
• If you're using Mycolog II to treat a child's diaper rash, avoid tight-fitting diapers and plastic pants.

Important reminders
If you're pregnant or breast-feeding, check with your doctor before using this medication.

If you have severe diabetes, also talk to your doctor before using Mycolog II. In rare instances, the drug can raise blood and urine glucose levels.

Mysoline

Mysoline is prescribed to treat seizure disorders. The generic name for this product is primidone.

How to take Mysoline
Mysoline is available in tablets and an oral suspension. Take it exactly as prescribed by the doctor. For best results, take the drug in regularly spaced doses.

Don't stop taking Mysoline suddenly. Check with your doctor, who may want you to reduce your dosage gradually to avoid potential withdrawal problems.

What to do if you miss a dose

Take the missed dose as soon as possible. But if it's within 1 hour of your next dose, skip the missed dose and take your next dose on schedule. Don't take a double dose.

What to do about side effects

Occasionally, Mysoline can make you feel drowsy or cause nausea, vomiting, double vision, or loss of coordination. Check with your doctor if you have any of these side effects, especially if they continue or become more severe.

What you must know about alcohol and other drugs

Check with your doctor about drinking alcoholic beverages; combining alcoholic beverages with Mysoline may lead to oversedation. For the same reason, check with your doctor before you take other medications that slow down your central nervous system, such as muscle relaxants, anesthetics, sleeping pills, and cold and flu remedies.

Your doctor may need to watch your progress closely if you're taking Dilantin (phenytoin) or Tegretol (carbamazepine), two other medications used to prevent seizures.

Special directions

• Tell your doctor if you have other medical problems, especially asthma or another lung disease, porphyria, and liver disease. These problems can affect your use of Mysoline.
• Because Mysoline can make you drowsy, don't drive or perform other potentially dangerous activities until you're sure of how it affects you.
• Before you have diagnostic tests on your liver, tell the doctor you're taking Mysoline; it may affect the test results.
• Keep all appointments for follow-up visits so your doctor can check your progress.

Important reminders

If you're pregnant or breast-feeding, don't use Mysoline unless your doctor tells you to do so.

If you're an older adult, you may be especially prone to Mysoline's side effects.

If you're an athlete, you should know that the U.S. Olympic Committee and the National Collegiate Athletic Association ban primidone and sometimes test for it.

N

Naftin

This medication is usually prescribed to treat fungus infections, such as athlete's foot, jock itch, and ringworm of the body. The generic name for this drug is naftifine.

How to apply Naftin

Naftin is a cream. Apply it twice a day unless your doctor tells you otherwise. Wash your hands first. Then apply enough cream to cover the affected skin and surrounding areas. Rub it in gently.

If you're using Naftin to treat *athlete's foot*, dry your feet carefully, especially between your toes, after bathing. Wear cotton socks and change them daily (more often if your feet sweat heavily). Avoid wearing wool socks or socks made of synthetic materials (such as nylon or rayon). After you have applied Naftin and it has disappeared into your skin, apply powder on the affected area. Make sure it's antifungal, talcum, or another bland, absorbent powder. Sprinkle it on your feet, between your toes, and in your socks and shoes once or twice a day.

If you're using Naftin to treat *jock itch*, dry your groin area carefully after bathing. Wear loose-fitting, cotton underwear. Avoid tight-fitting underwear made from rayon, nylon, or another synthetic material. After you have applied Naftin and it has disappeared into your skin, apply powder on your groin area. Make sure it's antifungal, talcum, or another bland, absorbent powder. Use the powder once or twice a day.

If you're using Naftin to treat *ringworm of the body,* dry yourself carefully after bathing. Try to prevent moisture buildup on the affected parts. Avoid excessive heat and humidity. Don't wear tight-fitting, poorly ventilated clothing. After you have applied the Naftin cream and it has disappeared into your skin, sprinkle an antifungal, talcum, or another bland, absorbent powder on the affected areas.

What to do if you miss an application   Apply the missed dose as soon as you remember. However, if it's almost time for your next regular application, skip the one you missed and resume your regular schedule.

What to do about side effects   You may notice burning or stinging on the treated area. These side effects usually go away over time as your body adjusts to the medication. But you should check with your doctor if they persist or become bothersome.

Special directions   • Keep Naftin away from your eyes, nose, and mouth.
• Use Naftin for the full treatment time prescribed. If you stop using it too soon, your symptoms may return. In fact, the doctor will probably instruct you to keep using the cream for 1 to 2 weeks after your symptoms go away. Be diligent in using it; don't skip doses.
• Call your doctor if your skin condition doesn't improve within 1 month or if it gets worse.

Nalfon

This medication helps relieve the inflammation, swelling, stiffness, and joint pain of rheumatoid arthritis or osteoarthritis. The generic name for this product is fenoprofen.

How to take Nalfon   Take the drug with food or an antacid and a full glass (8 ounces) of water. Remain upright for 15 to 30 minutes after taking it to help prevent swallowing problems.

What to do if you miss a dose   If it's within hours of your regular dosage time, take the missed dose immediately. If it's later than that, skip the missed dose and take your next dose at the regular time. Don't take a double dose.

What to do about side effects   Serious side effects, including ulcers or bleeding, can occur with or without warning. Stop taking Nalfon and call your doctor *right away* if you notice any of these warning signs: severe cramps, pain, or burning in your stomach; severe, continuing nausea, heartburn, or indigestion; or vomit tinged with blood or material that looks like coffee grounds.

You may experience dizziness, headache, drowsiness, heartburn, nausea, vomiting, itching, and black, tarry stools while taking Nalfon. If these symptoms persist or become severe, call your doctor.

Because Nalfon can make you drowsy or dizzy, make sure you know how you react to it before driving or performing other activities that require you to be fully alert.

If Nalfon makes you more sensitive to sunlight, wear a hat and sunglasses and use a sunblock outdoors.

What you must know about alcohol and other drugs
Avoid alcoholic beverages; they increase your risk of stomach problems.

Don't take aspirin or Tylenol (acetaminophen) with Nalfon for more than a few days (unless your doctor directs otherwise); these medications may increase your risk of serious side effects.

Be sure to tell your doctor about other medications you're taking, particularly anticoagulants (blood thinners) and sulfonylureas (drugs for diabetes). They can affect the way Nalfon works in your system.

Special directions
If you have other medical problems, let your doctor know. They may affect your use of Nalfon.

Important reminders
If you're pregnant or breast-feeding, consult your doctor about taking this medication.

If you're an older adult, you may be especially prone to side effects from Nalfon.

Nasalcrom

This drug's generic name is cromolyn. Nasalcrom, the brand name for the nasal solution and powder forms of this medication, is used to relieve allergies. The inhalation solution, capsule, and aerosol forms, known by the trade name Intal, are used to prevent asthma attacks and bronchospasm.

How to use Nasalcrom
To use Nasalcrom, first clear your nasal passages by blowing your nose.

If you're using the *nasal solution* or *powder,* you'll need a special inhaler. Read and follow the package instructions.

If you're using the *solution for inhalation,* use this medication only in a power-operated nebulizer with an adequate flow rate and a face mask or mouthpiece. Make sure you understand exactly how to use it. Hand-operated nebulizers aren't used with this medication.

If you're using capsules for inhalation, never swallow them. Read the directions before using the special inhaler.

If you're using the *inhalation aerosol,* read the directions before using. Keep the spray away from your eyes.

Don't use Nasalcrom more often than prescribed. If you have hay fever, it may take at least 1 week before you feel better. If you have chronic allergic rhinitis, it may take up to 1 month.

What to do if you miss a dose

Take the missed dose as soon as possible. Then take any remaining doses for that day at regularly spaced intervals. Don't take a double dose.

What to do about side effects

If you're using the Nasalcrom powder, *call for emergency help* if you start to wheeze and have difficulty breathing after using it.

Any form of chromolyn can make you cough or cause soreness or dryness of the mouth and throat. If these symptoms persist, call your doctor.

If your mouth or throat feels dry or irritated after using this medication, try gargling after each dose.

What you must know about other drugs

If you have asthma, you may be taking this medication along with an adrenocorticoid, such as Cortone Acetate (cortisone) or Deltasone (prednisone). If so, don't stop taking the adrenocorticoid, even if your asthma seems better, unless your doctor tells you to do so.

Special directions

Tell your doctor if you have other medical problems, especially asthma or diseases of the heart, kidney, or liver.

Important reminder

If you're pregnant or breast-feeding, check with your doctor before using this medication.

Navane

This medication is used to treat nervous, mental, and emotional illnesses. Its generic name is thiothixene.

How to take Navane
Take only the amount of medication your doctor has prescribed. You may have to use Navane for several weeks before you feel its full effect.

If you're taking the *liquid concentrate,* use the bottle dropper to measure the exact dose. Then dilute the dose in half a glass (4 ounces) of water, milk, soda, or tomato or fruit juice. Don't let the drug touch your skin; it could cause a rash.

Don't suddenly stop taking Navane unless you have a severe reaction to it or your doctor tells you to.

What to do if you miss a dose
Take the missed dose as soon as possible. But if it's within 2 hours of your next dose, skip the missed dose and take your next dose as scheduled.

What to do about side effects
Call your doctor *right away* if you have uncontrolled movements of your mouth, tongue, cheeks, jaw, or arms and legs. Also call if you have a fever, a sore throat, fast heartbeat, rapid breathing, profuse sweating, fainting or dizziness, difficulty urinating, or blurred vision.

Tell your doctor if you become constipated, have a dry mouth, or notice changes in skin color after being in the sun.

Because Navane makes your skin more sensitive to sunlight, avoid direct exposure to the sun.

Because it also reduces sweating, be careful not to become overheated.

Navane can make you drowsy as well as affect your vision, so don't drive or perform any activities that require you to be fully alert and to see clearly. The drowsiness should become less noticeable after several weeks.

What you must know about alcohol and other drugs
Don't drink alcoholic beverages while taking Navane. Doing so could cause you to become oversedated.

Call your doctor before taking other medications. Avoid drugs that make you drowsy, such as allergy medications, pain relievers, and muscle relaxants.

Special directions
- Tell your doctor if you're allergic to any medications.
- Tell the doctor if you have a history of a blood or bone marrow disorder; Navane can make this kind of medical problem worse. You should also tell the doctor if you've ever been in a coma, had a head injury, or had a circulation problem.
- Other conditions your doctor should be made aware of include heart or lung problems, seizures, glaucoma, enlarged prostate, Parkinson's disease, urine retention, tumors, low calcium level, or kidney or liver disease.

Important reminders
Before beginning a course of Navane, let the doctor know if you are breast-feeding or think you may be pregnant.

Athletes should be aware that the U.S. Olympic Committee and the National Collegiate Athletic Association ban the use of thiothixene.

NebuPent

This inhaled medication is prescribed to prevent or treat *Pneumocystis carinii* pneumonia. It's generic name is pentamidine. The injection form of pentamidine is Pentam.

How to take NebuPent
Take NebuPent exactly as directed by your doctor.

For the *inhalant,* use the aerosol device until the chamber is empty. This may take as long as 45 minutes.

If you're using the *injection* form of the drug, lie down during the injection; the medication can cause your blood pressure to drop suddenly, making you feel lightheaded or dizzy.

Continue to take the medication as directed, even after you begin to feel better. If you stop too soon, your infection may return.

What to do if you miss a dose
If you miss a dose of the *inhalant,* take the missed dose as soon as possible. If you miss an *injection,* check with your doctor about when to receive the next dose.

What to do about side effects
Call your doctor *right away* if you experience any of the following signs and symptoms:

- decreased urination
- sore throat and fever
- easy bleeding or bruising
- symptoms of low blood sugar: anxiety; chills; cold sweats; cool, pale skin; headache; increased hunger; nervousness; shakiness
- symptoms of low blood pressure: blurred vision, confusion, dizziness, fainting or light-headedness, and unusual tiredness or weakness.

Also check with your doctor if you develop diarrhea, loss of appetite, nausea, or vomiting.

If you're giving yourself injections, let your doctor know if you have pain, redness, or swelling at the injection site. Use warm compresses to relieve soreness.

What you must know about other drugs

It's important to tell the doctor about other medications you're taking. You may be at risk for kidney damage if you take NebuPent with certain antibiotics; with Fungizone (amphotericin B), a drug for fungal infections; with Platinol (cisplatin), a cancer medication; or with Retrovir (zidovudine), an AIDS medication.

Special directions

- Tell your doctor if you have other medical problems, especially anemia, asthma, diabetes, bleeding disorders, low blood pressure, or kidney, heart, or liver disease.
- If you're using NebuPent, don't smoke; smoking can cause coughing and difficulty breathing.

Important reminder

If you're pregnant or breast-feeding, check with your doctor before using this medication.

NegGram

This medication is usually prescribed to treat infections of the urinary tract. Its generic name is nalidixic acid.

How to take NegGram

NegGram is available in tablets as well as in an oral suspension.

Check the label carefully and take only the amount prescribed.

If you're taking the *oral suspension,* use a specially marked measuring spoon (not a household teaspoon).

For best results, take NegGram with a full glass (8 ounces) of water on an empty stomach (1 hour before or 2 hours after meals). However, if NegGram upsets your stomach, you may take it with food or milk.

Take NegGram for the full prescribed time, even if you feel better after a few days. Don't skip doses.

What to do if you miss a dose

Take the missed dose as soon as you remember. But if it's almost time for your next dose and the doctor has prescribed three or more doses a day, space the missed dose and the next dose 2 to 4 hours apart, or double your next dose. Then resume your regular schedule.

What to do about side effects

Call the doctor *immediately* if you experience vision changes (including double vision, blurring, decreased vision, halos around lights, too-bright appearance of lights, or changes in color vision), seizures, hallucinations, mood changes, pale skin, pale stools, sore throat, fever, severe stomach pain, yellow skin or eyes, unusual bleeding or bruising, or unusual weakness or fatigue.

You may also experience abdominal pain, nausea, and vomiting. These side effects usually go away over time as your body adjusts to NegGram. But you should check with your doctor if they persist or become severe.

Because NegGram can make you dizzy or impair your vision, avoid activities that require you to be fully alert and clear-sighted (driving a car, for instance).

If NegGram makes you sensitive to sunlight, avoid direct exposure, wear protective clothing and sunglasses, and use a sunblock.

What you must know about other drugs

Check with your doctor or pharmacist before taking a blood thinner with NegGram. The combination can increase NegGram's potential to cause bleeding.

Special directions

• Make sure your doctor knows about your medical history, especially if you've had seizures, liver or kidney problems, or brain or spinal cord damage. Also tell the doctor if you have a glucose-6-phosphate dehydrogenase (G6PD) deficiency or hardening of the brain arteries.

• Call your doctor if your symptoms don't improve within 2 days or if they get worse.

Important reminders   If you're pregnant or breast-feeding, check with your doctor before taking this medication.

NegGram is not recommended for use in infants or children.

Nembutal

This drug is prescribed to relax you. It belongs to a group of medications called barbiturates, which act by slowing down the central nervous system. The generic name for Nembutal is pentobarbital.

How to take Nembutal   Nembutal comes in capsule, elixir, and suppository forms. Take it exactly as your doctor directs. Because it can become habit-forming, don't take it for a longer time than your doctor recommends.

To use the *suppository,* first remove the foil wrapper; then moisten the suppository with cold water. Next, lie down on your side and use your finger to push the suppository well up into your rectum. Wash your hands afterward.

What to do if you miss a dose   If you're taking Nembutal regularly, take the missed dose as soon as possible. However, if it's almost time for your next dose, skip the missed dose and go back to your regular schedule. Don't take a double dose.

What to do about side effects   Get emergency help *immediately* if you think you may have taken an overdose. Overdose symptoms include the following: severe drowsiness, confusion, or weakness; shortness of breath; slow heartbeat; slow or troubled breathing; slurred speech; or staggering.

Check with your doctor if you become drowsy or lethargic or feel as though you have a hangover.

Because Nembutal can make you drowsy or lightheaded, don't drive or perform activities that require you to be fully alert until you know how the medication affects you.

What you must know about alcohol and other drugs

Don't drink alcoholic beverages while you're taking Nembutal. The combination may cause oversedation.

For the same reason, check with your doctor before taking other central nervous system depressants, such as many allergy and cold medications, narcotic pain relievers, and sleeping pills.

Also let the doctor know if you're using adrenocorticoids (cortisone-like medications), blood thinners, Fulvicin (griseofulvin) or other antifungal medications, or birth control pills.

Special directions

• Tell your doctor if you have other medical problems. They may affect your use of Nembutal.

• After prolonged use, don't stop taking Nembutal suddenly; check with your doctor and follow his or her advice for gradual withdrawal from the drug.

Important reminders

If you're pregnant or breast-feeding, check with your doctor before using this medication.

If you're an older adult, you may be especially prone to side effects from Nembutal.

If you're an athlete, you should know that the U.S. Olympic Committee and the National Collegiate Athletic Association ban the use of pentobarbital and sometimes test for the drug.

Neo-Synephrine (nasal)

This medication will help relieve your stuffy nose. The generic name for this drug is phenylephrine.

How to use Neo-Synephrine

Neo-Synephrine comes in nose drops, a nose spray, and a nose jelly. Follow your doctor's directions exactly when using it. If you bought your medication without a prescription, read the package directions carefully. Before you use this medication, blow your nose gently.

To use the *nose drops,* tilt your head back and squeeze the drops into each nostril. Keep your head tilted back for a few minutes. Rinse the dropper with hot water, dry it with a clean tissue, and recap the bottle.

To use the *nose spray,* hold your head upright and spray the medication into each nostril. Sniff briskly while squeezing the bottle. Spray once or twice; then wait a few minutes for the medication to work. Blow your nose and repeat until the complete dose is taken.

To use the *nose jelly,* place a pea-size amount of the jelly up each nostril. Sniff it well back into the nose.

Don't use Neo-Synephrine longer than directed; doing so can make your condition worse.

What to do if you miss a dose

Take the missed dose right away if you remember it within 1 hour or so. However, if you don't remember until later, skip the missed dose and take your next dose on schedule. Don't take a double dose.

What to do about side effects

Check with your doctor if your heart starts to pound irregularly or too rapidly. These symptoms suggest that you've used too much Neo-Synephrine.

When you use this medication, your nose may burn, sting, or feel dry. Let your doctor know if these symptoms continue or become bothersome.

Special directions

• Tell your doctor if you have other medical problems, especially heart or blood vessel disease, high blood pressure, glaucoma, diabetes, an overactive thyroid, or diseases of the liver or pancreas.

• Before you have a hearing test, tell the doctor that you're using Neo-Synephrine. It may affect the test results.

Important reminders

Check with your doctor before giving this medication to a child. Children are especially prone to Neo-Synephrine's side effects.

If you're an athlete, you should know that the U.S. Olympic Committee bans and tests for phenylephrine. Using the drug can lead to disqualification in most athletic events.

Neo-Synephrine (ophthalmic)

These eyedrops will relieve the redness of your eyes. They're also used to treat some other eye problems and to enlarge the pupils before eye examinations. The drug's generic name is phenylephrine.

How to instill Neo-Synephrine eyedrops

Follow your doctor's directions exactly. If you bought this medication without a prescription, carefully read the package directions before using.

Don't use more of the eyedrops or use them more often than your doctor or the package directions order. To use the eyedrops, follow these steps:

• Wash your hands.

• Tilt your head back and pull your lower eyelid away from the eye to form a pouch.

• Squeeze the drops into the pouch and gently close your eye for 1 to 2 minutes.

• Wash your hands again.

What to do if you miss a dose

Instill the missed dose as soon as possible. However, if it's almost time for your next dose, skip the missed dose and instill your next dose on schedule. Don't instill a double dose.

What to do about side effects

Check with your doctor if you have high blood pressure.

When you instill the eyedrops, your eyes may burn, sting, water, or become more sensitive to light. Check with your doctor if these symptoms continue or become bothersome.

Because your eyes may be more sensitive to light while you're using Neo-Synephrine eyedrops, wear sunglasses that block ultraviolet light when you're in a bright room or outside on sunny days.

What you must know about other drugs

Tell your doctor about other medications you're taking. Your doctor may want you to avoid certain medications to prevent harmful interactions. In particular, medications to avoid or use with your doctor's supervision are those for high blood pressure, Parkinson's disease, and depression or other psychiatric problems.

Special directions
- Tell your doctor if you have other medical problems, especially heart or blood vessel disease, high blood pressure, glaucoma, diabetes, an overactive thyroid, or diseases of the liver or pancreas.
- Before you have a hearing test, tell the doctor that you're using Neo-Synephrine eyedrops because it may affect the test results.

Important reminders
If you're giving Neo-Synephrine eyedrops to a child, check with the doctor first because children are especially prone to this drug's side effects.

Older adults are also especially prone to Neo-Synephrine's side effects.

If you're an athlete, you should know that the U.S. Olympic Committee bans the use of phenylephrine eyedrops.

Niacor

The doctor may prescribe Niacor to treat niacin deficiency or to help lower blood cholesterol and fat levels. The generic name for the drug is niacin. Another brand name is Slo-Niacin.

How to take Niacor
Niacor is available in regular and extended-release tablets and capsules as well as in an oral suspension. It should be taken with milk or meals if it causes diarrhea or stomach upset.

If you're taking the *extended-release tablets,* swallow them whole. If the tablets are scored, you may break them before swallowing, but don't crush or chew them.

If you're taking the *extended-release capsules,* swallow them whole; don't chew, crush, or break them. If they're too large to swallow, mix the contents with jelly or jam and swallow without chewing.

Take the medication only as directed and check with your doctor before you stop taking it.

Avoid taking large doses of Niacor except under your doctor's direction.

What to do if you miss a dose   If you're taking Niacor without a doctor's recommendation, missing 1 or 2 days won't hurt you. If the doctor has prescribed Niacor to help bring down your cholesterol level, take the missed dose as soon as possible. However, if it's almost time for your next dose, skip the missed dose and resume your regular schedule. Never take a double dose.

What to do about side effects   If you're taking the extended-release medication, call your doctor *immediately* if you have darkened urine, light gray stools, appetite loss, severe stomach pain, or yellow skin or eyes.

You may feel dizzy or faint, especially when getting up quickly from a lying or sitting position. This effect should decrease after 1 or 2 weeks.

If you're taking high doses of Niacor, you may have stomach pain, diarrhea, nausea, vomiting, dizziness, faintness, fever, frequent urination, itching, joint pain, muscle aches or cramps, lower back or side pain, unusual weakness or fatigue, or a fast, slow, or irregular heartbeat. Also, a feeling of warmth, skin flushing or redness, and headache may occur. Call your doctor if side effects persist or become more severe.

Special directions   • If your medical history includes diabetes, bleeding problems, glaucoma, gout, liver disease, low blood pressure, or a stomach ulcer, check with your doctor before using Niacor.

• If you're taking Niacor to lower your cholesterol level, follow any special diet your doctor recommends (such as a low-fat, low-cholesterol diet).

• If you're taking Niacor as a vitamin supplement, keep in mind that such supplements aren't meant to replace a varied, well-balanced diet that includes meat, eggs, and dairy foods — products that are rich in niacin.

Important reminder   If you're pregnant or breast-feeding, check with your doctor before taking Niacor.

Nicoderm

This skin patch is prescribed to help you stop smoking. You should use it only as part of a comprehensive stop-smoking program. The generic component of Nicoderm is nicotine. Another brand name is Habitrol.

How to use Nicoderm

Nicoderm comes in a stick-on patch that's available by prescription only.

Follow the package instructions carefully; they spell out just when and how often to apply a new patch and how long to leave it on. Typically, you should apply a new patch daily, preferably at the same time each day.

To apply the patch, choose a hairless part of your body, such as the outer part of your upper arm, or your stomach or back above the waist. The chosen site should be free from cuts and irritation.

Press the patch firmly to your skin. Then wash your hands with water only.

To avoid skin irritation, apply each new patch to a different site. Wait at least 1 week before reusing a site.

Discard patches properly — and always where children and animals can't reach them. Used patches contain enough nicotine to poison children and pets.

Continue to use this drug for the full time prescribed by your doctor. Don't stop using it suddenly.

What to do if you miss an application

Apply a new patch as soon as you remember. Then change the patch at the regular time.

If the patch falls off, apply a new one; then change it at your usual time.

What to do about side effects

Call your doctor *immediately* if you have symptoms of nicotine overdose: severe headache, vomiting, diarrhea, dizziness, weakness, or confusion.

The first patch you apply may cause mild itching, tingling, and burning. These problems should go away within 1 hour. If the skin under the patch becomes red or swollen or if a rash appears, remove the patch and call your doctor; you could be allergic to it.

What you must know about other drugs

Check with your doctor or pharmacist to find out if the dosages of any drugs you're taking need to be changed.

Special directions

• Don't use Nicoderm if you're allergic to any component in the patch.

• Make sure your doctor knows about your medical history, especially if you have high blood pressure, ulcers, kidney or liver disease, heart rhythm problems, or angina (chest pain) or if you've recently had a heart attack.

• To prevent nicotine overdose, be sure to stop smoking completely before starting Nicoderm.

• Follow the other parts of your stop-smoking program.

Important reminders

If you're pregnant, don't use Nicoderm. If you become pregnant while using it, stop using the patch until you've talked to your doctor.

If you're breast-feeding, check with your doctor before using Nicoderm.

Nilstat (oral)

Your doctor has prescribed oral Nilstat to treat your fungal infection. The generic name for this form of Nilstat is oral nystatin. Another brand name is Mycostatin.

How to take oral Nilstat

Oral Nilstat comes in tablets, lozenges, an oral solution, and a dry powder to mix with water. When taking it, follow your doctor's directions exactly.

If you're taking the *lozenges,* hold the lozenge in your mouth to allow it to dissolve slowly. Don't chew or swallow lozenges whole.

If you're taking the *oral solution,* place half of the dose in each side of your mouth. Then swish the dose in your mouth, gargle, and swallow.

If you're using the *dry powder,* follow these steps:

• Read the prescription label to find out what proportions of water and powder to use for each dose.

• Thoroughly mix the powder and water.

• Take the medication a mouthful at a time. Swish each portion in your mouth for as long as possible, gargle, and then swallow.

Continue to take oral Nilstat as directed, even if your symptoms disappear. If you stop too soon your infection may return.

What to do about side effects

Check with your doctor if you experience diarrhea, nausea, vomiting, or stomach pain.

Special directions

• To prevent recurrence of this type of fungal infection, take good care of your teeth and mouth. Don't overuse mouthwash or wear poorly fitting dentures; this can lead to infection.
• Check with your doctor or pharmacist about how to store the medication you're using. Keep Nilstat lozenges in the refrigerator. Don't allow the oral solution to freeze.

Important reminder

If you're giving oral Nilstat to a child under age 5, avoid the lozenges to prevent choking.

Nilstat (topical)

This medication is prescribed to treat a fungal infection of the skin or vagina. The generic name for this form of Nilstat is topical nystatin. Another brand name is Mycostatin.

How to apply topical Nilstat

For a skin infection, Nilstat comes in cream, ointment, and powder forms. For a vaginal infection, it's available as vaginal tablets. Follow your doctor's directions for applying the medication.

If you have a *skin infection,* apply just enough cream or ointment to cover the affected area. If you're using the powder on your feet, sprinkle it between your toes, on your feet, and in socks and shoes.

Don't cover the treated skin with a bandage, wrap, or other tight dressing unless directed to do so by your doctor.

If you have a *vaginal infection,* you'll probably insert the tablets with an applicator. Check with your doctor about how to use the applicator. Keep using this medication, even if you begin to menstruate.

Continue to use topical Nilstat for as long as your doctor directs, even if your symptoms disappear. If you stop taking it too soon your infection may return.

What to do about side effects

Check with your doctor if you have skin or vaginal irritation that wasn't present before you began using topical Nilstat.

If you're using the vaginal tablets, expect some vaginal drainage. Wear a sanitary napkin to protect your clothing.

Special directions

• Let your doctor know if you have any allergies, especially to foods, other medications, or preservatives.

• If you have a vaginal infection, practice good health habits to prevent reinfection. Wear cotton panties (or panties or pantyhose with cotton crotches) instead of synthetic underclothes, and wear only freshly washed underwear.

Important reminder

If you're pregnant and have a vaginal infection, check with your doctor before using the applicator to insert the vaginal tablets.

Nitro-Dur

This skin patch is prescribed to help you during attacks of angina (chest pain). The generic name of this patch is transdermal nitroglycerin. Another brand name is Transderm-Nitro.

How to use Nitro-Dur

Nitro-Dur comes in a stick-on patch. Read the prescription label carefully to find out how often to apply it. Don't use it more often than prescribed.

To apply the patch, choose a clean, dry skin area with little or no hair. The area should be free from cuts, scars, or irritation. Don't choose the lower part of your arm or leg because the drug won't work as well at these sites.

Always remove the previous patch before applying a new one.

To prevent skin irritation or other problems, apply each new patch to a different skin area.

If you think this medication isn't working properly, don't trim or cut the patch to adjust the dosage. Instead, check with your doctor.

If you've been using this medication for several weeks or more, don't suddenly stop using it; this may bring on angina attacks. Your doctor may instruct you to reduce your dosage gradually before you stop treatment completely.

What to do if you miss an application   Apply a new patch as soon as possible. Then resume your regular schedule.

What to do about side effects   Call your doctor *right away* if you get a severe or prolonged headache, dry mouth, or blurred vision.

Nitro-Dur may cause a fast pulse rate, flushing of your face and neck, headache, nausea, vomiting, and restlessness. Also, it may make you feel dizzy or light-headed when you get up from a sitting or lying position. These side effects usually subside as your body gets used to the medication. Check with your doctor if these effects persist or become more severe.

What you must know about alcohol and other drugs   Either avoid alcoholic beverages or drink them only in moderation. Alcohol will increase your chances for feeling dizzy or light-headed when you rise quickly.

Check with your doctor or pharmacist before taking other heart or blood pressure medications. Combined with Nitro-Dur, these medications can lower your blood pressure too much.

Special directions   Make sure your doctor knows about your medical history, especially if you have glaucoma, kidney or liver disease, an overactive thyroid, or severe anemia — or if you've recently had a heart attack, stroke, or head injury.

Important reminder   If you're an older adult, you may be especially sensitive to the side effects of Nitro-Dur.

Nitrol

This medication is prescribed to prevent angina (chest pain) attacks — or at least to reduce the number of times they occur. Its generic name is nitroglycerin ointment.

How to apply Nitrol

Read the label on your prescription tube carefully, and apply only the amount prescribed at each dose.

Measure the prescribed amount of ointment onto the special application paper provided. Spread it lightly over the area specified by the doctor — usually your upper arm or chest. *Don't rub it into your skin.* For best results, spread the ointment over an area about the size of the application paper (roughly 3½ by 2¼ inches (8.9 by 5.7 centimeters). Cover the ointment with the application paper and tape it in place.

You may want to cover the paper (including the side edges) with plastic wrap to protect your clothes from stains. Check with your doctor first, though; the covering will make your skin absorb more medication and may increase the chance for side effects.

If you've been using Nitrol for several weeks or more, don't suddenly stop using it; this can actually bring on angina attacks. Your doctor will advise you on how to reduce your dosage gradually.

What to do if you miss an application

Apply the missed dose as soon as possible. However, if your next scheduled application is within 2 hours, skip the one you missed and resume your regular schedule. Don't increase the amount you apply.

What to do about side effects

Call your doctor *right away* if you get a severe or prolonged headache, dry mouth, or blurred vision.

Nitrol may cause a headache, fast pulse rate, flushing of the face and neck, nausea, vomiting, and restlessness. It can also make you feel dizzy or light-headed when rising from a sitting or lying position. These side effects usually go away over time as your body gets used to the medication. Check with your doctor if they persist or become more severe.

To prevent skin irritation and other problems, apply each dose to a different skin site.

What you must know about alcohol and other drugs

Drink alcoholic beverages in moderation, if at all, because they will increase your chances of feeling dizzy or light-headed when you get up quickly.

Check with your doctor before taking other heart or blood pressure medications. Combined with Nitrol, these medications may lower your blood pressure too much.

Special directions

Make sure your doctor knows about your medical history, especially if you have glaucoma, kidney or liver disease, an overactive thyroid, or severe anemia or if you've recently had a heart attack, stroke, or head injury.

Important reminder

If you're an older adult, you may be especially sensitive to Nitrol and prone to side effects.

Nitrostat

This tablet form of the generic drug nitroglycerin is prescribed to prevent or relieve angina (chest pain) attacks.

How to take Nitrostat

Place one tablet under your tongue, between your lip and gum, or between your cheek and gum. Let it dissolve there. Don't chew, crush, or swallow it.

To *prevent* an angina attack, take a tablet 5 to 10 minutes before becoming involved in physical exertion or in an emotionally stressful situation that has caused an attack in the past.

To *relieve* angina, place one tablet in your mouth when you start to feel an attack coming on. If your pain doesn't go away within 5 minutes, take a second tablet. If you still have pain after another 5 minutes, take a third tablet. If three tablets don't provide relief, call your doctor and have someone take you to the nearest hospital. Never take more than three tablets.

Nitrostat works best when you take it while sitting or standing. Sitting is safer than standing because you may become dizzy or light-headed soon after taking a tablet.

If you get dizzy or light-headed while sitting, take a few deep breaths and bend forward with your head between your knees.

What to do about side effects

Call your doctor *right away* if you get a severe or prolonged headache, dry mouth, or blurred vision.

This medication may cause a fast pulse rate, flushing of your face and neck, headache, nausea, vomiting, and restlessness. It may also make you feel dizzy or light-headed when you get up from a sitting or lying position. These side effects usually go away over time as your body adjusts to the medication. If they persist or worsen, call your doctor.

What you must know about alcohol and other drugs

Drink alcoholic beverages in moderation, if at all. Alcohol will increase your chances of feeling dizzy or light-headed when you get up quickly.

Check with your doctor or pharmacist before taking other heart or blood pressure medications. When combined with Nitrostat, these drugs can decrease your blood pressure too much.

Special directions

• Make sure your doctor knows about your medical history, especially if you have kidney or liver disease or an overactive thyroid — or if you've recently had a heart attack.
• Don't eat, drink, smoke, or use chewing tobacco while the tablet is dissolving in your mouth.
• Get new tablets after 3 months, even if you have some left in the container.
• If you've been taking this medication regularly for several weeks or more, don't stop using it suddenly; this could actually bring on angina attacks. Ask your doctor how to reduce your dosage gradually to avoid problems.

Important reminder

If you're an older adult, you may be especially vulnerable to the side effects of Nitrostat.

Nizoral (oral)

Your doctor has prescribed Nizoral to treat your fungal infection. The generic name for this drug is oral ketoconazole.

How to take Nizoral

Take Nizoral exactly as prescribed and for the full time prescribed, even if your symptoms disappear. If you don't, your symptoms may return.

If necessary, take the tablets with food to decrease stomach upset. If you have achlorhydria (absence of stomach acid), your doctor may have you dissolve each tablet in a weak acid solution so your body can absorb it. A pharmacist will prepare the solution for you. After dissolving the tablet, add it to 1 to 2 teaspoons of water in a glass. Drink it through a straw placed far back in your mouth and away from your teeth. Then swish about half a glass (4 ounces) of water around in your mouth and swallow it.

What to do if you miss a dose

Take the missed dose as soon as possible. But if it's almost time for your next dose, space the missed dose and the next dose 10 to 12 hours apart. Then resume your normal schedule.

What to do about side effects

If you develop dark urine, pale stools, severe weakness, yellowing of your skin or the whites of your eyes, or loss of appetite, contact your doctor immediately.

Nausea, vomiting, and diarrhea may occur when you first start taking the tablets but should disappear as your body adjusts to the medication. If these symptoms persist, tell your doctor.

What you must know about alcohol and other drugs

Don't drink alcoholic beverages while you're taking Nizoral and for at least 1 day after you stop taking it; when combined with Nizoral, alcohol can aggravate liver or stomach problems. Many medications can interact with Nizoral, so tell your doctor about other medications you may be taking.

Special directions

• Tell your doctor about any medical problems you have. They can affect your use of Nizoral.

• If your symptoms don't improve in a few weeks or if they get worse, talk to your doctor.

Important reminders If you're pregnant or think you may be, check with your doctor before taking this medication.

Don't breast-feed while you're taking Nizoral and for 24 to 48 hours after you stop taking it.

Nizoral (topical)

Your doctor has prescribed Nizoral to treat your fungal infection. The generic name for this drug is topical ketoconazole.

How to apply Nizoral Apply Nizoral exactly as prescribed and for the full time prescribed, even if your symptoms disappear. If you don't, your symptoms may return.

To apply the cream, first wash your hands. Then apply enough to cover the affected area and surrounding skin. Rub it in gently. Keep the medication away from your eyes. Wash your hands again after applying the cream.

What to do if you miss a dose Skip the missed dose and apply the next dose at the regularly scheduled time.

What to do about side effects Nizoral cream may cause skin irritation, itching, and stinging. Call your doctor if these effects continue.

What you must know about alcohol and other drugs Don't drink alcoholic beverages while you're taking Nizoral and for at least 1 day after you stop taking it; when combined with Nizoral, alcohol can aggravate liver or stomach problems. Many medications can interact with Nizoral, so tell your doctor about other medications you may be taking.

Special directions • Tell your doctor if you're allergic to any antifungal medications or to other medications, foods, dyes, or preservatives.

• If you're using Nizoral to treat a *skin infection*, keep your skin clean and dry.

• If you're using this medication to treat *ringworm of the groin (jock itch)*, wear loose-fitting cotton underwear and use a bland, absorbent powder (such as talcum) on your skin between the times you apply Nizoral.

• If you're using this medication to treat *athlete's foot*, wear clean cotton socks and change them often to keep your feet dry. Wear sandals or shoes with lots of air holes. Remember to apply talcum or another absorbent powder between your toes, on your feet, and in your socks and shoes once or twice a day, between the times you apply Nizoral.

Important reminders   If you're pregnant or think you may be or if you're breast-feeding, check with your doctor before using Nizoral.

Noctec

Your doctor has prescribed Noctec to calm you and help you sleep. The generic name for this drug is chloral hydrate.

How to take Noctec   Noctec comes in capsule, syrup, and suppository forms. Follow the directions on the label exactly.

Take the *capsule* form after meals. Swallow it whole, and drink a full glass (8 ounces) of liquid to minimize possible stomach upset. For the same reason, mix a *syrup* dose in half a glass (4 ounces) of liquid before taking it. If you're taking Noctec to help you sleep, take it 15 to 30 minutes before bedtime.

If you're using a *suppository* and it's too soft to insert, chill it briefly or run cold water over it before removing the foil wrapper. To insert it, first wash your hands; then remove the wrapper and moisten the suppository with cold water. Lie on your side and use your finger to push the suppository gently into your rectum.

Take this medication only as directed. Overuse can lead to dependency.

Don't stop taking Noctec without consulting your doctor; he or she may adjust the dosage to prevent withdrawal effects.

What to do if you miss a dose

Skip the missed dose. Take your next dose on schedule. Don't take a double dose.

What to do about side effects

If you experience serious side effects, such as extreme drowsiness, swallowing or breathing difficulties, or seizures, stop taking Noctec and get emergency medical care *immediately*.

Common side effects include drowsiness, dizziness, a hangover-like feeling, and nausea. If these effects persist or worsen, tell your doctor.

Because Noctec can cause drowsiness, make sure you know how you react to it before you drive or perform other activities that require you to be fully alert.

What you must know about alcohol and other drugs

Avoid drinking alcoholic beverages while taking Noctec. The combination can cause oversedation.

Tell your doctor about other medications you're taking. Certain drugs that cause drowsiness (for example, allergy and cold medications, pain relievers, muscle relaxants, and anesthetics) increase the effects of Noctec. And Noctec increases the effects of anticoagulants (blood thinners).

Special directions

• Tell your doctor if you have other medical problems, including drug dependency or heart, liver, stomach, intestinal, kidney, blood, and emotional disorders. These conditions can affect the use of Noctec.

• Also, let your doctor know if you've ever had allergic reactions to drugs or foods.

• Check with the doctor before taking new medications or if you develop new medical problems.

Important reminder

If you're pregnant or breast-feeding, check with your doctor before taking this medication.

Nolvadex

This medication is used to help treat breast cancer. It blocks the effects of the hormone estrogen which, in turn, may improve your condition. The generic name for this drug is tamoxifen.

How to take Nolvadex
Follow your doctor's instructions exactly. Don't take more of the medication than prescribed, and be careful not to miss a dose. Take the medication even if it makes you feel nauseated.

If you're taking *enteric-coated tablets*, swallow them whole; don't crush or break a tablet before taking it.

What to do if you miss a dose
Skip the dose entirely, and take your next regular dose as scheduled. Call your doctor to let him or her know you missed a dose.

If you vomit shortly after taking a dose of Nolvadex, call your doctor. Depending on the circumstances, your doctor may tell you to take the dose again or to wait until the next scheduled dose.

What to do about side effects
Nolvadex causes some patients to become nauseated and vomit. It can also cause hot flashes, weight gain, bone pain, and changes in your menstrual cycle. Let your doctor know if these symptoms become a problem.

Watch for easy bruising or bleeding. If these symptoms develop, call your doctor.

To help control hot flashes, don't drink alcoholic beverages or smoke while you're taking Nolvadex. Drink lots of fluids, wear layers of clothing that you can easily remove if you get too warm, and use fans or an air conditioner to control indoor temperature.

Nolvadex causes women to become more fertile. But because you should not become pregnant while taking the drug, use a barrier method of contraception.

What you must know about other drugs
Birth control pills can change the effects of Nolvadex; therefore, a barrier method of contraception is recommended.

Special directions
• Before taking Nolvadex, tell your doctor if you've ever had cataracts or other eye problems.
• Try to eat a high-calorie diet. If you become nauseated, sip fluids throughout the day.

Important reminder
Tell your doctor immediately if you think you've become pregnant while taking Nolvadex.

Noroxin

This medication usually is prescribed for bacterial infections of the urinary tract. Its generic name is norfloxacin.

How to take Noroxin

Noroxin comes in tablets. Follow your doctor's instructions exactly. Take your tablet with a full glass (8 ounces) of water on an empty stomach, either 1 hour before or 2 hours after meals. Also, try to drink several extra glasses of water every day.

For best results, take the medication at evenly spaced times during the day and night. For example, if you take two doses daily, you might take one dose at 8 a.m. and the other at 8 p.m.

Continue to take your medication, even after you begin to feel better. If you stop too soon, your infection may return.

What to do if you miss a dose

Take the missed dose as soon as possible. But if it's almost time for your next dose, skip the missed tablet and go back to your regular dosing schedule. Don't take a double dose.

Try not to forget a dose; Noroxin works best when there is a constant amount in your blood or urine.

What to do about side effects

Call your doctor *right away* if you start to wheeze, have difficulty breathing, or break out in hives or a rash.

Check with your doctor if you become dizzy, drowsy, or unusually tired. Also tell the doctor if you develop constipation, heartburn, nausea, a dry mouth, headache, or trouble sleeping.

Because Noroxin can make you drowsy, make sure you know how you react to it before you drive or perform other activities that require you to be fully alert.

Noroxin can increase your sensitivity to light, so wear sunglasses and use a sunblock while outdoors on bright days. Call your doctor if you have a severe reaction from the sun.

What you must know about other drugs

Tell your doctor about other medications you're taking. Some medications, such as antacids or the ulcer medication Carafate (sucralfate), should not be taken at the same time as Noroxin. Instead, take them at least 2 hours after you take your Noroxin tablets.

Your doctor also needs to know if you're taking Macrodantin (nitrofurantoin), another medication for urinary tract infections, or Benemid (probenecid), a gout medication.

Special directions

Tell your doctor if you have other medical problems, especially kidney disease or a history of seizures.

Important reminders

If you're pregnant or breast-feeding, don't use Noroxin unless your doctor instructs you to do so.

Don't give this medication to infants, children, or adolescents because it may cause bone problems.

Norpace

Norpace is used to correct an irregular heartbeat or to slow an overactive heart. Its generic name is disopyramide.

How to take Norpace

This medication comes in both capsules and extended-release capsules. Read the label on your prescription bottle and follow the directions exactly.

If you're taking the *extended-release capsule,* swallow it whole; don't break, crush, or chew it.

Check with your doctor before you stop taking Norpace. Stopping suddenly can cause a serious change in heart function.

What to do if you miss a dose

Take the missed dose as soon as possible unless you are within 4 hours of the next scheduled dose. In that case, skip the missed dose and take your next dose on schedule. Don't take a double dose.

What to do about side effects

Call your doctor *right away* if you experience increasing shortness of breath, sudden weight gain (3 pounds [1.5 kilograms] or more in 1 week), or swelling of your ankles or fingers. Also check with the doctor if you experience blurred vision, constipation, or dryness of your eyes, nose, or mouth, especially if any of these symptoms persists or becomes severe.

Norpace can make you dizzy, light-headed, or faint, especially when you get up from a lying or sitting position. Getting up slowly may help relieve the problem.

Because Norpace can make you dizzy, make sure you know how you react to it before you drive, use machines, or perform other activities that could be dangerous if you're not fully alert.

Norpace can make you sweat less. To prevent becoming overheated, exercise moderately, especially during hot weather; don't overexert yourself.

What you must know about alcohol and other drugs Don't drink alcoholic beverages until you've checked with your doctor. When combined with Norpace, alcohol can make your blood sugar level drop dangerously low and make you faint or dizzy.

Tell your doctor about other medications you're taking. Other heart medications used to correct irregular heartbeats or slow an overactive heart may alter the effects of Norpace beyond a safe level. And Dilantin (phenytoin), a seizure medication, may reduce the effectiveness of Norpace.

Special directions Tell your doctor if you have other medical problems, especially myasthenia gravis, glaucoma, difficulty urinating, other heart conditions, or liver or kidney disease.

Important reminders If you're pregnant or breast-feeding, check with your doctor before taking Norpace.

If you have diabetes or congestive heart failure, be alert for symptoms of low blood sugar while taking this medication. These symptoms include headache, shakiness, cold sweats, excessive hunger, and weakness. If these symptoms occur, eat or drink a sugary food and call your doctor *right away.*

Norplant

This medication is a contraceptive used to prevent pregnancy. Its generic component is levonorgestrel.

How to use Norplant

The doctor will make a small cut in your upper arm, implant six tablets there, and close the skin over them. The tablets will start to work and won't require any action on your part. Their contraceptive effect lasts for 5 years.

Call the doctor right away if one of the tablets falls out; this could reduce the contraceptive effect.

What to do about side effects

Call your doctor if you have pain in your stomach or muscles or if you notice discharge from your breasts or vagina.

You should expect changes in your menstrual bleeding pattern. For instance, your menstrual period may stop or it may last longer than usual. You may have spotting, scanty or irregular bleeding, or frequent bleeding episodes. These irregularities usually correct themselves over time. If they don't, call your doctor.

What you must know about other drugs

Check with your doctor before taking Tegretol (carbamazepine) or Dilantin (phenytoin). These drugs can make Norplant less effective.

Special directions

• Before you get the implants, make sure your doctor knows about your medical history, especially if you've had thrombophlebitis or a thromboembolic disorder; seizures; liver, kidney, or heart disease; breast cancer; or unusual genital bleeding that hasn't been diagnosed. You should also let the doctor know if you've ever had depression or an emotional disorder. Norplant can make these conditions worse.

• Because Norplant can cause you to retain fluid, the doctor may want you to limit salt in your diet if you've had heart or kidney disease. Follow any specially prescribed diet that's recommended.

• Don't assume you're pregnant if you miss a menstrual period. However, if your period still doesn't come after 6 or more weeks (following a pattern of regular periods), this could mean you're pregnant.

- Have a physical exam at least every year so the doctor can check for any problems caused by Norplant.
- Your implants must be removed if you become pregnant, develop phlebitis or a thromboembolism, have jaundice, or must stay in bed for a long time.
- Call your doctor if you notice a change in vision — for instance, if you wear contact lenses and suddenly have vision changes or can't tolerate your lenses.

Important reminders If you're breast-feeding, let your doctor know about it before the implants are inserted.

If you suspect you're pregnant — either before or after receiving the implants — be sure to tell your doctor right away.

Norpramin

Your doctor has prescribed Norpramin to help relieve your depression. The generic name for this drug is desipramine.

How to take Norpramin Norpramin comes in capsules and tablets. Follow your doctor's instructions exactly. Don't take more medication than prescribed or take it more often than directed. Take your dose with food, even a bedtime dose, unless your doctor has told you to take it on an empty stomach.

Don't stop taking this medication suddenly; check with your doctor who may want to wean you from it gradually.

What to do if you miss a dose If you normally take one dose a day at bedtime and you miss a dose, call your doctor about what to do. Don't take the missed dose in the morning. It may cause disturbing side effects during waking hours.

If you take more than one dose a day, take the missed dose as soon as possible. However, if it's almost time for your next dose, skip the missed dose and take your next dose on schedule. Don't take a double dose.

What to do about side effects Check with your doctor if the medication makes you feel drowsy, dizzy, or light-headed, especially when you get up suddenly from a lying or sitting position. Also call if you experience an irregular or fast heartbeat, blurred vision, dry mouth, constipation, difficulty urinating, or unusual sweating.

Because Norpramin can make you feel dizzy or faint, make sure you know how you react to it before you drive or perform other activities that require you to be fully alert.

If Norpramin makes you feel faint when rising, try getting up slowly.

What you must know about alcohol and other drugs

Check with your doctor about drinking alcoholic beverages while taking Norpramin.

Also tell your doctor if you're taking other medication. Norpramin may not work well if taken with barbiturates (sedatives). And taking it with the ulcer drug Tagamet (cimetidine) may increase the risk of side effects.

Other drugs you may need to avoid while taking this medication are Ritalin (methylphenidate), Adrenalin (epinephrine), and certain drugs used to treat depression and other psychiatric disorders.

Special directions

• Tell your doctor if you have other medical problems, especially heart, liver, or kidney disease; breathing problems; an overactive thyroid; diabetes; or an enlarged prostate.

• Before you have any medical tests, tell your doctor you're taking Norpramin; the drug can affect some test results.

Important reminders

If you're pregnant or breast-feeding, check with your doctor before you take this medication.

If you have diabetes, be aware that Norpramin can affect your blood sugar levels. If you notice a change in the results of your blood or urine glucose tests, call your doctor.

Norvasc

Your doctor has prescribed Norvasc to help relieve your angina (chest pain) or to treat your high blood pressure. This drug's generic name is amlodipine besylate.

How to take Norvasc
Norvasc comes in tablet form. Be sure to follow the label directions carefully.

What to do if you miss a dose
If you take one dose daily, take the missed dose as soon as possible. But if you miss a daily dose completely, skip the missed dose and go back to your regular schedule. Don't take a double dose.

What to do about side effects
Norvasc may cause tiredness, headache, or sleepiness. You may also experience swelling, dizziness, flushing, or an irregular heartbeat. You may also feel nauseated or have abdominal pain. Notify your doctor if any of these effects persists or becomes severe.

Until you know how Norvasc affects you, don't drive, use machinery, or do anything else that requires alertness.

If you start having more frequent angina attacks or you feel very dizzy when you arise from a sitting or standing position, notify your doctor. Call your doctor also if you notice swelling of your hands and feet or shortness of breath.

What you should know about other drugs
Tell you doctor if you're taking other hypertensives. If you take sublingual nitroglycerin for acute angina you may continue to take it as needed. Make sure that your doctor is aware you're continuing nitrate therapy.

Special directions
• Tell your doctor about your medical history, especially if you have liver disease or heart or artery problems such as congestive heart failure or coronary artery disease.
• Remember to keep taking this medication even if you feel better.

Important reminders
Tell you doctor if you're pregnant or breast-feeding.
If you're an older person you may be more sensitive to Norvasc.

O

Orap

Prescribed to treat the symptoms of Tourette's syndrome, Orap helps reduce the vocal outbursts and uncontrolled, repeated body movements (tics) that can disrupt everyday living. The generic name for this drug is pimozide.

How to take Orap

Follow your doctor's instructions exactly when taking Orap tablets. Don't use more medication than prescribed or take it more often than recommended.

Don't stop taking this medication suddenly. Check with your doctor, who may want you to reduce your dosage gradually to avoid withdrawal symptoms.

What to do if you miss a dose

Take the missed dose as soon as possible. Then take any remaining doses for the day at regularly spaced intervals. Don't take a double dose.

What to do about side effects

Get emergency help *at once* if you start to experience seizures, difficulty breathing, fast heartbeat, high fever, heavy sweating, severe muscle stiffness, loss of bladder control, or extreme fatigue.

Call your doctor right away if you have difficulty speaking or swallowing, loss of balance, mood changes, muscle spasms, or unusual changes in your body movements.

Check with your doctor if Orap makes you feel faint, dizzy, or drowsy or if you have blurred vision, constipation, mouth dryness, a rash, or breast swelling or soreness.

Because Orap can make you dizzy or drowsy, make sure you know how you react to it before you drive or perform other activities that require you to be fully alert.

What you must know about alcohol and other drugs

Avoid drinking alcoholic beverages while taking Orap. The combination may make you overly drowsy.

For the same reason, don't use other medications that

depress the nervous system, including tranquilizers, sleeping pills, and many cold and flu medications.

Tell your doctor about prescription and nonprescription medications you're taking. To prevent harmful interactions, you need to avoid a variety of other medications, including certain drugs for depression, mental illness, and stomach or abdominal cramps.

Special directions

• Tell your doctor if you have other medical problems, especially breast cancer or diseases of the heart, kidneys, or liver. Also let the doctor know if you've ever had tics other than those caused by Tourette's syndrome. Other medical problems may affect your use of Orap.

• Before you have surgery, dental work, or emergency care, tell the doctor you're taking Orap.

Important reminders

If you're pregnant, check with your doctor before using this medication.

If you're an older adult, you may be especially prone to side effects from Orap.

Orasone

This medication is used to relieve severe inflammation and to treat a number of diseases. Its generic name is prednisone. Another brand name is Deltasone.

How to take Orasone

Orasone comes in tablets, an oral solution, and a syrup. Take it exactly as prescribed — no more or less and no longer. To prevent stomach upset, take your dose with food.

Never stop taking this medication suddenly. Doing so could be fatal. Check with your doctor if you plan to stop using Orasone; he or she will advise you about reducing your dosage gradually.

What to do if you miss a dose

If you take one dose every other day, take the missed dose as soon as possible if you remember it the same morning. If not, wait and take it the next morning. Then skip a day and resume your regular dosing schedule.

If you take one dose daily, take the missed dose as soon as possible. If you don't remember until the next day, skip the missed dose and take your next dose on schedule. Don't take a double dose.

If you take several doses a day, take the missed dose as soon as possible; then go back to your regular dosing schedule. If you don't remember until your next dose is due, double the next dose.

What to do about side effects

Orasone can act on your metabolism to make your potassium levels too low or your blood sugar level too high. Call your doctor *at once* if you have symptoms of a low potassium level: dizziness, tiredness, weakness, leg cramps, nausea, or digestive upset. Also call the doctor if you have symptoms of high blood sugar: frequent urination and thirst.

Call your doctor *right away* if you have bloody or black, tarry stools — or if you have difficulty sleeping.

Be aware that Orasone can also affect your mood and cause euphoria.

What you must know about other drugs

Tell your doctor if you're taking other medications. Check before you take aspirin or Indocin (indomethacin); these pain relievers increase the risk of stomach distress when taken with Orasone. Also check with your doctor before you have vaccinations.

If you take barbiturates (sedatives) or medications for seizures or tuberculosis, your doctor may need to adjust your Orasone dosage.

Special directions

• Tell your doctor if you have other medical problems, especially ulcers, high blood pressure, diabetes, and kidney, liver, or bone disease. These problems can affect your use of Orasone.
• Before you have medical tests, tell the doctor you're taking Orasone; it can have an affect on the test results.

Important reminders

If you're pregnant or breast-feeding, check with your doctor before taking Orasone.

If you're an athlete, be aware that the U.S. Olympic Committee and the National Collegiate Athletic Association have restrictions on the use of prednisone.

Orinase

Your doctor has prescribed Orinase to help control your diabetes. Taken by mouth, it works by stimulating the pancreas to produce more insulin. The generic name for this drug is tolbutamide.

How to take Orinase

Take each dose with food. If your doctor has prescribed one dose a day, take it with breakfast. If he's prescribed two doses a day, take one dose with breakfast and the second dose with your evening meal.

Keep taking the medication, even if you feel well. Orinase relieves the symptoms of diabetes; it doesn't cure it.

What to do if you miss a dose

Take the missed dose as soon as possible. But if it's almost time for your next dose, skip the missed dose and take your next dose as scheduled. Don't take a double dose.

What to do about side effects

Taking too much Orinase can cause hypoglycemia, which can produce symptoms such as drowsiness, headache, nervousness, cold sweats, and confusion. If these symptoms occur, eat or drink something sweet, such as orange juice, and call your doctor.

Orinase may increase your sensitivity to sunlight. Take precautions to protect your skin when outdoors.

What you must know about alcohol and other drugs

Avoid drinking alcoholic beverages while you're taking Orinase. The combination could produce unpleasant side effects. And be aware that many foods and drugs contain alcohol.

Tell your doctor if you're taking any other medication. Orinase can interfere with the way certain medications work and vice versa. It's especially important that your doctor know if you're taking a blood thinner; diet pills; medication for asthma, colds, allergies, high blood pressure, or tuberculosis; sulfa medication; aspirin; steroids; or a thiazide diuretic (a type of water pill).

Special directions

• Tell your doctor if you've ever had an allergic reaction to an oral diabetes medication or to a diuretic.

• Because some medical conditions prohibit you from taking Orinase, tell the doctor if you have a disorder that affects your liver, kidneys, adrenal glands, pituitary gland, or thyroid gland.

• Follow your doctor's instructions for testing your blood or urine for glucose. Also closely follow your prescribed diet and exercise regimen.

• At all times, wear a medical identification bracelet stating you have diabetes and listing your medication.

Important reminder Tell your doctor if you're breast-feeding or pregnant. He or she may want to prescribe a different medication.

Ortho-Novum

Known as an oral contraceptive or birth control pill, Ortho-Novum prevents pregnancy by changing your body's hormonal balance. The generic component of this medication is estrogen with progestin. Another brand name is Triphasil.

How to take Ortho-Novum Ortho-Novum comes in variously colored tablets. The color indicates the tablet's strength. Read and follow the directions carefully. Usually, you take a certain color tablet at the same time every day. The tablets are arranged in order in the container. Follow this order; don't take a tablet out of sequence.

To prevent nausea, take each tablet with food or just after eating.

Based on your needs, the doctor will prescribe a certain dosing schedule: *one-phase, two-phase,* or *three-phase.* Here's how the schedules work.

One-phase schedules *If you're on a 20- or 21-day schedule,* take a tablet of the same strength for 20 or 21 days.

If you're on a 28-day schedule, take one tablet for 21 days and a different color tablet (containing inactive ingredients) for 7 more days.

Two-phase schedules *If you're on a 21-day schedule,* take a tablet of one strength (first color) for 10 days, then a different tablet (second color) for the next 11 days.

If you're on a 24-day schedule, take a tablet of one strength (first color) for 17 days, then a different tablet (second color) for the next 7 days.

If you're on a 28-day schedule, take a tablet of one strength (first color) for 10 days of the cycle, a different tablet (second color) for the next 11 days, then a tablet with inactive ingredients (third color) for 7 days.

Three-phase schedules *If you're on a 21-day schedule,* take a tablet in the order directed by your prescription. For example, you may take the first tablet (first color) for 6 or 7 days, a different tablet (second color) for the next 5 to 9 days, and another tablet (third color) for 5 to 10 days, for a total of 21 tablets.

If you're on a 28-day schedule, follow a 21-day schedule; then take a tablet with inactive ingredients (fourth color) for the next 7 days, for a total of 28 tablets.

What to do if you miss a dose If you forget to take your medication, consult your doctor and review the guide that follows.

One-phase and two-phase schedules *If you're on a 20-, 21-, or 24-day one-phase or two-phase schedule* and you miss one dose, take it when you remember it. If you don't remember it until the next day, take the missed dose and your scheduled dose; you can take two tablets on the same day. Then resume your normal schedule.

If you miss two doses in a row, take two tablets a day for the next 2 days; then resume your normal schedule. Use another birth control method to protect you for the rest of your cycle, and consult your doctor.

If you miss three or more doses in a row, stop taking the tablets, and use another birth control method until you have your period or until the doctor tells you you're not pregnant. Resume your normal schedule with the next cycle.

If you're on a 28-day cycle and you miss any of the first 21 tablets (which contain active ingredients), follow the instructions for the 21-day schedule and the number of doses you missed.

Three-phase schedules   *If you're on a three-phase schedule* and miss a dose during the 21-day period, take the missed tablet when you remember it. If you don't remember it until the next day, take the missed dose and the regular dose for that day. In this case, you can take two doses in the same day; then resume your regular schedule. Use another birth control method for the rest of your cycle, and consult your doctor.

If you miss two doses in a row, take two doses for the next 2 days; then resume your normal schedule. Use another birth control method, and consult your doctor.

If you miss three doses in a row, don't take any tablets. Instead, use another birth control method until you have your period or until your doctor confirms that you're not pregnant. Resume your normal schedule as directed.

If you're on a 28-day cycle and you miss any of the first 21 tablets, follow the directions for the 21-day schedule, depending on how many doses you missed. Pregnancy isn't a risk if you miss any of the last seven tablets. But you must take the first tablet of the next month's cycle on your regularly scheduled day to prevent pregnancy.

What to do about side effects   Seek *emergency* care if you cough up blood or experience sudden shortness of breath, severe headache, vision changes, slurred speech, unexplained weakness in your arms or legs, or pain in your stomach, chest, groin, or leg.

When you begin taking Ortho-Novum, you may experience some vaginal bleeding. If so, consult your doctor.

Special directions   • You may need to take this medication for about 1 month before it works effectively. During this time, you may need to use an additional birth control method.
• Before having any dental work or surgery, tell the dentist or doctor that you're taking Ortho-Novum.

Important reminders   If you become pregnant, stop taking this medication at once and notify your doctor.

Also consult your doctor if you're breast-feeding.

Orudis

This medication relieves fever, pain, swelling, and joint stiffness. Its generic name is ketoprofen.

How to take Orudis

Take Orudis capsules exactly as your doctor has prescribed. Overuse can aggravate side effects.

For best results, continue taking the medication regularly. You may not feel its full effects for several weeks.

Take the capsules with a full glass (8 ounces) of water either 30 minutes before or 2 hours after meals. Avoid lying down for 15 to 30 minutes after you take them. If stomach upset occurs, take the capsules with food or milk.

What to do if you miss a dose

Take the missed dose as soon as possible. But if it's almost time for your next dose, skip the missed dose and take the next one as scheduled.

What to do about side effects

If you develop a hivelike rash or itching, stop taking Orudis and call your doctor *immediately* — you may be experiencing an allergic reaction. Although rare, an allergic reaction can be serious. If you become restless, begin to wheeze, have difficulty breathing, or get puffy around your eyes, get emergency medical care *immediately.*

Orudis can cause ulcers and internal bleeding. Stop taking the medication and call your doctor *at once* if you have stomach pain; pass black, tarry stools; have severe nausea, heartburn, or indigestion; or vomit coffee ground–like matter.

Abdominal cramps, nausea, diarrhea, constipation, gas, headache, nervousness, dizziness, and drowsiness can occur. These symptoms usually disappear as your body adjusts to the medication. If they persist or become more severe, tell your doctor.

Because Orudis can make you dizzy or drowsy, make sure you know how you react to it before you drive or perform other activities that require you to be fully alert.

What you must know about alcohol and other drugs

Don't drink alcoholic beverages while taking Orudis; doing so could increase stomach problems.

Tell your doctor about other drugs you're taking, especially Probalan (probenecid) and blood thinners.

Special directions

• Tell the doctor if you have other medical problems. Some conditions can affect your use of Orudis.

• If you're on a special diet, let your doctor know about it; Orudis may contain sugar or sodium.

Important reminders

If you're pregnant or breast-feeding, check with your doctor before taking this medication.

If you're an older adult, you may be especially susceptible to side effects when taking Orudis.

P

Parlodel

By regulating certain hormones, Parlodel relieves menstrual problems, enhances fertility in some women, and stops breast milk production. It's also used for Parkinson's disease, acromegaly (overproduction of growth hormone), and pituitary disorders. The generic name for this drug is bromocriptine.

How to take Parlodel

Parlodel comes in capsules and tablets. Read the medication label carefully and follow the directions exactly. If Parlodel upsets your stomach, try taking it with meals or with milk.

What to do if you miss a dose

Take the missed dose as soon as possible if you remember within 4 hours of the scheduled dosing time. If more than 4 hours have passed, skip the missed dose and resume your normal schedule. Don't take a double dose.

What to do about side effects

Contact your doctor if you suddenly become short of breath or experience chest pain, blurred vision, headache, or severe nausea and vomiting.

Common side effects include dizziness, headache, abdominal cramps, and light-headedness. If these symptoms persist or become severe, call the doctor.

Because Parlodel can make you feel dizzy or lightheaded, make sure you know how you react to it before you drive or perform activities that require you to be fully alert.

If you feel dizzy or faint when rising from bed or a chair, get up slowly.

To relieve dry mouth, use sugarless hard candy or gum, ice chips, or a saliva substitute. Persistent dryness increases the risk of tooth decay and other mouth disorders.

What you must know about alcohol and other drugs

Avoid alcoholic beverages when taking Parlodel. The combination can cause unwanted side effects.

Tell your doctor about any other prescription and non-prescription medications you're taking. Some drugs can intensify or decrease Parlodel's effect to the point that your doctor may need to make dosage changes.

Special directions

• Tell your doctor if you have other medical problems, particularly uncontrolled high blood pressure, liver disease, or emotional illness. They can affect your use of Parlodel.

• Have regular checkups so your doctor can monitor your condition as well as the drug's effects.

• It may be several weeks before Parlodel becomes effective. Don't stop taking it or reduce your dosage without consulting your doctor.

• When the doctor starts you on Parlodel to treat your infertility, you may be advised to use birth control measures (other than oral contraceptives) at first. Once you've become established on the drug, you can determine when to stop using birth control.

Important reminders

If you're pregnant or breast-feeding, consult your doctor before taking Parlodel.

Older adults may be more sensitive to this drug and its side effects.

Pamelor

Your doctor has prescribed Pamelor to treat your depression. The generic name for this drug is nortriptyline.

How to take Pamelor

Pamelor comes in capsules and an oral solution. Follow the label directions exactly.

To lessen stomach upset, take the medication with food unless your doctor has told you to take it on an empty stomach.

If you're taking the *oral solution,* use the dropper provided to measure each dose. Dilute each dose with about a half cup (4 ounces) of water, milk, or orange juice. Then drink the liquid.

Check with your doctor before you stop taking this medication.

What to do if you miss a dose

If you take one dose a day at bedtime, don't take the missed dose the next morning; it may cause side effects during waking hours. Check with your doctor about what to do.

If you take more than one dose a day, take the missed dose as soon as possible. If it's almost time for your next dose, skip the missed dose and take your next dose as scheduled. Don't take a double dose.

What to do about side effects

Check with your doctor if you have blurred vision, dry mouth, increased sweating, constipation, dizziness, drowsiness, rapid or irregular heartbeat, or difficulty urinating.

Because Pamelor can make you drowsy, make sure you know how it affects you before you drive or perform other activities that require you to be fully alert.

If Pamelor makes your mouth feel dry, use sugarless gum or hard candy, ice chips, or a saliva substitute.

What you must know about alcohol and other drugs

Don't drink alcoholic beverages while taking Pamelor; the combination may cause oversedation.

For the same reason, don't use other medications that slow the central nervous system, such as sleeping pills, sedatives, tranquilizers, and cold, flu, and allergy medications.

Be sure to tell your doctor about any other medications you're taking. In particular, he or she needs to know if you take barbiturates (for seizures or sedation); Tagamet (cimetidine), an ulcer medication; Sus-Phrine (epinephrine), for asthma or severe allergic reactions; or medications for depression or other emotional problems.

Special directions

Tell your doctor if you have other medical problems. They can affect your use of Pamelor.

Important reminders   If you're pregnant or breast-feeding, don't use Pamelor unless you've discussed the risks and benefits with your doctor.

Children and older adults are especially prone to Pamelor's side effects.

Paxipam

Your doctor has prescribed Paxipam to relieve your tension and anxiety. The generic name for this drug is halazepam.

How to take   Take Paxipam tablets exactly as your doctor prescribes.
Paxipam   Overuse could lead to dependency and increased risk of overdose.

Don't stop taking Paxipam suddenly or you may experience withdrawal symptoms. Rather, follow your doctor's instructions for gradually decreasing your dosage.

What to do if you   Take the missed dose as soon as you remember it if it's
miss a dose   within an hour or so after the scheduled time. Otherwise, skip the missed dose and take the next dose as scheduled. Don't take a double dose.

What to do about   If you think you've taken an overdose or if you experi-
side effects   ence severe side effects such as prolonged confusion, severe drowsiness, difficulty breathing, slow heartbeat, slurred speech, staggering, or severe weakness, get emergency care *immediately.*

Paxipam can cause drowsiness, dizziness, difficulty thinking clearly, a hangover-type feeling, nausea, vomiting, and mouth dryness. These side effects commonly disappear as your body adjusts to the medication; if they continue or become more severe, notify your doctor.

Because Paxipam can cause drowsiness or dizziness, make sure you know how you react to it before you drive or perform other activities that require you to be fully alert.

To minimize dizziness, rise slowly after sitting or lying down.

Relieve mouth dryness with sugarless hard candy or gum, ice chips, mouthwash, or a saliva substitute. If dryness continues for more than 2 weeks, tell your doctor or dentist because it increases your risk of tooth and gum problems.

What you must know about alcohol and other drugs

Don't drink alcoholic beverages while taking Paxipam; this combination could cause an overdose.

Also, tell your doctor about any other prescription or nonprescription medications you're taking. They can add to Paxipam's effects and lead to overdose.

Special directions

• Because many medical problems can affect the use of Paxipam, tell your doctor about your medical history.

• After you stop taking this medication, your body may need time to adjust. Call your doctor if you experience irritability, nervousness, or trouble sleeping.

Important reminders

If you're pregnant or breast-feeding, check with your doctor before taking Paxipam.

Children and older adults may be especially prone to this drug's side effects.

If you're an athlete, be aware that the U.S. Olympic Committee and the National Collegiate Athletic Association ban the use of halazepam.

Pediazole

Your doctor has prescribed Pediazole to treat your ear infection. This drug is a combination of the generic products erythromycin and sulfisoxazole.

How to take Pediazole

Pediazole comes as an oral liquid. When taking it, follow your doctor's instructions exactly. You should use a specially marked measuring spoon — not a household teaspoon — to measure your dose. Take the medication with food or extra water, if possible, to help prevent side effects.

Because Pediazole works best if you have a constant amount in your blood, take it in evenly spaced doses during the day and night. If you need to take four doses a day, schedule each dose 6 hours apart. Talk to your doctor, nurse, or pharmacist if this schedule disrupts your sleep or other activities.

Continue to take your medication, even if you start to feel better in a few days. If you stop taking it too soon, your infection may return.

What to do if you miss a dose

Take the missed dose as soon as possible unless it's almost time for your next dose. In that case (if you take three or more doses a day), space the missed dose and the next dose 2 to 4 hours apart. Then return to your regular dosing schedule.

What to do about side effects

If you become short of breath or have difficulty breathing, stop taking Pediazole and get emergency medical care *at once*. You may be experiencing a serious allergic reaction.

If you have a persistent fever, a sore throat, or joint pain — or if you notice that you have started to bleed easily — stop taking Pediazole and call your doctor as soon as possible.

You may experience some abdominal pain, nausea, vomiting, or diarrhea. Check with your doctor about these symptoms, especially if they continue or become more severe.

What you must know about other drugs

Tell your doctor about any other medications you're taking. Taking Pediazole with oral blood thinners could put you at risk for bleeding. Taking it with the asthma medication Theo-Dur (theophylline) or the allergy drug Seldane (terfenadine) can also cause unwanted effects.

Pediazole can decrease the effectiveness of birth control pills. If necessary, switch to a barrier type of birth control while you're taking it.

Special directions

• Drink lots of extra water to prevent side effects, such as kidney stones, caused by the sulfa in Pediazole.
• Tell your doctor about any allergy to sulfa drugs or erythromycin.

Important reminder

If you're pregnant or breast-feeding, let your doctor know before you take this medication.

Pepcid

Pepcid is used to treat ulcers as well as Zollinger-Ellison disease (a disease in which the stomach produces too much acid). The generic name for this medication is famotidine.

How to take Pepcid

Pepcid comes in tablets as well as in powder for oral suspension. Take it carefully, as prescribed.

If you're taking Pepcid once a day, take it at bedtime unless your doctor directs otherwise. If you're taking it twice a day, take one dose in the morning and one at bedtime. If you're taking it more than twice a day, take your dose with meals and at bedtime for best results.

What to do if you miss a dose

Take the missed dose as soon as possible. If it's almost time for your next regular dose, skip the missed dose and take your next dose on schedule. Don't take a double dose.

What to do about side effects

If you have a headache (a common side effect) that persists or becomes severe, contact your doctor.

Special directions

• Be sure to tell your doctor if you have other medical problems, especially kidney or liver disease, because certain disorders can affect the way Pepcid works for you.

• It may be several days before Pepcid begins to relieve your stomach pain. Meanwhile, unless your doctor directs otherwise, you can take antacids to help relieve the pain. However, wait 30 minutes to 1 hour after taking the antacid before taking Pepcid.

• Tell your doctor that you're taking Pepcid before you undergo any skin tests for allergies or tests to determine how much acid your stomach produces.

• If you smoke, now is the time to stop — or at least try not to smoke after taking the last dose of your medication each day. Cigarette smoking tends to decrease Pepcid's effect, especially at night.

• Contact your doctor if your ulcer pain continues or gets worse.

Important reminders   If you're pregnant or breast-feeding, check with your doctor before taking this medication.

If you're an older adult, you may be especially sensitive to Pepcid's side effects.

Percocet

This medication combines two generic pain relievers: oxycodone (a narcotic analgesic) and acetaminophen. Another brand name for this drug is Tylox.

How to take Percocet   Percocet is available in capsules, tablets, and an oral solution. Take it exactly as directed. Taking more than the prescribed amount can lead to dependency or overdose. If you think this medication isn't helping you, check with your doctor.

What to do if you miss a dose   Take the missed dose as soon as you remember it. However, if it's almost time for your next dose, skip the missed dose and take your next dose on schedule. Don't take a double dose.

What to do about side effects   Call for emergency help *immediately* if you think you may have taken an overdose. Symptoms include cold, clammy skin; confusion; seizures; difficulty breathing; severe dizziness or drowsiness; increased sweating; slow heartbeat; stomach cramps; and weakness.

Call your doctor *at once* if you experience:
• black, tarry stools
• bloody or dark urine
• easy bruising or bleeding
• facial swelling
• an irregular heartbeat or breathing
• mental depression
• skin problems
• a sore throat or fever.

Also check with your doctor if this medication makes you feel dizzy or faint or if it causes nausea or vomiting.

Because Percocet can make you dizzy or drowsy, make sure you know how it affects you before you drive a car or perform any activities that require you to be fully alert.

What you must know about alcohol and other drugs

Don't drink alcoholic beverages while taking Percocet; the combination can lead to oversedation.

For the same reason, avoid other medications that depress the central nervous system, including many cold and flu remedies, muscle relaxants, sleeping pills, and seizure medications.

Check with your doctor before you take aspirin, aspirin-containing products, or nonsteroidal anti-inflammatory drugs, such as Motrin (ibuprofen) and Naprosyn (naproxen).

Special directions

• Tell your doctor if your medical history includes alcohol or drug abuse, emotional problems, brain disease or head injury, or diseases of any of the major organs.

• Tell your doctor or dentist that you're taking this medication before you have surgery.

Important reminders

If you're pregnant or breast-feeding, check with your doctor before using Percocet.

Children and older adults may be especially vulnerable to side effects from this medication.

If you're an athlete, you should know that the U.S. Olympic Committee bans the use of oxycodone and tests for it.

Percodan

Percodan combines two generic pain relievers: oxycodone (a narcotic analgesic) and aspirin. Another brand name for this drug is Roxiprin.

How to take Percodan

Percodan comes in tablets. Take it exactly as directed. Don't take more than the prescribed amount; this could lead to dependency or overdose. If Percodan isn't relieving your pain, check with your doctor.

What to do if you miss a dose

Take the missed dose as soon as you remember it. However, if it's almost time for your next dose, skip the missed dose and take your next dose on schedule. Don't take a double dose.

What to do about side effects

Call for emergency help *immediately* if you think you may have taken an overdose. Symptoms include cold, clammy skin; confusion; seizures; severe dizziness or drowsiness; increased sweating or thirst; slow heartbeat; severe stomach pain; vision problems; and weakness.

Call your doctor *right away* if you notice:
- black, tarry stools
- confusion
- dark urine
- facial swelling
- an irregular heartbeat or breathing
- mental depression
- rashes or other skin problems
- unusual tiredness or weakness
- vomit that looks like coffee grounds.

Check with your doctor if you feel faint or dizzy or if you have stomach upset.

Because Percodan can make you drowsy, make sure you know how it affects you before you drive or perform other activities that require you to be fully alert.

What you must know about alcohol and other drugs

Don't drink alcoholic beverages while taking Percodan. The combination can cause oversedation.

For the same reason, avoid taking other drugs that depress the central nervous system, including many cold and flu remedies, muscle relaxants, and sleeping pills.

Check with your doctor before you take other medications, especially blood thinners, Tylenol (acetaminophen), aspirin or aspirin-containing products, diabetes medications, Probalan (probenecid, a gout medication), and Retrovir (zidovudine).

Special directions

Tell your doctor if you have other medical problems. They can affect your use of Percodan. Also mention if you're allergic to any medication.

Important reminders

If you're pregnant or breast-feeding, check with your doctor before taking Percodan.

If you're an older adult, you may be especially vulnerable to this drug's side effects.

If you're an athlete, you should know that the U.S. Olympic Committee bans the use of oxycodone and tests for it.

Persantine

Used to prevent blood clots after heart valve replacement surgery, this medication is also used to treat a variety of heart and blood vessel problems. Its generic name is dipyridamole.

How to take Persantine

Persantine comes in tablets. Read the label on your prescription bottle carefully and take the tablets exactly as ordered. This medication works best when taken in regularly spaced doses, as directed by your doctor.

Take each dose with a full glass (8 ounces) of water at least 1 hour before or 2 hours after meals. If the drug upsets your stomach, your doctor may advise you to take it with food or milk.

What to do if you miss a dose

Take the missed dose as soon as possible. But if it's within 4 hours of your next scheduled dose, skip the missed dose and go back to your regular dosing schedule. Don't take a double dose.

What to do about side effects

Check with your doctor if Persantine makes you dizzy or nauseated. Also call if you get a headache or a rash or if you have chest pain.

Persantine can make you feel dizzy, light-headed, or faint, especially when rising. Getting up slowly may help. If this problem continues or gets worse, check with your doctor.

What you must know about other drugs

Tell your doctor if you're taking Persantine along with a blood thinner or aspirin; these combinations increase the risk of bleeding. Don't take aspirin or any product containing aspirin unless the same doctor who prescribed the Persantine specifically tells you to do so.

If you've been instructed to take aspirin together with Persantine, take only the amount of aspirin ordered by your doctor.

If you need a medication to relieve pain or a fever, discuss the issue with your doctor before beginning a course of Persantine. Your doctor may not want you to take extra aspirin.

Special directions

• Tell your doctor if you have other medical problems, especially chest pain or low blood pressure.

• Keep all appointments for follow-up visits so your doctor can check your progress.

• If you visit a dentist or doctor other than the one who prescribed Persantine, be sure to tell him or her that you take it. Also mention whether or not you're taking it with a blood thinner or aspirin.

Important reminder

If you're pregnant or breast-feeding, check with your doctor before taking Persantine.

Phillips' Milk of Magnesia

This medication is used to relieve constipation. Its generic name is magnesium hydroxide.

How to take Phillips' Milk of Magnesia

This medication is available as an oral solution, an oral suspension, and granules. You can buy it without a prescription. If you're treating yourself, read the label carefully; it tells you how much to take at each dose. If your doctor prescribed this drug or gave you special instructions on how to use it and how much to take, follow his instructions.

If you're taking the *oral suspension,* shake it well and take your dose with a full glass (8 ounces) of fruit juice or water.

Schedule your dose so that the bowel movement it produces won't interfere with your sleep or activities. Phillips' Milk of Magnesia usually produces a watery stool in 3 to 6 hours. However, it may take longer if you take a small dose with food.

Don't take this or any other laxative regularly; you could become dependent on it. And don't take it if you have missed a bowel movement for only 1 or 2 days.

Laxatives are meant only for short-term relief of constipation. Don't take this medication for more than 1 week unless your doctor directs you to do so.

What to do about side effects

Call your doctor as soon as possible if you become confused, dizzy, or light-headed; if you develop an irregular heartbeat; or if you experience muscle cramps or unusual tiredness or fatigue.

Diarrhea, abdominal cramps, gas, nausea, and increased thirst may occur. These side effects usually subside as your body adjusts to the medication. But you should check with your doctor if they persist or become more intense.

What you must know about other drugs

Check with your doctor or pharmacist if you're taking Achromycin (tetracycline). Phillips' Milk of Magnesia can make this drug less effective.

Don't take Phillips' Milk of Magnesia within 1 to 2 hours of taking another medication by mouth (tablet, capsule, or liquid). It may make that other medication less effective.

Special directions

• Don't take Phillips' Milk of Magnesia if you have kidney failure, a colostomy or an ileostomy, abdominal pain, nausea, vomiting, fecal impaction, or intestinal obstruction. It can make these conditions worse.

• To help prevent the need for a laxative, eat a high-fiber diet, exercise regularly, and increase your fluid intake. Good sources of dietary fiber include bran and other cereals as well as fresh fruits and vegetables.

• If you have a sudden change in bowel habits that lasts for more than 2 weeks or returns every now and then, contact your doctor before using this medication. You may have a more serious problem.

Important reminder

Don't give laxatives to children unless the doctor has specifically directed you to do so.

Pilocar

This medication is used to treat glaucoma and other eye conditions. Its generic name is pilocarpine.

How to use Pilocar

Pilocar comes in eyedrops, eye gel, and an eye system. Use it exactly as directed by your doctor. Don't take more of it or take it more often than prescribed. Before you use the medication, wash your hands. Then follow these steps:

If you're using *eyedrops,* first tilt your head back. Use your index finger to pull the lower eyelid away from the eye, forming a pouch. Squeeze the drops into the pouch and gently close your eyes for 1 to 2 minutes. Don't blink.

If you're using *eye gel,* first pull the lower eyelid away to form a pouch. Squeeze a thin strip of gel into the pouch. Gently close your eyes for 1 to 2 minutes.

Right after using the eyedrops or eye gel, wash your hands to remove any medication that might be on them. Also, take care to keep your medication bottle germfree. Don't let the applicator tip touch any surface, including your eye.

Before you use the *eye system,* read the patient instructions carefully. If you have any questions, check with your doctor.

What to do if you miss a dose

If you forget to use the eyedrops or eye gel, make up the missed dose as soon as possible. But if it's almost time for your next application, skip the one you missed and continue the applications on schedule.

What to do about side effects

When you use this medication, it may make your brow or head hurt or cause eye pain. For a short time after you use it, your vision may be blurred or you may notice a change in your near or distant vision, especially at night. If these symptoms persist or intensify, check with your doctor.

If you're using the eyedrops or eye gel, make sure your vision is clear before you drive or perform other activities that might be dangerous if you can't see well.

What you must know about other drugs
Tell your doctor about other medications you're taking. To prevent harmful interactions, you need to avoid drugs such as ophthalmic Neo-Synephrine (phenylephrine, used to treat eye redness) and Carbacel (carbachol, a medication for glaucoma).

Special directions
Tell your doctor if you have other medical problems, especially asthma, other eye problems, heart disease, difficulty urinating, stomach ulcers, an overactive thyroid, or Parkinson's disease.

Premarin

This female hormone is used to relieve menopausal symptoms, to treat certain breast cancers, and to help prevent brittle bone disease (osteoporosis). Its generic name is estrogen.

How to take Premarin
Premarin comes in tablets, capsules, and vaginal cream. Follow your doctor's instructions for using it. For best results, take your medication at the same time each day.

If you take *tablets* or *capsules,* you may need to take them with food to control nausea.

If you're using the *vaginal cream,* your doctor may want you to apply it at bedtime so it will be absorbed better. If you're not using it at bedtime, lie down for 30 minutes after use.

What to do if you miss a dose
If you miss a *tablet* or *capsule,* take it as soon as possible. But if it's almost time for your next dose, skip the missed dose and take your next dose on schedule. Don't take a double dose.

If you forget to apply a dose of *vaginal cream* and don't remember until the next day, skip the missed dose and go back to your regular dosing schedule.

What to do about side effects
Be alert for symptoms of blood clots, a rare but serious complication. Call for emergency help *immediately* if you have any of the following symptoms:
- sudden or severe headache
- sudden loss of coordination

- vision changes, such as loss of sight, blurred vision, or seeing flashing lights
- numbness or stiffness in your legs
- pain in your chest, groin, or legs
- shortness of breath.

Also call your doctor *right away* if you experience rapid weight gain; breast swelling, pain, or lumps; or unusual vaginal bleeding. If you're using the vaginal cream, call your doctor if you develop swelling, redness, or itching in the vaginal area.

Check with your doctor if you feel nauseated or lose your appetite or if your stomach becomes cramped or bloated.

What you must know about other drugs

Because many medications can interfere with Premarin therapy, make sure your doctor is aware of all other medications (both nonprescription and prescription) that you're taking.

Special directions

- Tell your doctor about other medical problems you have, especially breast disease, cancer, diabetes, high blood pressure, porphyria, gynecologic problems, or diseases of the major organs. Mention if you've ever had blood clots or a stroke. Also tell the doctor if you have female relatives who've had breast or female organ cancer.
- Keep all appointments for follow-up care so your doctor can check your progress and detect side effects early.
- Be sure to perform regular breast self-exams and see your doctor for routine breast exams.

Important reminders

If you're pregnant or breast-feeding, don't use Premarin.

If you have diabetes, be aware that Premarin may affect your blood sugar level. Check with your doctor if you notice any changes.

Prilosec

This medication is used to treat duodenal ulcers, severe or chronic heartburn, and other problems involving an excess of stomach acid. Its generic name is omeprazole.

How to take Prilosec   Prilosec comes in delayed-release capsules. Take them exactly as directed. Don't break, chew, or crush the capsules; swallow them whole.

Take Prilosec for the full treatment period, even after you feel better.

What to do if you miss a dose   Take the missed dose as soon as possible. However, if it's almost time for your next dose, skip the missed dose and take your next scheduled dose. Don't take a double dose.

What to do about side effects   Call your doctor *immediately* if you have any of the following:
- bloody or cloudy urine
- difficult, frequent, or painful urination
- easy bruising or bleeding
- fever
- persistent sores or ulcers in the mouth
- a sore throat
- unusual tiredness.

Check with your doctor if you get a cough, a headache, back or chest pain, or a rash. Also let the doctor know if you have digestive troubles, such as abdominal or stomach pain, constipation, diarrhea, gas, heartburn, nausea, or vomiting.

What you must know about other drugs   Tell the doctor about any other medications you are taking. Some drugs are more likely to cause side effects when taken with Prilosec. These include blood thinners, the muscle relaxant Valium (diazepam), and the seizure medication Dilantin (phenytoin).

Special directions   • Tell your doctor about other medical problems you have, especially liver disease. Also mention if you're allergic to anything, such as foods or dyes.

• Keep appointments for follow-up exams so your doctor will know when you can stop taking this medication.

• After you start therapy, several days may pass before you experience pain relief. Until then, you can take antacids with Prilosec unless your doctor advises otherwise.

Important reminder If you're pregnant or breast-feeding, check with your doctor before taking this medication.

Prinivil

Prinivil is used to treat high blood pressure. Its generic name is lisinopril. Another brand name is Zestril.

How to take Prinivil Prinivil comes in tablets. Read the label on your prescription bottle carefully and take only the amount prescribed.

Continue to take Prinivil as directed, even if you feel well. You may have to continue this or another medication for the rest of your life to keep your blood pressure under control.

You may not notice the effects of this medication for several weeks. If you don't think it's working or if you have unpleasant side effects, check with your doctor. Don't stop taking Prinivil abruptly.

What to do if you miss a dose Take the missed dose as soon as possible. However, if it's almost time for your next dose, skip the missed one and resume your regular schedule. Don't take a double dose.

What to do about side effects Call the doctor *right away* if you suddenly have trouble breathing or swallowing or if you experience dizziness, light-headedness, nausea, vomiting, diarrhea, loss of taste, fever, chills, hoarseness, or swelling of the face, mouth, hands, or feet. Severe nausea, vomiting, or diarrhea can cause you to lose too much water, which can precipitate a severe drop in your blood pressure.

Because Prinivil can make you feel dizzy, make sure you know how you react to it before you drive a car or perform other potentially hazardous activities.

Prinivil can also make you cough. If the coughing continues or becomes bothersome, call your doctor.

What you must know about other drugs Check with your doctor or pharmacist before taking other drugs, especially nonprescription medications (such as remedies for colds, asthma, cough, hay fever, or appetite control). These drugs can change the way Prinivil works or cause high blood pressure and other medical problems.

Taking diuretics (water pills) or Indocin (indomethacin, an arthritis drug) with Prinivil can cause your blood pressure to drop too low or your potassium level to rise too high.

Drugs and nutritional supplements that contain potassium or salt substitutes can also cause your potassium level to rise too high and your heart to beat abnormally.

Special directions • Make sure your doctor knows about your medical history, especially if you have diabetes; heart, kidney, or liver disease; a kidney transplant; or lupus.
• Follow any special diet the doctor has prescribed.

Important reminder If you're pregnant or breast-feeding, check with your doctor before taking Prinivil.

Pro-Banthine

Pro-Banthine is prescribed for the relief of stomach cramps, spasms, and acid stomach. The generic name for this drug is propantheline.

How to take Pro-Banthine Take Pro-Banthine tablets exactly as directed, 30 to 60 minutes before meals. And take your bedtime dose at least 2 hours after your last meal of the day. Swallow the tablets whole; don't chew or crush them.

What to do if you miss a dose If you forget to take a dose, don't make it up. Just start your schedule all over again with the next dose. Never take a double dose.

What to do about side effects Call your doctor *right away* if you develop difficulty urinating or swallowing, dizziness, drowsiness, eye pain, headaches, nervousness, rapid heartbeat or palpitations, or a rash.

Because Pro-Banthine can make you drowsy, make sure you know how you react to it before you drive or perform other activities that require you to be fully alert.

Call the doctor if you have constipation, decreased sweating, heartburn, nausea, or vomiting — or if your eyes are unusually sensitive to bright light.

If your eyes are sensitive to sunlight, protect them by wearing sunglasses or a wide-brimmed hat.

Your body sweats less while you're taking this medication. To avoid heatstroke, avoid strenuous exercise and limit outdoor exercise during hot weather.

Avoid eating spicy or acidic foods while you're on Pro-Banthine; they can upset your stomach.

To prevent constipation, drink lots of extra water or other fluids.

What you must know about alcohol and other drugs

Avoid alcoholic beverages; they can worsen your condition.

Make sure your doctor knows all the medications you're taking and consult with him or her (or your pharmacist) before you take other medications. Certain drugs can interact with Pro-Banthine and cause problems.

Special directions

Tell your doctor if you have other medical problems, especially glaucoma, difficulty urinating, myasthenia gravis, or diseases of the digestive tract, heart, liver, or kidneys. These problems can affect your use of Pro-Banthine.

Important reminders

If you're pregnant or breast-feeding, check with your doctor before taking this medication.

Older adults may be especially prone to Pro-Banthine's side effects.

Prolixin

Prolixin is prescribed to treat emotional problems. The generic name for this drug is fluphenazine. Another brand name is Permitil.

How to take Prolixin

Follow your doctor's instructions exactly. You can take Prolixin with food or a full glass (8 ounces) of water or milk to minimize possible stomach upset.

If your medication comes in a bottle, measure each dose with the special dropper. Dilute the medication in a half glass (4 ounces) of orange juice, grapefruit juice, or water. Avoid spilling the medication on your skin; it can cause irritation and a rash.

What to do if you miss a dose

If you take one dose a day and miss the dose, take it as soon as possible. Then take your next dose at the regular time. But if you don't remember the missed dose until the next day, skip it and take your next scheduled dose.

If you take more than one dose a day and miss a dose, take the missed dose as soon as you remember it if it's within an hour or so of the scheduled time. But if you don't remember it until later, skip the missed dose and take your next dose as scheduled. Don't take a double dose.

What to do about side effects

Contact your doctor *immediately* if you learn that your blood count is abnormal or if you develop an infection or fever, rapid heartbeat, rapid breathing, and profuse sweating.

Also call your doctor *immediately* if you start to have uncontrollable movements such as lip smacking, mouth puckering, cheek puffing, wormlike tongue movements, chewing motions, and arm or leg twitches.

Prolixin can cause dizziness, light-headedness, or faintness when you rise from a bed or a chair; blurred vision; dry mouth; constipation; urine retention; and mild sensitivity to sunlight. Contact your doctor if these side effects persist or become more severe.

Because Prolixin can make you dizzy or affect your vision, make sure you know how you react to it before you drive or perform any activities that require you to be fully alert and have clear vision.

Relieve a dry mouth with sugarless hard candy or gum, ice chips, or a saliva substitute.

Protect yourself against overexposure to sunlight.

What you must know about alcohol and other drugs

Avoid alcoholic beverages and other medications that affect your nervous system.

Tell your doctor about all other prescription and nonprescription medications you're taking. They can interact with Prolixin and cause problems.

Special directions Before taking Prolixin, tell your doctor about any other medical problems you have. Some conditions can affect your use of Prolixin.

Important reminders If you're pregnant or breast-feeding, check with your doctor before taking this medication.

Children and older adults are especially sensitive to Prolixin.

If you're an athlete, be aware that the National Collegiate Athletic Association and the U.S. Olympic Committee ban the use of fluphenazine.

Propulsid

Your doctor has prescribed Propulsid to help relieve your heartburn. This drug's generic name is cisapride.

How to take Propulsid This medication is available in tablet form. Take Propulsid 15 minutes before meals and at bedtime. Be sure to follow the label directions carefully.

What to do if you miss a dose If you miss a dose, take the missed dose as soon as you remember. If it's almost time for your next dose, skip the missed dose, and return to your regular schedule. Don't take a double dose.

What to do about side effects Propulsid may make you feel anxious or nervous and may cause headache, abnormal vision, or wakefulness. You may also experience diarrhea, abdominal pain, nausea, constipation, gassiness, or stomach upset. This medication may also cause a rash or itching and may cause vaginitis, urinary tract infection, or frequent urination as well as head-cold symptoms such as coughing, runny nose, sinus pain, muscle aches, and fever. Notify your doctor if any of these side effects persists or becomes severe.

What you must know about alcohol and other drugs Check with your doctor before drinking alcohol or taking other drugs that make you sleepy, such as Valium (diazepam). Propulsid may speed up the action of other medications, so talk to your doctor before you combine this medication with any other drug.

Tell your doctor if you take a blood thinner such as Coumadin (warfarin) because you may need a dosage adjustment. Propulsid may speed the absorption of Tagamet (cimetidine) and Zantac (ranitidine), but it may decrease the effectiveness of anticholinergics such as Atropisol (atropine) and Cogentin (benztropine).

Special directions Let your doctor know if you have any gastrointestinal problems such as bleeding before you take Propulsid.

Important reminders Be sure to tell your doctor if your pregnant or breast-feeding.

If you're an older adult you may need a dosage adjustment because Propulsid will tend to stay in your blood longer.

Propyl-Thyracil

To stop your thyroid gland from producing too much thyroid hormone, your doctor has prescribed Propyl-Thyracil. This drug's generic name is propylthiouracil.

How to take Propyl-Thyracil Propyl-Thyracil comes in tablets. Take them exactly as directed. Don't use more medication than prescribed or use it longer than recommended.

Take your tablets with meals to prevent stomach upset unless your doctor gives you other instructions. Also, if you're taking more than one dose a day, try to take your medication at evenly spaced times day and night.

Don't stop taking Propyl-Thyracil until you've discussed it with your doctor.

What to do if you miss a dose Take the missed dose as soon as possible. However, if it's almost time for your next dose, take both doses together. Then go back to your regular dosing schedule. If you miss more than one dose, check with your doctor.

What to do about side effects

Call your doctor *right away* if your skin starts to turn yellow, you gain unexpected weight, or your feet and ankles start to swell. Also call your doctor *at once* if you have fever, chills, a sore throat, or mouth sores.

This medication may cause nausea, vomiting, or easy bruising or bleeding. If these side effects occur, check with your doctor; your dosage may need to be adjusted.

What you must know about other drugs

Check with your doctor before you use other prescription or nonprescription medications. In particular, your doctor may want you to avoid iodine-containing medications — Pima (potassium iodide), for example, as well as certain cough medicines. Using these medications with Propyl-Thyracil can lead to a goiter or can decrease thyroid activity too much.

Special directions

• Tell your doctor if you have other medical problems, especially an infection or liver disease. These problems can affect your use of Propyl-Thyracil.

• Check with your doctor *right away* if you're injured or get an infection or illness of any kind. The doctor may want you to stop taking Propyl-Thyracil or to change your dosage.

• Before you have medical tests, tell the doctor you're taking Propyl-Thyracil; it can affect the test results.

• Ask your doctor if it's okay for you to eat iodine-containing foods such as iodized salt and shellfish.

Important reminder

If you're pregnant or breast-feeding, check with your doctor before using this medication.

ProSom

Your doctor has prescribed ProSom to help you sleep. The generic name for this drug is estazolam.

How to take ProSom

ProSom comes in tablets. Take them exactly as directed; no more and no longer. Too much of this drug can lead to dependency or can lessen or negate the effects of the medication.

Check with your doctor if you think the medication isn't working well, especially if you've been taking it every night for several weeks.

What to do if you miss a dose

Skip the missed dose and go back to your regular dosing schedule. Don't take a double dose.

What to do about side effects

If you think you've taken an overdose or you're experiencing severe side effects — prolonged confusion, severe drowsiness, trouble breathing, slow heartbeat, continuing slurred speech, staggering, severe weakness — call for emergency help *immediately*.

If this medication makes you drowsy in the daytime or dizzy, check with your doctor, especially if these symptoms continue or bother you.

What you must know about alcohol and other drugs

Don't drink alcoholic beverages while taking this medication; the combination can cause oversedation.

For the same reason, avoid other central nervous system depressants (medications that slow down the nervous system), such as tranquilizers, other sleep medications, muscle relaxers, and cold, allergy, and flu medications.

Other medications that can cause oversedation if combined with ProSom include Tagamet (cimetidine), an ulcer medication; birth control pills; Antabuse (disulfiram), a medication for alcoholism; and Laniazid (isoniazid), a tuberculosis medication.

Because ProSom may not work well in combination with certain drugs, be sure to tell your doctor what medications you're taking.

Special directions

• Tell your doctor if you have other medical problems, such as a history of alcohol or drug dependence, brain disorders, asthma or other lung diseases, kidney or liver disease, depression, myasthenia gravis, seizures, porphyria, or breathing problems while sleeping.

• Check with your doctor at least every 4 months to determine if you need to continue taking ProSom.

• After you stop taking ProSom, your body may need time to adjust. Call your doctor if you experience any irritability, nervousness, or trouble sleeping.

Important reminders If you're pregnant or breast-feeding, check with your doctor before taking this medication.

If you're an older adult, you may be especially prone to daytime drowsiness, so take care to prevent falls.

Proventil

Proventil is prescribed for bronchial asthma, chronic bronchitis, emphysema, and other lung disorders. It relieves coughing, wheezing, shortness of breath, and breathing difficulties by improving the flow of air in the lungs. The generic name for this drug is albuterol. Another brand name is Ventolin.

How to take Proventil Proventil comes in syrup, tablets, extended-release tablets, or an aerosol. It also comes in a solution for use in a nebulizer.

Take Proventil exactly as directed; don't increase the amount or frequency of your doses without consulting your doctor.

If you're taking the *extended-release tablets*, don't break or chew them. Swallow them whole.

Use your nebulizer or other breathing device exactly as you were shown. Don't take more than two inhalations at a time, unless the doctor tells you otherwise. Wait 1 to 2 minutes after the first inhalation to make sure you need another. If you use up your breathing device in less than 2 weeks, you may be taking too much medication.

If you're taking two aerosol medications — such as Proventil and an adrenocorticoid drug or Atrovent (ipratropium) — inhale the Proventil, wait about 5 minutes, and then use the other aerosol. Taking Proventil first opens your air passages and helps the next medication work better.

What to do if you miss a dose
Take a missed dose as soon as possible; then take any remaining doses for that day at regularly spaced intervals. Don't take a double dose.

What to do about side effects
You may experience tremors, nervousness, dizziness, difficulty sleeping, headaches, or an unusual taste in your mouth. If these symptoms persist, call your doctor.

What you must know about other drugs
Tell your doctor what other medications you're taking; some drugs can affect the way Proventil works. For example, when taken with Proventil, some medications for depression can affect the heart and blood vessels. Likewise, some heart medications can keep Proventil from working properly.

Special directions
If you still have trouble breathing after using Proventil, or if your condition is worse, contact your doctor.

Important reminders
If you have diabetes, be aware that Proventil can increase your blood sugar level. Contact your doctor if you notice a change in your blood or urine test results.

Tell your doctor if you become pregnant while taking this medication.

If you're an athlete, you should know that the U.S. Olympic Committee permits the use of inhalation aerosol and inhalation solution forms of albuterol.

Provera

Provera is usually prescribed to treat abnormal bleeding of the uterus caused by hormonal imbalance, to treat amenorrhea (absence of menstruation), or to help treat cancer of the endometrium or kidney. The generic name for this drug is medroxyprogesterone.

How to take Provera
Provera comes in tablets. Check the label carefully and take only the prescribed amount at each dose.

What to do if you miss a dose
Take the missed dose as soon as possible. However, if it's almost time for your next dose, skip the missed dose

and resume your regular schedule. Don't take a double dose.

What to do about side effects

Rarely, this medication may cause a blood clot — a life-threatening emergency. If you have any of the following symptoms, stop taking the Provera and get medical help *immediately:* pain in the chest, groin, or leg; sudden shortness of breath or loss of coordination; sudden or severe headache; sudden slurring of speech; sudden vision loss or change in vision; or weakness, numbness, or pain in the arm or leg.

If Provera causes changes in your vaginal bleeding pattern, such as spotting, breakthrough bleeding, or prolonged bleeding, report these side effects to your doctor *promptly.*

Brush and floss your teeth and massage your gums carefully and regularly to help prevent your gums from bleeding. See your dentist regularly.

What you must know about other drugs

Check with your doctor or pharmacist before taking Rifadin (rifampin), a tuberculosis drug; it may make Provera less effective.

Special directions

• Don't take this medication if you have a history of blood clots, severe liver disease, breast or genital cancer, or undiagnosed abnormal vaginal bleeding. Provera can make these disorders worse.

• Tell your doctor about any other medical problems you have, especially heart or kidney disease, fluid retention, seizures, migraine headaches, depression, or breast or genital cancer.

• Contact your doctor if your menstrual period doesn't start within 45 days of your last period or if vaginal bleeding lasts an unusually long time.

• Have regular medical checkups so the doctor can check your progress, adjust your dosage if needed, and detect any side effects.

Important reminders

If you're pregnant, you shouldn't take this medication. If you become pregnant while taking it, stop taking it immediately because it may harm your fetus.

If you're breast-feeding, check with your doctor before taking Provera.

If you have diabetes, report symptoms of high blood sugar (such as increased thirst and urination) to the doctor.

Prozac

Prozac is prescribed to help relieve depression. The generic name for this drug is fluoxetine.

How to take Prozac Take this drug exactly as prescribed. It may be 4 weeks or longer before you begin to feel its effects.

What to do if you miss a dose Skip the missed dose and take your next regular dose as scheduled. Never take a double dose.

What to do about side effects If you develop a rash or hives, stop taking this medication and call your doctor *immediately* — you may be having an allergic reaction.

This medication may cause nervousness, anxiety, insomnia, headache, drowsiness, shakiness, dizziness, nausea, diarrhea, dry mouth, loss of appetite, stomach upset, weight loss, itching, and weakness. If you have any of these symptoms and they persist or worsen, contact your doctor.

Because Prozac can cause drowsiness, make sure you know how it affects you before you drive or perform other activities that require you to be fully alert.

If the medication makes you feel dizzy, light-headed, or faint when getting up from a bed or chair, rise slowly. If the problem persists or worsens, consult your doctor.

To relieve a dry mouth, use sugarless gum or hard candy, ice chips, or a saliva substitute. Dryness that persists for longer than 2 weeks increases your chance for dental problems. Consult your doctor or dentist.

What you must know about alcohol and other drugs Avoid drinking alcoholic beverages while taking Prozac.

Also avoid taking other medications that affect the central nervous system (such as cough, cold, and allergy medications; narcotics; muscle relaxants; sleeping pills; and seizure medications).

Tell your doctor about any other medications you're taking. Taking Prozac with Valium (diazepam), Coumadin (warfarin), or Lanoxin (digoxin) can cause serious side effects.

Special directions
• Before taking Prozac, tell your doctor if you have other medical problems, especially diabetes, kidney or liver disease, or a seizure disorder.
• Schedule regular checkups so your doctor can monitor your progress, check for side effects, and adjust your dosage as needed.

Important reminders
If you have diabetes, be aware that Prozac can affect your blood sugar levels. Report changes in your at-home blood or urine glucose tests to your doctor.

If you're breast-feeding, check with your doctor before taking Prozac.

Pulmozyme

Your doctor has prescribed Pulmozyme to help reduce the number of respiratory infections you get. This drug's generic name is dornase alfa recombinant.

How to take Pulmozyme
You'll probably receive this liquid medication in containers called ampules. To take Pulmozyme, insert an ampule into a nebulizer. Then put mouthpiece of the nebulizer in your mouth. As you squeeze the nebulizer and inhale, the medication will be sprayed into your mouth and will flow into your lungs. Carefully follow the label directions to determine how many times to squeeze the nebulizer.

What to do if you miss a dose
Take the missed dose as soon as you remember. If it's almost time for your next dose, skip the missed dose and return to your regular schedule. Don't take a double dose.

What to do about side effects
Pulmozyme may cause chest pain, rash, voice alteration, pharyngitis, laryngitis, or pink eye. If a side effect is persistent or becomes severe, contact your doctor.

What you must know about other drugs Don't mix other drugs with Pulmozyme in your nebulizer. They could reduce Pulmozyme's effect, or Pulmozyme could change the way the other drugs work.

Special directions • Remember to keep Pulmozyme refrigerated and protect it from strong light. Throw out the medicine if it looks cloudy or discolored. Pulmozyme contains no preservative so throw out the opened ampule after you take the prescribed dose.
• Keep the nebulizer clean and follow any other directions you received on how to care for the nebulizer.

Important reminder Be sure to tell your doctor if you're pregnant or breastfeeding.

Pyridium

This medication will help to ease the pain of your infected or irritated urinary tract. The generic name for this drug is phenazopyridine.

How to take Pyridium Pyridium comes in tablets. Take it exactly as prescribed by your doctor. If you bought it without a prescription, read the package instructions carefully before taking it.
To prevent stomach upset, take the tablets with meals or a snack.
You can stop using this medication after 3 days if your pain is gone, unless your doctor gives you other instructions.

What to do if you miss a dose Take the missed dose as soon as possible. However, if it's almost time for your next dose, skip the missed dose and take your next dose on schedule. Don't take a double dose.

What to do about side effects Check with your doctor *right away* if you have any of these symptoms: bluish skin, shortness of breath or difficulty breathing, a rash, unusual tiredness or weakness, or yellow eyes or skin.
Let your doctor know if Pyridium makes you dizzy or nauseated or if it gives you a headache.

Because Pyridium can make you dizzy, make sure you know how you react to it before you drive or perform other activities that require you to be fully alert.

Don't be surprised if the medication turns your urine reddish orange. This is to be expected and won't cause any harm.

Special directions
• If you have kidney or liver disease, tell your doctor; these problems can affect your use of Pyridium.
• Before you have medical tests, tell the doctor that you're taking this medication; it can affect the test results.
• If you have another urinary tract problem in the future, don't use any leftover Pyridium without first checking with your doctor.

Important reminder
If you have diabetes, be aware that this medication can cause false test results with urine glucose or urine ketone tests. Check with your doctor for more information, especially if your diabetes isn't well controlled.

Q

Questran

Your doctor has prescribed Questran to lower your blood cholesterol level and to remove substances called bile acids from your body. This drug's generic name is cholestyramine. Another brand name is CholyBar.

How to take Questran

Questran comes as a powder and a chewable bar.

If you're taking the *powder* form of this medication, first mix it with liquid. Never take it in its dry form because you might choke. To mix it, follow these steps:

• Place the prescribed dose in 2 ounces (60 milliliters) of any beverage and stir thoroughly.

• Add an additional 2 to 4 ounces (60 to 80 milliliters) of the beverage and again mix thoroughly (it won't dissolve). Drink the liquid.

• After drinking all the liquid, rinse the glass with a little more liquid and drink that also.

You may also mix the powder with milk in hot or regular breakfast cereals or in thin soups. Or add it to pulpy fruits, such as crushed pineapple or fruit cocktail.

If you're using the *chewable bar* form of this medication, chew each bite well before swallowing.

Don't stop taking Questran without first checking with your doctor.

What to do if you miss a dose

Take the missed dose as soon as possible. But if it's almost time for your next dose, skip the missed dose and take the next dose on schedule. Don't take a double dose.

What to do about side effects

While you're taking Questran, you may experience constipation, nausea, or rashes. Check with your doctor if these symptoms persist or become bothersome.

What you must know about other drugs

Tell your doctor about other medications you're taking. Many medications may not be absorbed well if taken at the same time as Questran. Examples include Tylenol (acetaminophen), certain blood thinners, beta blockers such as Calan (verapamil), corticosteroids such as Decadron (dexamethasone), Lanoxin (digoxin), fat-soluble vitamins (A, D, E, and K), iron preparations, some water pills, and thyroid hormone. If possible, take Questran 2 hours before or 2 hours after taking any other medication to prevent this problem.

Special directions

• Because Questran can make certain medical problems worse, tell your doctor if you have gallbladder disease or a history of constipation or digestive problems.

• Also let your doctor know if you're allergic to tartrazine (a yellow food dye) because the powder form of this medication contains tartrazine.

• This medication may not work well if you're very overweight, so you may be advised to go on a reducing diet. However, check with your doctor before starting any diet.

Important reminders

If you're pregnant or breast-feeding, check with your doctor before taking Questran.

If you're an older adult, you may be especially prone to this medication's side effects.

R

Reglan

This medication may be prescribed to prevent nausea and vomiting after treatment with anticancer medications, to help diagnose stomach or intestinal problems, to treat certain gastrointestinal disorders, or to help relieve nausea, vomiting, and bloating after meals. The drug's generic name is metoclopramide.

How to take Reglan

Reglan is available in tablets and as a syrup. Carefully check the label. Take only the amount prescribed.

Take this medication 30 minutes before meals and at bedtime unless your doctor tells you otherwise.

What to do if you miss a dose

Take the missed dose as soon as you remember. However, if it's almost time for your next dose, skip the missed dose and resume your regular dosage schedule. Don't take a double dose.

What to do about side effects

Call your doctor *promptly* if you experience a fever, chills, sore throat, loss of balance, odd tongue movements, arm or leg stiffness, a shuffling walk, or difficulty swallowing or speaking.

If you're taking high doses, you may experience a paniclike sensation, lower leg discomfort, or unusual restlessness, nervousness, or irritability within minutes of taking a dose. Report these effects to the doctor *as soon as possible*.

Reglan can make you drowsy or less alert, so avoid potentially hazardous activities, such as driving a car or using dangerous tools, until you know how it affects you.

Drowsiness usually goes away over time. If it persists or becomes bothersome, check with your doctor.

What you must know about other drugs

Avoid sedatives (drugs that relax you and make you feel sleepy), antihistamines such as Benadryl (diphenhydramine), and other central nervous system depressants while taking this drug because of the risk of oversedation.

Check with your doctor before taking a narcotic pain reliever or an anticholinergic drug (used to treat spastic disorders of the stomach or intestine). These drugs can prevent Reglan from working properly.

Special directions
- Tell your doctor if you're allergic to Novocain (procaine) or Pronestyl (procainamide).
- Tell your doctor about other medical problems you have, especially stomach bleeding, breast cancer, intestinal blockage, Parkinson's disease, seizures, or severe kidney or liver disease.
- Don't take this medication for more than 12 weeks.

Important reminders
If you're an older adult, you may be especially sensitive to this medication if you take it for a long time. Children are more sensitive than adults to the effects of Reglan.

If you're an athlete, you should know that the U.S. Olympic Committee and the National Collegiate Athletic Association ban the use of metoclopromide.

Relafen

This medication is usually prescribed to reduce the joint pain, swelling, and stiffness caused by arthritis. The drug's generic name is nabumetone.

How to take Relafen
This medication is available in tablets.

Carefully check the prescription label. Take only the prescribed amount.

If Relafen gives you heartburn, check with your doctor to see if you may take it with food or an antacid.

What to do if you miss a dose
Take the missed dose as soon as you remember. However, if it's almost time for your next regular dose, skip the missed dose and resume your regular dosage schedule. Never take a double dose.

What to do about side effects
Call your doctor *right away* if you see blood in your urine, if you start urinating less often, or if you have diar-

rhea, black stools, a sore throat, wheezing, dizziness, light-headedness, drowsiness, ringing in your ears, vision changes, swollen ankles, or a rash.

You may experience stomach or abdominal cramps or pain, headache, heartburn, indigestion, nausea, or vomiting. These side effects usually go away as your body adjusts to the medication. Check with your doctor if they persist or become bothersome.

Because Relafen may make you drowsy, avoid driving, operating machinery, or other activities that require alertness.

What you must know about alcohol and other drugs

Don't drink alcoholic beverages while you're taking this drug. Alcohol may increase Relafen's depressant effects on the central nervous system.

Check with your doctor or pharmacist before taking other drugs. Many drugs increase the chance for serious side effects when taken with Relafen. Especially avoid taking aspirin or steroids because these drugs increase the risk of gastrointestinal side effects.

Special directions

• You shouldn't take this medication if you're allergic to aspirin.

• Be sure your doctor knows about your medical history, especially if you have gastrointestinal disease, stomach ulcers, kidney disease, or heart or blood vessel disease.

• Take all doses at the prescribed times. Don't postpone taking a dose to make the medication last longer than intended.

• Keep taking this drug even if your symptoms don't get better right away. Relafen may take about 1 month to achieve its full effect.

• If you're taking this medication for a long time, be sure to get regular medical checkups so the doctor can evaluate your progress.

Important reminders

If you're pregnant or breast-feeding, check with your doctor before taking this medication.

If you're an older adult, you may be especially sensitive to Relafen's side effects.

Reserpine

Your doctor has prescribed Reserpine to lower your high blood pressure. This drug's generic name is also reserpine.

How to take Reserpine

Reserpine comes in tablets. Follow your doctor's directions for taking your medication exactly, even if you feel well. If Reserpine upsets your stomach, take it with meals or milk.

Don't stop taking Reserpine suddenly without checking first with your doctor.

What to do if you miss a dose

Don't take the missed dose or double the next one. Instead, take your next dose on schedule.

What to do about side effects

Call your doctor *right away* if you start having nightmares. Also call if you feel drowsy, dizzy, depressed, faint, or unusually nervous. Tell the doctor if you start to gain weight unexpectedly or if you have a dry mouth, a stuffy nose, a slow heartbeat, or stomach upset.

If you're male, let your doctor know if you become impotent while taking this medication.

Make sure you know how you react to Reserpine before you drive, operate machinery, or perform other activities that require alertness.

If Reserpine makes your mouth dry, use sugarless gum or hard candy, ice chips, or a saliva substitute.

To prevent dizziness, get up slowly when you rise from a sitting or lying position.

What you must know about alcohol and other drugs

Don't drink alcoholic beverages except with your doctor's okay because combined use with Reserpine may cause oversedation. For the same reason, check with your doctor before you take medications that slow down the central nervous system, such as cold, flu, and allergy remedies; sleeping pills; and tranquilizers.

Tell your doctor if you're taking other medications, especially if you're taking Marplan (isocarboxazid) or other monoamine oxidase (MAO) inhibitors for emotional problems. Also check before you take new prescription or nonprescription medications.

Special directions Tell your doctor if you have other medical problems, especially asthma, allergies, a seizure disorder, stomach ulcers, depression, Parkinson's disease, pheochromocytoma, or heart or kidney disease. Other medical problems may affect the use of this medication.

Important reminders If you're pregnant or breast-feeding, don't use Reserpine without first discussing the risks and benefits with your doctor.

If you're an older adult, you may be especially prone to Reserpine's side effects, especially drowsiness and dizziness.

Restoril

Your doctor has prescribed Restoril to relieve nervousness and tension to help you sleep. The generic name of this sedative is temazepam.

How to take Restoril Follow your doctor's instructions exactly. Don't increase your dose, even if you think your current one isn't effective. Instead, call your doctor. Also, because Restoril can be habit-forming, don't take it for a longer time than your doctor recommends.

What to do about side effects Restoril may make you feel tired, drowsy, or dizzy. If the symptoms are severe or if you feel very tired or hungover the day after you've taken the medication, your dose may be too high. Call your doctor so your dosage can be adjusted.

Make sure you know how you react to Restoril before driving, operating machinery, or performing other activities that require alertness.

What you must know about alcohol and other drugs Avoid drinking alcoholic beverages when taking Restoril because combined use increases the depressant effects of both alcohol and the drug on the central nervous system. If you drink alcoholic beverages with Restoril, you could have an overdose.

For the same reason, avoid taking other depressant drugs unless your doctor says otherwise. Examples include many allergy or cold medications, narcotics, muscle relaxants, sleeping pills, and drugs for seizures.

Tell your doctor if you're taking Retrovir (zidovudine). Restoril could cause your body to absorb more Retrovir, so your doctor may need to lower your Retrovir dosage.

Special directions

• Restoril can make some medical problems worse. For this reason, be sure to tell your doctor if you have glaucoma, a history of alcohol or drug abuse, mental depression, myasthenia gravis, Parkinson's disease, chronic obstructive pulmonary disease, kidney or liver disease, or porphyria.

• Check with your doctor every month to make sure you still need to be taking this medication.

Important reminders

Don't take Restoril if you think you might be pregnant or if you're breast-feeding.

If you're an older adult, be aware that this medication could make you feel drowsy during the day, which could lead to falls.

If you're an athlete, you should know that the U.S. Olympic Committee and the National Collegiate Athletic Association ban the use of temazepam.

Retin-A

Primarily used to treat acne, Retin-A may also be used to treat fine wrinkles resulting from sun damage. This drug's generic name is tretinoin.

How to apply Retin-A

Retin-A comes as a cream, gel, or solution for topical use.

First wash your skin with a mild, nonallergenic soap and water. Gently pat dry. Wait 20 to 30 minutes to allow your skin to dry completely.

If you're applying the *cream* or *gel*, apply enough medication to cover the affected areas and rub in gently.

If you're applying the *solution*, use your fingertips, a gauze pad, or a cotton swab to cover the affected areas.

What to do if you miss an application

Skip the missed dose and apply your next dose as scheduled.

What to do about side effects

When you first start using Retin-A, your skin may turn red and you may notice a slight stinging or feeling of warmth. After a few days, your skin may scale or peel.

If you have severe burning or redness, swelling, blisters, or crusting or if your skin darkens or lightens noticeably, check with your doctor.

Retin-A will increase your skin's sensitivity to sunlight. Protect your skin from the sun by wearing a sunscreen, a hat, and protective clothing. If your face becomes sunburned, stop using the medication until the burn heals.

The medication may also increase your sensitivity to wind and cold. Protect yourself by covering all exposed skin when you go out.

What you must know about other skin products

Don't use solutions containing high concentrations of alcohol (such as skin freshener or aftershave lotion), menthol, spices, or lime (as in some perfumes) because they can interact with Retin-A and irritate your skin.

Special directions

• Tell your doctor if you're allergic to vitamin A or retinoic acid. Also mention whether you've had eczema.
• Avoid applying Retin-A close to your eyes or mouth, at the angles of your nose, on your mucous membranes, in an open wound, or to windburned or sunburned skin.
• While you're using Retin-A, don't use any of the following, unless your doctor tells you otherwise:
— abrasive or perfumed soaps or cleansers
— any other topical acne medication that makes the skin peel
— cosmetics or soaps that dry the skin
— medicated cosmetics
— any other topical skin medication.
You may, however, wear unmedicated cosmetics.
• Don't wash your face more than two or three times a day to keep from drying out your skin.

Important reminder

If you're pregnant or breast-feeding, talk with your doctor before using this medication.

Retrovir

This medication can help slow the progress of the human immunodeficiency virus (HIV). In turn, Retrovir helps slow HIV's destruction of the immune system. This drug does not cure HIV infection or acquired immunodeficiency syndrome (AIDS). Nor will it keep you from spreading HIV to others. This drug's generic name is zidovudine.

How to take Retrovir

Retrovir comes in capsule, syrup, and injection forms. Take it only as your doctor directs. Don't take more or less of it, and don't take it more often or longer than directed. Take it for the full length of treatment, even if you begin to feel better. And don't stop taking it without checking with your doctor first.

You need to take Retrovir every 4 hours around the clock — even during the night. Take your medication at the same times every day.

If you're taking the *syrup*, measure your dose in a specially marked spoon. A household teaspoon may not hold the correct amount.

What to do if you miss a dose

Take the missed dose as soon as possible. But if it's almost time for your next dose, skip the missed dose and take your next dose as scheduled. Don't take a double dose.

What to do about side effects

Retrovir may cause some serious side effects, including bone marrow problems. Call your doctor *right away* if you develop any of the following: fever, chills, or sore throat; pale skin; unusual tiredness or weakness; or unusual bleeding or bruising.

Also let your doctor know if you develop a severe headache, muscle soreness, nausea, or trouble sleeping.

If the medication makes you dizzy, don't drive or perform any activity that could be dangerous if you're not fully alert.

Because Retrovir may cause blood problems and slow healing, be careful not to injure yourself. Use a soft toothbrush, and use toothpicks or dental floss cautiously so you don't injure your gums.

What you must know about other drugs
Taking certain drugs while you're taking Retrovir may increase your risk of dangerous side effects. That's why you need to tell your doctor about any other drugs you're taking — even nonprescription ones like Tylenol (acetaminophen).

Special directions
• Because other medical problems may affect the use of Retrovir, tell the doctor if you have anemia, other blood disorders, or liver disease.
• Remember to keep your follow-up appointments. You need to have your blood checked frequently — at least every 2 weeks — to monitor the effectiveness and potential side effects of your medication.

Important reminders
If you become pregnant, let your doctor know at once. If you're breast-feeding, you should stop while you're taking the drug.

Rheumatrex

This medication is often prescribed to treat psoriasis or rheumatoid arthritis. (It's also used to treat cancer. However, these instructions don't apply to that use.) This drug's generic name is methotrexate.

How to take Rheumatrex
This medication is available in tablets. Carefully check the prescription label. Take only the prescribed amount.

What to do if you miss a dose
Don't take the missed dose or double the next dose. Resume your regular dosage schedule and call your doctor.

What to do about side effects
Call your doctor *immediately* if you have diarrhea; reddened skin; red spots on the skin; stomach pain; mouth or lip sores; black, tarry stools; bloody urine or stools; blurred vision; seizures; cough; hoarseness; fever; chills; lower back or side pain; painful urination; shortness of breath; or unusual bleeding or bruising.

Check with your doctor *promptly* if you have dark urine, dizziness, drowsiness, headache, unusual fatigue or weakness, or yellow eyes or skin.

Hair loss may occur. However, after you finish Rheumatrex treatment, your normal hair growth should return.

If nausea and vomiting occur, check with your doctor. If you vomit shortly after taking a dose, ask the doctor whether you should take the dose again or wait until the next scheduled dose.

Practice birth control during and at least 3 months after treatment ends. Rheumatrex may cause birth defects if either the mother or the father takes it at the time of conception or if the mother takes it during pregnancy.

What you must know about alcohol and other drugs

Avoid drinking alcoholic beverages, which may increase unwanted effects on the liver. Check with your doctor or pharmacist before taking other drugs, including nonprescription medications. Especially avoid taking aspirin and other drugs used for pain and inflammation because they may increase the risk of serious side effects.

Special directions

• Tell your doctor about other medical problems you have, especially a stomach ulcer, colitis, an immune system disease, liver or kidney disease, or a blood disorder.
• Don't get immunizations during treatment except with your doctor's approval. Also, avoid people who've recently taken oral polio vaccine.

Important reminders

If you're pregnant, don't take this medication because it may harm the fetus. If you think you've become pregnant while taking Rheumatrex, call your doctor right away.

If you're breast-feeding, check with your doctor before taking Rheumatrex because it may cause serious side effects in your baby.

If you're an older adult, you may be especially sensitive to the side effects of Rheumatrex.

Rhythmol

Your doctor has prescribed Rhythmol to correct your irregular heartbeat to a normal rhythm. This drug's generic name is propafenone.

How to take Rhythmol

Rhythmol comes in tablets. Take this medication exactly as prescribed, even if you feel well. Don't take more or less of it than directed.

For best results, take Rhythmol at evenly spaced times day and night around the clock. To prevent stomach upset, take your medication with food.

What to do if you miss a dose

If you remember the missed dose within 4 hours, take it as soon as possible. But if you don't remember until later, skip it and take your next dose on schedule. Don't take a double dose.

What to do about side effects

Call your doctor *right away* if you have chest pain, palpitations, a fast or irregular heartbeat, difficulty breathing, or unusual weakness and fatigue.

This medication also may make you dizzy or cause taste changes. Let your doctor know if these side effects continue or become bothersome.

Make sure you know how you react to Rhythmol before you drive, operate machinery, or perform other activities that require alertness.

This medication may make you more sensitive to light, so cover up outdoors and limit your sun exposure.

What you must know about other drugs

To prevent harmful drug interactions, tell your doctor if you're taking other medications, in particular blood thinners, other heart medications such as Lanoxin (digoxin), the ulcer drug Tagamet (cimetidine), or high blood pressure medications.

Special directions

• Tell your doctor if you have other medical conditions, especially asthma, bronchitis, emphysema, and kidney or liver disease. Also reveal if you've had other heart problems, such as a recent heart attack, or if you have a pacemaker. Other medical problems may affect the use of this medication.

• Tell your doctor or dentist that you're taking this medication before you have surgery or emergency treatment.

• Your doctor may want you to carry a medical identification card or wear a medical identification bracelet stating that you're taking Rhythmol.

Important reminder   If you're pregnant, check with your doctor before taking this medication.

Rid

This medication is used to treat head, body, and pubic lice infestations. This medication's generic components are pyrethrins and piperonyl butoxide.

How to apply Rid   If this medication was prescribed, follow your doctor's directions exactly. If you bought it without a prescription, carefully read the package instructions.

If you're using the *gel* or *solution,* follow these steps: Apply enough medication to thoroughly wet the skin or dry hair and scalp. Let the medication remain on the treated area for exactly 10 minutes. Wash the treated area with warm water and soap or regular shampoo. Rinse thoroughly and dry with a clean towel.

If you're using the *shampoo,* follow these steps: Apply enough medication to thoroughly wet the dry hair and scalp. Let the medication remain on the treated scalp for exactly 10 minutes. Then work the shampoo into a lather, using a small amount of water. Rinse well and dry with a clean towel.

Wash your hands right after using this medication.

If you're using Rid on your hair, follow up by combing your hair with a nit-removal comb to remove dead lice and eggs (nits) from your hair.

Repeat the treatment 1 week to 10 days after the first treatment, as directed.

Keep this medication away from your eyes, mouth, and nose. Also, apply it in a well-ventilated room so you don't inhale the vapors.

What to do about   With repeated use, Rid may irritate your skin. Call your
side effects   doctor if you develop a rash or an infection.

Special directions   • If you have hay fever or are allergic to ragweed, check with your doctor before you use Rid. If you have a skin problem, such as severe inflammation or rawness, see your doctor before applying the drug.

• To prevent the spread of lice, machine wash all clothing, bedding, towels, and washcloths in very hot water. Then dry them using the hot cycle of a dryer for at least 20 minutes. Clothing or bedding that can't be washed should be dry-cleaned and sealed in a plastic bag for 2 weeks.

• Wash all hairbrushes and combs in very hot soapy water for 5 to 10 minutes.

• Clean the house or room by thoroughly vacuuming upholstered furniture, rugs, and floors.

• If more than one person lives in your household, all members should be checked for lice and, if they're infested, treated.

Rifadin

Your doctor has prescribed Rifadin to treat your tuberculosis. This drug's generic name is rifampin. Another brand name is Rimactane.

How to take Rifadin

Take this medication exactly as directed for as long as the doctor prescribes. Take it 1 hour before or 2 hours after meals. However, if Rifadin upsets your stomach, your doctor may tell you to take it with food.

What to do if you miss a dose

Take the missed dose as soon as possible. But if it's almost time for your next dose, skip the missed dose and take your next dose on schedule. Don't take a double dose.

What to do about side effects

Call your doctor *immediately* if you have any of the following: appetite loss, bloody or cloudy urine, bone and muscle pain, breathing problems, chills, dizziness, headache, nausea, or vomiting.

Also call the doctor promptly if you experience shivering, sore throat, unusual bleeding or bruising, fever, joint pain and inflammation (especially in the feet), abdominal pain, yellowish skin or eyes (jaundice), dark urine, or light-colored stools.

You may experience diarrhea, itching, reddened skin or a rash, a sore mouth or tongue, and stomach cramps.

As your body adjusts to Rifadin, some of these side effects may subside.

Because Rifadin may make you drowsy, make sure you know how you react to it before you drive or perform other activities that might be dangerous if you're not fully alert.

What you must know about alcohol and other drugs

Avoid drinking alcoholic beverages while taking Rifadin because the combination may damage your liver.

Tell your doctor if you're taking other prescription or nonprescription medications because Rifadin decreases the effectiveness of many other medications. For instance, if you're taking an oral contraceptive, you may need to use another method of birth control. If you're taking a heart medication, a blood thinner, or diabetes medication, the doctor may need to change the dosage.

Rifadin will turn your body fluids and secretions reddish orange or reddish brown. It can permanently discolor soft contact lenses, but doesn't affect hard lenses.

Take precautions to avoid injuries or accidental bleeding because Rifadin affects the blood's clotting ability.

Special directions

• Tell your doctor if you have other medical problems, especially liver disease or alcoholism, because they may affect the use of this medication.
• Call your doctor if your symptoms seem worse or don't subside after 2 to 3 weeks of therapy.

Important reminders

Avoid becoming pregnant while taking Rifadin because it can cause birth defects.

If you're pregnant or breast-feeding, don't use this medication without careful discussion with your doctor.

Riopan

This medication is used to relieve heartburn or acid indigestion or to treat symptoms of a stomach or duodenal ulcer. This drug's generic name is magaldrate.

How to take Riopan

This medication is available in regular and chewable tablets and an oral suspension.

If you buy Riopan without a prescription and are treating yourself, carefully follow the instructions on the label. If your doctor prescribed this medication or gave you special dosage instructions, follow those instructions carefully.

If you're using the *chewable tablets,* chew them completely before swallowing. Drink a glass of milk or water afterward.

If you're using the *oral suspension,* shake it well before pouring your dose. Sip water or juice after taking it.

What to do if you miss a dose

If you're taking this medication on a regular schedule, take the missed dose as soon as possible. However, if it's almost time for your next dose, skip the missed dose and resume your regular dosage schedule. Never take a double dose.

What to do about side effects

Constipation or diarrhea may occur. If these symptoms persist or are bothersome, call your doctor.

If you have cramping, bloating, nausea, vomiting, or pain in your stomach or lower abdomen, stop taking Riopan and call your doctor promptly.

What you must know about other drugs

Check with your doctor or pharmacist before taking other medications. Taken in combination, Riopan and another medication might each change the way the other works.

As a general rule, don't take Riopan within 1 to 2 hours of taking another oral medication (such as a tablet, capsule, or liquid). Riopan may make the other medication less effective.

If you're taking Achromycin (tetracycline), Nizoral (ketoconazole), or Hiprex (methenamine), wait 3 hours after a dose before you take Riopan.

If you're taking Inversine (mecamylamine), check with your doctor before taking Riopan because Riopan may increase the risk of side effects.

Special directions

• You shouldn't take Riopan if you have a colostomy or an ileostomy, ulcerative colitis, diverticulitis, chronic diarrhea, kidney problems, a low blood phosphate level, appendicitis, Alzheimer's disease, or unexplained bleeding from the rectum or gastrointestinal tract.

• Check with your doctor if Riopan doesn't improve your stomach problem.
• Don't take this medication for more than 2 weeks unless your doctor tells you to.
• Be aware that the chewable tablets contain sugar.

Important reminder If you're an older adult, check with your doctor before taking Riopan.

Ritalin

This drug is usually given to treat attention-deficit disorder in children. It's sometimes used to treat narcolepsy (sudden episodes of sleeping) in adults. This drug's generic name is methylphenidate.

How to give Ritalin Ritalin is available in regular and sustained-release tablets. Carefully check the prescription label. Administer only the amount prescribed.

If the doctor has prescribed the *sustained-release tablets,* make sure your child swallows them whole and doesn't break, crush, or chew them first.

To help the drug work better, you should give it to your child 30 to 45 minutes before meals. However, if the drug causes loss of appetite, give it after meals.

Give your child the last daily dose 6 hours before bedtime so it won't cause difficulty sleeping.

What to do about a missed dose Give the missed dose as soon as possible; then give remaining doses for that day at regularly spaced intervals. Never give a double dose.

What to do about side effects Call your doctor *right away* if your child has a fast heartbeat, bruising, chest pain, fever, joint pain, a rash, hives, uncontrolled body movements, vision changes, seizures, a sore throat, or unusual weakness or fatigue.

Appetite loss, nervousness, or difficulty sleeping may occur at first. Check with the doctor if these symptoms persist or become bothersome.

Depression, unusual behavior, or unusual weakness or fatigue may occur after your child stops taking this drug. Report these side effects to the doctor.

What you must know about other drugs

Check with the doctor or pharmacist before giving your child Symmetrel (amantadine), amphetamines, asthma medications, or any nonprescription medications. Serious problems could occur when these drugs are combined with Ritalin.

Don't give your child Ritalin within 14 days of a monoamine oxidase (MAO) inhibitor such as Marplan (isocarboxazid), a drug for depression.

Special directions

• Make sure the doctor knows about your child's medical history. Ritalin increases the chance of seizures and may worsen Tourette's syndrome, glaucoma, high blood pressure, psychosis, severe anxiety, agitation, depression, or tics. Also, a child with a history of drug abuse or dependence is more likely to become dependent on Ritalin.

• If your child has been taking this drug in large doses for a long time, the doctor may want to reduce the dosage gradually before stopping it completely.

Don't let your child perform activities requiring alertness or good coordination until you know the effects of the drug.

After long-term treatment, the doctor may recommend drug-free periods to reduce the risk of a slowed growth rate.

Important reminder

If your child has diabetes, the doctor may need to adjust the dosage of diabetes medication.

Robaxin

This medication is usually prescribed to relax muscles and to relieve pain and discomfort caused by muscle injury (such as sprains and strains). The drug's generic name is methocarbamol.

How to take Robaxin Robaxin is available in tablets. Carefully check the prescription label and take only the amount prescribed. If you have trouble swallowing tablets, you may crush the tablets and mix them with food or liquid.

What to do if you miss a dose Take the missed dose if you remember within 1 hour or so. Otherwise, skip the missed dose and resume your regular dosage schedule. Don't take a double dose.

What to do about side effects Call your doctor *right away* if you develop a fever, a fast heartbeat, skin rash or redness, itching, hives, shortness of breath, troubled breathing, wheezing, tightness in the chest, stinging or burning of the eyes, red or bloodshot eyes, or a stuffy nose.

You may experience vision changes (including blurring or double vision), dizziness, light-headedness, or drowsiness. These effects usually go away as your body adjusts to the medication. But you should check with your doctor if they persist or become bothersome.

Robaxin may make you drowsy or less alert and may affect your vision, so avoid potentially hazardous activities, such as driving a car or using dangerous tools.

This medication may discolor your urine. This effect goes away once you stop taking the medication.

You may notice a metallic taste.

What you must know about alcohol and other drugs Avoid alcoholic beverages, sedatives, antihistamines such as Benadryl (diphenhydramine), and other central nervous system depressants while taking Robaxin because of the risk of oversedation.

Special directions • Tell your doctor about other medical problems you have, especially allergies, kidney disease, seizures, or a blood disease caused by an allergy to another medication. Also tell the doctor if you've ever abused or been dependent on drugs.

• To prevent stomach upset, take this drug with meals or milk.

• If you're taking this medication for more than a few weeks, have regular medical checkups so the doctor can evaluate your progress and detect any unwanted side effects.

Important reminders If you're breast-feeding, check with your doctor before taking Robaxin.

If you're an athlete, you should know that the U.S. Olympic Committee and the National Collegiate Athletic Association ban the use of methocarbamol and test for its presence.

Robitussin

This medication will help relieve your cough by loosening mucus or phlegm in your lungs. It's helpful for coughs due to colds but not for long-term coughs, such as those associated with asthma, emphysema, or smoking. This drug's generic name is guaifenesin.

How to take Robitussin Robitussin is available without a prescription; however, your doctor may suggest the proper dosage for your specific condition. The drug comes in tablets, capsules, extended-release tablets and capsules, an oral liquid, and a syrup.

Carefully read and follow the directions and precautions on the medication label. You may take a dose every 4 hours. Don't take more than the recommended total daily dosage.

Drink a full glass (8 ounces) of water with each dose to help loosen phlegm. Also, drink at least eight full glasses during the day unless your doctor orders otherwise.

If you're taking the *extended-release tablet* or the *extended-release capsule*, swallow it whole. Don't crush, break, or chew it.

You shouldn't use this medication for longer than the directions recommend, unless your doctor directs otherwise.

What to do if you miss a dose If you're taking this medication regularly, take the missed dose as soon as possible. But if it's almost time for the next dose, skip the missed dose and take your next dose at its scheduled time. Don't take a double dose.

What you must know about other drugs You should check with your doctor before using other medications — especially nonprescription cough or cold medications — because they can increase Robitussin's effects and cause an overdose.

Special directions
- If your cough doesn't improve within 7 days or you develop a fever, rash, persistent headache, or sore throat, check with your doctor.
- Because this medication may cause dizziness or drowsiness, don't drive, operate machinery, or perform other activities requiring alertness until you know how you respond to it.
- Occasionally throughout the day, take several deep breaths and then cough to help bring up phlegm.
- Avoid fumes, smoke, and dust because they can irritate your lungs.

Important reminder If you're pregnant or think you may be, check with your doctor before taking this medication.

Rogaine

This medication is prescribed to stimulate hair growth. Its generic name is minoxidil.

How to apply Rogaine This medication is available as a topical solution.

Carefully follow the dosage instructions on the label of your prescription applicator. Use only the amount prescribed. Applying more medication won't speed hair growth or cause more hair to grow. In fact, using too much might cause unwanted side effects.

Apply the medication once in the morning and again at bedtime. Before applying the morning dose, shampoo your hair and dry it thoroughly with a towel. Then, starting at the center of the bald area, use the applicator to spread the medication.

After applying your bedtime dose, let the medication dry for at least 30 minutes. This allows more to be absorbed by your scalp and less by your pillowcase.

What to do if you miss a dose

Apply the missed dose as soon as possible; then resume your regular dosage schedule. However, if it's almost time for your next dose, skip the missed dose and go back to your regular schedule. Don't apply the medication twice or try to make up for a missed dose some other way.

What to do about side effects

Call your doctor *right away* if you have difficulty breathing, chest pain, a fast or irregular heartbeat, flushing, headache, dizziness, faintness, rapid weight gain, swelling of the feet or lower legs, or numbness or tingling in your hands, feet, or face.

Check with your doctor if your scalp gets sunburned or starts burning or itching, if your face swells, or if you notice a rash.

Your skin may become reddened or dry and flaky, and you may have increased hair growth on your face, arms, and back. These side effects usually go away over time as your body adjusts to the medication. But you should check with your doctor if they persist or become bothersome.

What you must know about other drugs

Don't apply other drugs to your scalp while using Rogaine. Other drugs may prevent Rogaine from working properly or cause unwanted side effects.

Special directions

• Make sure your doctor knows about your medical history, especially if you have heart disease or high blood pressure or you've had other skin problems, irritation, or sunburn on your scalp.

• If you apply Rogaine by hand, wash your hands thoroughly when you're finished.

• Don't use a hair dryer during treatment because this might make the medication less effective.

• Stop using Rogaine temporarily if your scalp becomes irritated or sunburned — but check with the doctor first.

• You may have to use Rogaine for 4 or more months before you see results, and you must use it every day. If you stop using it, hair growth stops and you can expect to lose any new hair within a few months.

Roxicodone

Your doctor has prescribed this narcotic medication to help relieve your pain. This drug's generic name is oxycodone.

How to take Roxicodone

Roxicodone is available in tablets and an oral solution. Follow the directions exactly as ordered. Don't take more Roxicodone than directed because it may cause an overdose or become habit-forming.

Check with your doctor before you stop taking this medication.

What to do if you miss a dose

Take the missed dose as soon as possible. However, if it's almost time for your next dose, skip the missed dose and take your next dose on schedule. Don't take a double dose.

What to do about side effects

Confusion, seizures, difficulty breathing, severe dizziness or drowsiness, slow heartbeat, and weakness are possible signs of an overdose. If you have any of these side effects, call for emergency medical help *right away.*

This medication can make you sleepy or drowsy or can create a false sense of well-being. And it can cause nausea, vomiting, constipation, or difficulty urinating. Check with your doctor if you develop any of these symptoms, especially if they continue or become severe.

Make sure you know how Roxicodone affects you before driving, operating machinery, or performing other activities requiring alertness.

Roxicodone may also make you feel faint, dizzy, or light-headed, especially when you get up suddenly from a lying or sitting position. To prevent falls, get up slowly from these positions.

What you must know about alcohol and other drugs

Don't drink alcoholic beverages while taking Roxicodone because the combination can lead to oversedation.

For the same reason, check with your doctor before taking medications that slow the central nervous system—for example, many allergy and cold medications, sleeping pills, and muscle relaxants.

If you regularly take blood thinners, aspirin, or products containing aspirin, check with your doctor before using Roxicodone. Combined use may lead to abnormal or prolonged bleeding.

Special directions

• Tell your doctor if you have other medical problems. They may affect the use of this medication.
• Tell your doctor or dentist before you have surgery that you're taking this medication.

Important reminders

If you're pregnant or breast-feeding, check with your doctor before using this medication.

If you're an athlete, you should know that the U.S. Olympic Committee bans the use of oxycodone and tests for its presence.

S

To keep your transplant functioning normally, your doctor has prescribed Sandimmune. This drug's generic name is cyclosporine.

How to take Sandimmune

Sandimmune comes in liquid and capsules. If you take the *liquid* form, measure your dose precisely. Each milliliter of liquid contains 100 milligrams of Sandimmune. Store the liquid at room temperature to prevent it from becoming too thick.

If you wish, mix your dose in a glass container with fruit juice (preferably at room temperature) or milk to make it taste better. Stir it well and drink it immediately. Then rinse the glass with a little more liquid and drink that too to make sure you take all the medication.

If you take the *capsules,* you should know that they come in two strengths: 25 milligrams and 100 milligrams. You may be taking some of both strengths to obtain an exact dose. Swallow the capsules whole. Don't chew or open them.

Take your dose at the same time each day, preferably in the morning. Take it with meals if it causes nausea.

What to do if you miss a dose

If you forget to take a dose or if you vomit soon after taking it, call your doctor *right away*. Follow his or her instructions for getting back on schedule. Never skip a dose or take two doses together.

What to do about side effects

Call your doctor *right away* if you:
- have chills or a fever
- need to urinate frequently
- notice your heart beating irregularly
- feel unusually weak or tired or if your legs feel unusually heavy or weak
- see blood in your urine
- have a seizure
- experience breathing problems.

Also check with your doctor if you have:
- diarrhea or stomach pain with nausea and vomiting
- swollen, tender, or bleeding gums
- headaches or dizziness (indicating a rise in blood pressure)
- shaky or trembling hands
- a change in hair texture.

If Sandimmune causes unwanted hair growth, remove it with a depilatory such as Nair.

What you must know about other drugs

Check with your doctor before you take other medications, including nonprescription preparations. Also tell your doctor before you have any immunizations (vaccinations) while you're being treated with Sandimmune.

Special directions

- Tell your doctor if you have other medical problems, especially high blood pressure or liver or kidney disease.
- Keep all appointments for follow-up tests so your doctor can detect side effects early.
- See your dentist regularly, and inform him or her that you're taking Sandimmune.

Important reminder

If you're pregnant or breast-feeding, check with your doctor before taking Sandimmune.

Sectral

Sectral will help control your high blood pressure or correct your irregular heartbeat. This drug's generic name is acebutolol.

How to take Sectral

Sectral comes in long-acting capsules. Carefully read the medication label, and follow the directions exactly. Don't break, chew, or crush the capsule. Swallow it whole.

Always check your pulse rate before taking Sectral. If it's under 50 beats a minute, call your doctor and don't take the dose.

What to do if you miss a dose

Take the missed dose as soon as you remember. But if it's within 4 hours of your next dose, skip the dose you missed and take your next dose at the regular time. Don't take a double dose.

What to do about side effects

Call the doctor *right away* if you have trouble breathing or swallowing. Also call your doctor if you feel very tired or light-headed (a symptom of low blood pressure).

Make sure you know how you react to this medication before driving or performing activities requiring alertness.

If you feel tired after taking Sectral, plan frequent rest periods.

What you must know about other drugs

Tell the doctor what other medications you're taking because they can affect how Sectral works. For example, taking Sectral with Lanoxin (digoxin) can slow your heart too much, whereas taking it with Indocin (indomethacin) can reduce Sectral's effect.

If you take medication for diabetes, check your blood sugar levels carefully because Sectral can hide signs of low blood sugar levels.

Special directions

• Tell your doctor about medical conditions you have, such as chronic lung disease, diabetes, heart or blood vessel disease, kidney or liver disease, depression, thyroid problems, or an unusually slow heartbeat.
• Tell your doctor and pharmacist if you're allergic to any medications, foods, preservatives, or dyes. Sectral may make allergic reactions worse and harder to treat.
• If you have diabetes, keep a fast-acting carbohydrate, such as a package of raisins, nearby in case your blood sugar level drops.
• Don't abruptly stop taking Sectral. Doing so may lead to heart problems.
• Before you have surgery, dental work, or emergency treatment, tell the doctor that you're taking Sectral.
• Check with your doctor or pharmacist before taking any nonprescription drugs.

Important reminders

Notify your doctor if you become pregnant while taking Sectral.

If you're an athlete, you should know that the National Collegiate Athletic Association and the U.S. Olympic Committee ban the use of acebutolol.

Seldane

This antihistamine can help relieve your allergy symptoms. Unlike most other antihistamines, Seldane usually doesn't cause drowsiness. This drug's generic name is terfenadine.

How to take Seldane
Follow your doctor's instructions precisely. Don't take more than the recommended dose, even if your symptoms don't subside. If you're giving the medication to a child, break the tablet as needed to obtain the right dose.

What to do if you miss a dose
If you're taking this medication on a regular schedule and you miss a dose, take the missed dose as soon as you remember. But if it's almost time for your next dose, skip the missed dose and take your next dose as scheduled. Don't take a double dose.

What to do about side effects
Some patients complain of a headache after taking Seldane. If this happens to you, take Tylenol (acetaminophen) or another mild pain reliever. If the headache is severe, call your doctor.

Drink plenty of fluids while you're taking Seldane, especially if you're congested. That's because Seldane has a drying effect. If you don't stay well hydrated, your secretions could become thick and difficult to cough up.

Special directions
• Tell the doctor if you've ever had an allergic reaction to Seldane or another antihistamine. Also tell the doctor if you have a history of asthma or another lung disorder because Seldane could aggravate these conditions.
• Expect to wait about an hour after taking this medication for your symptoms to subside.

Important reminder
If you're pregnant or breast-feeding, check with your doctor before taking this medication.

Ser-Ap-Es

This medication is prescribed to reduce high blood pressure. The generic components in Ser-Ap-Es are resperine, hydralazine, and hydrochlorothiazide.

How to take Ser-Ap-Es

Follow your doctor's directions exactly for taking this medication. If the tablets upset your stomach, take them with meals or milk.

Ser-Ap-Es may make you urinate more frequently. Scheduling your doses can help prevent this increase in urine from affecting your sleep. If you take one dose daily, take it in the morning after breakfast. If you take more than one dose daily, don't take the last dose after 6 p.m., unless your doctor gives you other instructions.

What to do if you miss a dose

Take the missed dose as soon as possible. But if it's almost time for your next dose, skip the missed dose and take your next dose on schedule. Don't take a double dose.

What to do about side effects

Call your doctor *right away* if you start having nightmares. Also call if you feel drowsy, dizzy, depressed, faint, unusually nervous, or weak. Also tell the doctor if you start to gain weight unexpectedly or if you have a dry mouth, a stuffy nose, a slow heartbeat, or an upset stomach.

Because this medication may make you drowsy or dizzy, make sure you know how you react to it before you drive or perform other activities that might be dangerous if you're not fully alert.

If you're male, let your doctor know if you become impotent while taking this medication.

What you must know about alcohol and other drugs

Don't drink alcoholic beverages unless your doctor approves because combined use with Ser-Ap-Es may cause oversedation. For the same reason, check with your doctor before you take medications that slow down the central nervous system, such as cold, flu, and allergy remedies; sleeping pills; and tranquilizers.

Tell your doctor if you're taking other medications. Also check before you take new prescription or nonprescription medications.

To prevent harmful drug interactions, tell your doctor if you take Eskalith (lithium), heart medication, or adrenocorticoids (cortisone-like medications). Also reveal if you take Marplan (isocarboxazid) or another monoamine oxidase (MAO) inhibitor for depression or other emotional problems.

Special directions   Tell your doctor if you have other medical problems, especially asthma, allergies, diabetes, a seizure disorder, stomach ulcers, gallstones, gout, depression, Parkinson's disease, pheochromocytoma, or heart, kidney, or liver disease. Other medical problems may affect the use of Ser-Ap-Es.

Important reminders   If you're pregnant or breast-feeding, don't use Ser-Ap-Es without discussing the risks and benefits with your doctor.

If you're an older adult, you may be especially prone to this medication's side effects.

Serevent

This medication is prescribed to help relieve asthma. The drug's generic name is salmeterol.

How to take Serevent   You'll use an inhaler to take Serevent. Follow the directions carefully on how to use your inhaler and remember to shake the container of Serevent well before using it. Carefully follow the label directions.

Serevent works the best if you space doses about 12 hours apart. Remember to take it even when you're feeling better. This drug isn't meant to be used for acute asthma attacks.

What to do if you miss a dose   Take the missed dose as soon as you remember. However, if it's almost time for your next dose, skip the missed dose, and return to your regular schedule. Don't take a double dose.

What to do about side effects

Serevent may give you a regular or sinus headache or may make you feel shaky. You may develop a cough, upper or lower respiratory infections, a rash, or other problems with your nose, throat, and sinuses. Serevent may also cause stomach pain or a fast or irregular heartbeat. If any of these effects persists or becomes severe, contact your doctor.

If you experience chest pain after using Serevent, stop using the medication and call your doctor.

What you must know about other drugs

Be careful using this drug if you're sensitive to sympathomimetic drugs such as Primatene Mist or Bronkaid (epinephrine) — you could react more strongly to Serevent. Tell your doctor if you take a beta blocker such as Inderal (propranolol) or methylxanthines such as Theo-Dur (theophylline). If you use Serevent often and take one of these drugs, you could develop heart problems.

Don't take Serevent if you take a monoamine oxidase (MAO) inhibitor such as Marplan (isocarboxazid) or tricyclic antidepressants such as Elavil (amitriptyline). The combination could cause severe heart problems.

Special directions

• Be sure to tell your doctor if you have any heart or blood pressure problems, a thyroid condition, or diabetes or if you suffer from seizures.

• Don't use Serevent more than the recommended twice a day. If you are still having breathing problems, call your doctor. You may need another medication to help your breathing problem.

• If you're already using another medication to help your breathing, such as Proventil (albuterol), talk to your doctor about coordinating your medications.

• If you have an asthma attack, use your asthma attack medication, not Serevent. If you're using your asthma attack medication more than four times a day, talk to your doctor; you may need to change medications.

• If you take Serevent to prevent breathing problems when you exercise, you should take it 30 to 60 minutes before you exercise.

Important reminders

If you're an older adult with a heart problem, watch carefully for side effects.

Tell your doctor if you're pregnant and discuss whether you should breast-feed while taking Serevent.

Sinemet

Sinemet is usually given to treat Parkinson's disease. This drug's generic name is levodopa with carbidopa.

How to take Sinemet This medication is available in tablets. Carefully check the label on your prescription bottle, which tells you how much to take. The doctor may prescribe three to six tablets daily. Take only the amount prescribed.

What to do if you miss a dose Take the missed dose as soon as possible. However, if your next scheduled dose is within 2 hours, skip the missed one and resume your regular dosage schedule. Never take a double dose.

What to do about side effects Call your doctor if you experience fatigue, headache, shortness of breath, insomnia, depression, mood or behavior changes, or unusual and uncontrolled body movements.

This medication may make you dizzy, especially when you first start taking it. Tell your doctor if you feel dizzy or light-headed when you get up from a lying or sitting position.

Before getting out of bed, change position slowly and dangle your legs for a few moments to avoid dizziness.

Avoid potentially hazardous activities, such as driving a car or using dangerous tools, until you know how this medication affects you. It may make you drowsy or less alert.

If Sinemet upsets your stomach, you may take it with food.

Contact your doctor if you believe your behavior or mood is changing.

What you must know about other drugs Check with your doctor or pharmacist before taking other prescription or nonprescription drugs because they can change the way Sinemet works.

Monoamine oxidase (MAO) inhibitors (drugs for depression) can cause very high blood pressure when taken within 14 days of Sinemet. Check with your doctor or pharmacist about stopping treatment.

Special directions

• Make sure your doctor knows about your medical history before you take this medication.
• The doctor may need to change your dosage, possibly several times, to find the right amount for you to take.
• Increase your physical activities gradually so your body can adjust to your changing balance, coordination, and circulation.
• You may not notice this drug's effects for several weeks. If you don't think it's working, don't stop taking it; call your doctor. Also, don't increase the dosage if your symptoms continue or get worse; check with the doctor.

Important reminders

If you're breast-feeding, check with your doctor before taking Sinemet.

If you have diabetes, the doctor may need to adjust your dosage of insulin or other diabetes medication. Also, you may need to switch to another type of urine glucose test.

Solfoton

This medication is used to prevent seizures caused by epilepsy and other disorders. It's also used as a sedative to produce relaxation — for example, before surgery. The drug's generic name is phenobarbital.

How to take Solfoton

Solfoton comes in tablets, capsules, an oral solution, and an elixir. Take it exactly as prescribed by your doctor. Don't increase your dose. Solfoton can become habit-forming.

If you're taking the *capsule or tablet* form, swallow it whole; don't chew or crush it.

If you're taking this medication for epilepsy, take it every day in regularly spaced doses, as prescribed.

What to do if you miss a dose

Take the missed dose as soon as possible. However, if it's almost time for your next dose, skip the missed dose and take your next dose on schedule. Don't take a double dose.

What to do about side effects

Call for emergency medical help *at once* if you think you may have taken an overdose. Symptoms of overdose include severe drowsiness, weakness, and confusion; slurred speech; and difficulty breathing.

Check with your doctor *right away* if you have any skin problems. Also let the doctor know if this medication makes you feel drowsy, sluggish, or hungover.

Because Solfoton can make you drowsy, make sure you know how you react to it before you drive or perform other activities that require you to be fully alert.

What you must know about alcohol and other drugs

Avoid drinking alcoholic beverages while taking Solfoton. The combination can lead to oversedation.

For the same reason, don't use other medications that depress the central nervous system, including tranquilizers, sleeping pills, and many cold and flu remedies.

To prevent harmful drug interactions, tell your doctor about other medications you're taking. Solfoton may not work well with blood thinners, birth control pills, or estrogen.

Special directions

• Tell your doctor if you have other medical problems, especially asthma, lung disease, or porphyria. Also reveal if you're depressed or in chronic pain.

• Before you have medical tests, tell the doctor you're taking Solfoton because it can affect the test results.

Important reminders

If you're pregnant or breast-feeding, don't take Solfoton without specific instructions from your doctor.

If you're an older adult, you may be especially sensitive to this drug's side effects.

If you're an athlete, you should know that the U.S. Olympic Committee and the National Collegiate Athletic Association ban the use of phenobarbital and sometimes test for it.

Soma

This medication relaxes your muscles and relieves the pain and discomfort of strains, sprains, and other muscle injuries. The drug's generic name is carisoprodol.

How to take Soma

Soma comes in tablet form. Follow the directions on your medication label exactly.

What to do if you miss a dose

If you remember within 1 hour or so, take the dose you missed right away. But if you don't remember until later, skip the missed dose and resume your normal dosage schedule. Don't take a double dose.

What to do about side effects

Common side effects include drowsiness, dizziness, and skin changes. If these symptoms persist or worsen, call your doctor.

Make sure you know how you react to Soma before you drive, operate machinery, or perform other activities requiring alertness and coordination.

What you must know about alcohol and other drugs

Tell your doctor if you're taking other medications. Avoid taking Soma with alcoholic beverages or other drugs that depress the central nervous system (such as sleeping pills and cold remedies). Doing so can cause increased drowsiness and dizziness.

Special directions

• Before you start to take Soma, tell your doctor if you have other medical problems. They may affect the use of this medication.

• If you're taking this medication for more than a few weeks, see your doctor regularly to check your progress.

Important reminders

If you become pregnant while taking Soma, tell your doctor.

If you're breast-feeding, be aware that Soma passes into breast milk and can cause drowsiness and stomach upset in breast-feeding infants. Discuss its use with your doctor.

If you're an athlete, be aware that the National Collegiate Athletic Association and the U.S. Olympic Committee ban the use of carisoprodol.

Sparine

This medication is used to treat nervous, mental, and emotional disorders. This drug's generic name is promazine.

How to take Sparine

Sparine comes in tablets and a syrup. Follow your doctor's directions exactly. Take your medication with food or a full glass (8 ounces) of water or milk.

What to do if you miss a dose

If you take more than one dose a day, take the missed dose right away if you remember within 1 hour or so. But if you don't remember until later, skip it and take your next dose on schedule. Don't take a double dose.

What to do about side effects

Call your doctor *right away* if you have fever, chills, headache, or extreme tiredness. Also call *at once* if you start sweating heavily or have a fast heartbeat or difficulty breathing.

Check with your doctor if you feel dizzy, your skin turns yellow, or you start to have blurred vision, dry mouth, constipation, or difficulty urinating.

Sparine can cause a movement disorder called tardive dyskinesia, so be sure to report any uncontrolled movements of your mouth, tongue, or other body parts.

Because Sparine may make you dizzy, make sure you know how you react to it before you drive or perform other activities requiring alertness.

This medication may make you more sensitive to light, so cover up outdoors and limit your sun exposure.

What you must know about alcohol and other drugs

Don't drink alcoholic beverages while taking Sparine because the combination can cause oversedation. For the same reason, avoid medications that slow down the central nervous system, including tranquilizers, sleeping pills, and cold and flu remedies.

Tell your doctor about other medications you're taking. In particular, your doctor needs to know if you're taking blood thinners or medications for Parkinson's disease, depression, manic-depressive disorder, or high blood pressure.

If you take antacids, take them at least 2 hours before or after you take Sparine.

Special directions Tell your doctor if you have other medical conditions, especially heart or blood disease, glaucoma, a seizure disorder, Parkinson's disease, or kidney, lung, or liver problems. These conditions and other medical problems may affect the use of Sparine.

Important reminders If you're pregnant or breast-feeding, check with your doctor before taking Sparine.

Children and older adults are especially prone to Sparine's side effects.

If you're an athlete, you should know that the U.S. Olympic Committee and the National Collegiate Athletic Association ban the use of promazine.

Sudafed

Used to relieve stuffiness of your nose or sinuses, Sudafed also relieves ear congestion caused by ear infection or inflammation. This drug's generic name is pseudoephedrine. Another brand name is Drixoral.

How to take Sudafed This medication comes in tablets, a syrup, an oral solution, and extended-release tablets and capsules. If this medication was prescribed, follow the doctor's directions exactly. If you bought the medication without a prescription, carefully follow the package instructions.

If you're taking the *extended-release tablets* or *capsules*, swallow them whole; don't chew, crush, or break them.

To prevent trouble sleeping, take your last dose for the day a few hours before bedtime.

What to do if you miss a dose If you remember within 1 hour or so, take the missed dose right away. If you don't remember until later, skip the missed dose and take your next dose on schedule. Don't take a double dose.

What to do about side effects

Check with your doctor if this medication makes you feel anxious, nervous, or restless or causes palpitations or trouble sleeping.

If Sudafed makes your mouth feel dry, use sugarless gum or hard candy, melt bits of ice in your mouth, or use a saliva substitute.

What you must know about other drugs

Check with your doctor before you use new prescription or nonprescription medications. Also, tell your doctor about other medications you're taking, especially medications for high blood pressure.

If you're taking a monoamine oxidase (MAO) inhibitor (a drug used to treat depression and other emotional problems) such as Marplan (isocarboxazid), don't use Sudafed because the combination can cause a life-threatening rise in blood pressure.

Special directions

• Tell your doctor if you have other medical problems, especially high blood pressure, heart disease, an overactive thyroid, diabetes, or difficulty urinating. Other medical problems may affect the use of this medication.

• If you don't feel better within 5 days or if you also have a high fever, check with your doctor. These signs may mean you have some other medical problem.

Important reminders

If you're pregnant or breast-feeding, check with your doctor before using Sudafed.

If you're an athlete, you should know that the U.S. Olympic Committee bans the use of pseudoephedrine and tests for the drug.

Surfak

This medication is a laxative used to treat constipation. The drug is known generically as docusate calcium.

How to take Surfak
Surfak comes in capsule form. If this medication was prescribed, follow the doctor's directions exactly. If you bought this medication without a prescription, carefully read the package directions before taking your first dose.

What to do if you miss a dose
Check with your doctor or pharmacist for how to handle a missed dose.

What to do about side effects
Although side effects aren't common, Surfak may irritate your throat or leave a bitter taste in your mouth. You may also have mild abdominal cramping or diarrhea. If these symptoms persist or become severe, call your doctor.

What you must know about other drugs
Don't take mineral oil while you're taking Surfak because it may cause your body to absorb too much mineral oil, causing unwanted effects.

If you're taking other medications, take them at least 2 hours before or 2 hours after taking Surfak because Surfak may interfere with the desired actions of the other medications.

Special directions
• Don't use Surfak (or any other laxative) if you have symptoms of appendicitis or an inflamed bowel, such as stomach or lower abdominal pain, cramping, bloating, soreness, nausea, or vomiting. Instead, check with your doctor as soon as possible.

• Drink at least six 8-ounce glasses of water or other liquids daily. This will help soften your bowel movements and relieve constipation.

• Don't take Surfak for more than 1 week unless your doctor has prescribed a special schedule for you. This is true even if you continue to have constipation.

• If you notice a sudden change in your bowel habits or function that lasts longer than 2 weeks or that occurs from time to time, check with your doctor. Your doctor will need to find the cause of your problem before it becomes more serious.

• Don't overuse Surfak. Otherwise, you may become dependent on this medication to produce a bowel movement. In severe cases, overuse of laxatives can damage the nerves, muscles, and other tissues of the bowel.

Important reminders If you're pregnant, check with your doctor before taking Surfak.

Don't give this medication to children under age 6 unless a doctor prescribes it.

Symmetrel

Used to prevent or treat type A influenza (flu), Symmetrel is also used to treat Parkinson's disease and the stiffness and shaking caused by some other medications. This drug's generic name is amantadine.

How to take Symmetrel
Symmetrel comes as capsules and a syrup. Follow the directions on your medication label exactly.

Take the doses at regular intervals both day and night. Pour the syrup into a measuring spoon — not a household teaspoon — for an accurate dose.

If you're taking Symmetrel to prevent or treat influenza, finish all of your medication. If you stop taking it too soon, your symptoms may recur.

What to do if you miss a dose
Take the missed dose as soon as possible. However, if you're within 4 hours of the next dose, skip the missed dose and go back to your regular dosage schedule. Don't take a double dose.

What to do about side effects
Contact the doctor *immediately* if you faint, have blurred vision, feel confused, have difficulty urinating, or experience seizures or hallucinations.

Common side effects include dizziness, distractibility, irritability, difficulty sleeping, and purplish red, lacy spots on your skin. If any of these side effects persists or becomes severe, contact your doctor.

Until you know how this medication affects you, avoid driving or other activities that require alertness and clear vision.

You may feel dizzy, light-headed, or faint if you get up suddenly from a lying or sitting position. Getting up slowly may help.

Symmetrel may cause mouth, nose, and throat dryness. Try using sugarless hard candy or gum, ice chips, or a saliva substitute. If dryness persists after 2 weeks, check with your doctor.

What you must know about alcohol and other drugs

Avoid alcoholic beverages while you're taking Symmetrel because they can increase the drug's side effects.

Special directions

• If you're taking this medication to prevent or treat the flu and your symptoms continue or worsen within a few days, contact your doctor.

• If you think Symmetrel is losing its effectiveness for you, call your doctor. Don't adjust the dosage on your own. And don't stop taking your medication suddenly. If you do, your Parkinson's disease or symptoms may become worse. The doctor may reduce your dose gradually.

Important reminders

If you're pregnant or breast-feeding, notify your doctor.

Older adults may be especially sensitive to Symmetrel's side effects.

Synalar

Your doctor has prescribed Synalar to help relieve redness, swelling, itching, and other skin discomfort. This drug's generic name is fluocinolone.

How to apply Synalar

Synalar is available as a cream, ointment, or topical solution. To apply it, follow your doctor's directions exactly. Use your finger to apply it to your skin. Then wash your hands. Don't bandage or wrap the area being treated unless your doctor directs you to do so.

What to do if you miss an application

Apply the missed dose as soon as possible. But if it's almost time for your next dose, skip the missed dose and apply the next dose on your regular schedule.

What to do about side effects

Although side effects from using Synalar are uncommon, the drug may produce such skin reactions as burning, itching, dryness, changes in color or texture, or a rash and inflammation (dermatitis). Consult your doctor if you have these side effects.

If you're applying Synalar to a child's diaper area, avoid using tight-fitting diapers or plastic pants, which could increase absorption of the medication through the skin and possibly cause side effects.

Special directions

- If you have other medical problems, be sure to let your doctor know. A change in your medication may be necessary while you're using Synalar.
- Don't get Synalar in your eyes. If you do, flush your eyes with water.
- If the doctor tells you to apply an occlusive dressing (an airtight covering, such as plastic wrap or a special patch) over Synalar, be sure to get complete directions for doing so.
- Don't use leftover medication for other skin problems without first consulting your doctor.

Important reminders

If you become pregnant while using Synalar, consult your doctor.

Don't apply this medication to your breasts before breast-feeding.

Children and adolescents using this medication should be checked closely. Synalar can affect growth and cause other unwanted effects.

If you're an older adult, you may be especially susceptible to certain side effects, such as skin tearing and blood blisters.

Synthroid

This thyroid hormone supplements the amount of hormone produced by your thyroid gland. Its generic name, which is also another brand name, is levothyroxine.

How to take Synthroid

Take Synthroid exactly as your doctor has prescribed. Don't take more or less of it, and don't take it more often than prescribed. Also, don't stop taking this medication without first talking with your doctor.

If you're taking Synthroid for an underactive thyroid gland, realize that it may take several weeks before you notice any change in your condition.

What to do if you miss a dose
Take the missed dose as soon as possible. But if it's almost time for your next dose, skip the missed dose and take your next dose as scheduled. Don't take two doses at the same time.

If you miss two or more doses in a row, call your doctor.

What to do about side effects
Call your doctor *right away* if you develop any of these symptoms:
- nervousness
- an inability to sleep
- hand tremors
- a rapid heartbeat or palpitations
- nausea
- headache
- fever
- sweating.

Also let your doctor know if you experience a change in your appetite, changes in your menstrual period, diarrhea, increased sensitivity to heat, leg cramps, irritability, or weight loss.

What you must know about other drugs
Some drugs, when taken with Synthroid, can cause undesirable effects. Let your doctor know if you're taking amphetamines, blood thinners, diet pills, medication for a high cholesterol level, medication for asthma or other breathing problems, or allergy or cold medication.

Before you take any other drugs, check with your doctor or pharmacist.

Special directions
- Because other medical problems may affect how much Synthyroid is prescribed, let your doctor know if you have diabetes, hardening of the arteries, heart disease, high blood pressure, or an underactive adrenal or pituitary gland.
- If you have heart disease, Synthroid may cause you to develop chest pain or shortness of breath when you exert yourself. If this occurs, take care not to overdo physical exercise.

Important reminder
Let your doctor know right away if you become pregnant or if you're breast-feeding.

T

Tagamet

This medication treats ulcers and may prevent their return. It may also be used to treat Zollinger-Ellison disease, an illness in which the stomach makes too much acid. This drug's generic name is cimetidine.

How to take Tagamet

Tagamet is available as an oral solution and tablets.

Carefully follow the directions on your prescription label. If you're taking this medication once a day, take it at bedtime unless otherwise directed. If you're taking two doses a day, take one in the morning and one at bedtime. If you're taking more than two doses a day, take them with meals and at bedtime for best results.

What to do if you miss a dose

Take the missed dose as soon as possible. But if it's almost time for your next dose, skip the missed dose and take your next dose as scheduled. Don't take a double dose.

What to do about side effects

Contact your doctor *immediately* if you develop signs and symptoms of infection or bleeding.

A common side effect is mild, temporary diarrhea. If this symptom doesn't go away or becomes severe, call your doctor.

What you must know about other drugs

Tell your doctor about other medications you're taking. Antacids may interfere with the absorption of Tagamet.

Also, Tagamet can interfere with the breakdown of other medications in your body, including Coumadin (warfarin), a blood thinner; Dilantin (phenytoin), a seizure medication; Theo-Dur (theophylline), an asthma medication; Inderal (propranolol), a heart and high blood pressure medication; and some sedatives.

Special directions

• Tell your doctor if you have other medical problems, especially kidney and liver disease.

• Several days may pass before Tagamet begins to relieve your stomach pain. In the meantime, you may take antacids unless your doctor has told you not to use them. Wait 30 minutes to 1 hour between taking the antacid and Tagamet.

• Tell the doctor that you're taking this medication before you have skin tests for allergies or tests to determine how much acid your stomach produces.

• Avoid cigarette smoking because it reduces the effectiveness of Tagamet.

• Contact your doctor if your ulcer pain continues or gets worse while taking Tagamet.

Important reminders

If you're pregnant or breast-feeding, talk to your doctor before you use Tagamet.

If you're an older adult, you may be especially prone to Tagamet's side effects.

Talwin

Your doctor has prescribed Talwin to relieve your pain. This drug's generic name is pentazocine.

How to take Talwin

Talwin comes in tablet and injection forms. If you're taking the *tablets,* carefully follow the prescription directions. If you're *injecting* yourself with Talwin at home, make sure you understand and follow your doctor's instructions exactly.

Don't take more Talwin or use it for a longer time than directed because it may become habit-forming. If you think this medication isn't helping your pain, check with your doctor.

What to do if you miss a dose

Take the missed dose as soon as you remember. However, if it's almost time for your next dose, skip the missed dose and take your next dose at the scheduled time. Don't take a double dose.

What to do about side effects

Get emergency help *at once* if you think you may have taken an overdose. Symptoms of overdose include seizures; confusion; severe nervousness, restlessness, dizziness, weakness, or drowsiness; and slow or troubled breathing.

Let your doctor know if you feel dizzy, light-headed, faint, or drowsy or if you have difficulty urinating or nausea and vomiting.

Because Talwin may make you drowsy or light-headed, don't drive or perform activities requiring alertness until you know how you respond.

What you must know about alcohol and other drugs Don't drink alcoholic beverages while taking Talwin. Combined use increases the depressant effects of the medication on the central nervous system. For the same reason, don't take other depressant medications, such as sleeping pills, tranquilizers, and cold and flu medications, unless your doctor tells you otherwise. And avoid other narcotic pain relievers, such as Darvon (propoxyphene).

Special directions • Tell your doctor if you have other medical problems, especially lung disease, colitis, or a history of seizures, emotional problems, or alcohol or drug abuse. Also reveal if you have any disease that affects a major organ, such as the heart, kidneys, and liver.

• Don't stop taking Talwin suddenly without checking first with your doctor. Your doctor may want you to reduce your dosage gradually to lessen the chance of withdrawal effects.

Important reminders If you're pregnant or breast-feeding, check with your doctor before using Talwin.

If you're an older adult, you may be especially prone to Talwin's side effects.

If you're an athlete, you should know that the U.S. Olympic Committee bans the use of pentazocine and tests for its presence.

Tambocor

This medication helps stabilize your heart rhythm. Tambocor's generic name is flecainide.

How to take Tambocor

This medication comes in tablet form. Take two daily doses 12 hours apart in the morning and evening unless your doctor orders otherwise.

What to do if you miss a dose

Take the missed dose of Tambocor as soon as possible if you remember within 6 hours of your regularly scheduled time. If it's later than that, skip the missed dose and resume your normal dosage schedule. Don't take a double dose.

What to do about side effects

Seek medical treatment *right away* if you experience any of these side effects: chest pain, irregular heartbeat, shortness of breath, swelling in your feet or lower legs, and trembling or shaking.

Tambocor may also cause dizziness, headache, and vision problems. If these symptoms persist or become severe, consult your doctor.

Because Tambocor may make you feel dizzy, light-headed, or sluggish, don't drive a car or perform activities requiring alertness until you know how this medication affects you.

What you must know about other drugs

Tell your doctor if you're taking other drugs, particularly other heart medications. These may produce unpredictable effects when taken with Tambocor.

Special directions

• Before taking Tambocor, discuss other medical problems you have with your doctor, especially kidney or liver disease, a recent heart attack, or a pacemaker.
• See your doctor regularly so he or she can check your progress and adjust your dosage as needed.
• Carry medical identification with you or wear a medical identification bracelet stating that you're taking Tambocor.
• Before you undergo any dental or surgical procedure or emergency treatment, tell the dentist or doctor that you're taking Tambocor.

- If you've been taking this medication regularly for several weeks, don't suddenly stop taking it. Check with your doctor, who can help you reduce the dosage gradually.

Important reminders   If you're pregnant or breast-feeding, check with your doctor before taking Tambocor.

If you're an older adult, you may be especially susceptible to Tambocor's side effects.

Tapazole

This medication is usually prescribed to treat an overactive thyroid gland. Tapazole's generic name is methimazole.

How to take Tapazole   This medication is available in tablets. Carefully check the prescription label and take only the amount prescribed.

If the doctor has prescribed more than one daily dose, take the doses at evenly spaced intervals throughout the day and night. If you need help in planning the best times to take the doses, call your doctor or pharmacist.

Take this medication at a consistent time every day in relation to meals. Either take all doses with meals or take all doses on an empty stomach. If this drug upsets your stomach, you may want to take it with meals.

What to do if you miss a dose   Take the missed dose as soon as possible. However, if it's almost time for your next regular dose, take both doses together; then resume your regular dosage schedule. If you miss two or more doses, check with your doctor.

What to do about side effects   Call your doctor *immediately* if you experience nausea, vomiting, fever, chills, a sore throat, malaise, unusual bleeding, or yellowing of the eyes.

What you must know about other drugs   Check with your doctor or pharmacist if you're taking Eskalith (lithium), Pima (potassium iodide), or Iophen (iodinated glycerol). These drugs may reduce your thyroid function too much and increase the chance for goiter (swollen thyroid gland) when taken with Tapazole. Avoid nonprescription cough remedies because they may contain iodine, which may make Tapazole less effective.

Special directions

- Tell your doctor about other medical problems you have, especially an infection or liver disease.
- To maintain the proper amount of this medication in your blood, don't skip any doses.
- When your thyroid function becomes normal, the doctor may reduce your dosage.
- Ask your doctor whether you can eat shellfish or use iodized salt. The iodine in these substances may make Tapazole less effective.
- If you're injured or get sick, you may need to stop taking this medication or you may need to take a different dosage for a while. Call your doctor for instructions.
- Contact your doctor if you have symptoms of an underactive thyroid, such as mental depression, intolerance to cold, or swelling. These symptoms may mean your dosage should be changed.
- This medication may take several weeks to work. Don't stop taking it without consulting your doctor.
- Tell the doctor or dentist before having any type of surgery.

Important reminders

If you're pregnant, make sure the doctor monitors you carefully during treatment.

If you're breast-feeding, check with your doctor before taking Tapazole.

Tavist

Your doctor has prescribed Tavist to relieve your hay fever or other allergy. This drug's generic name is clemastine.

How to take Tavist

Take Tavist exactly as ordered on your prescription label. Take it with food, water, or milk to lessen stomach irritation.

What to do if you miss a dose

If you take this medication regularly and you miss a dose, take the missed dose as soon as possible. But if it's almost time for your next dose, skip the missed dose and take your next dose on schedule. Don't take a double dose.

What to do about side effects

Call your doctor *immediately* if you've been told your blood count is abnormal or if you develop a fever, shortness of breath, or bleeding.

This medication may make you feel drowsy or cause dryness of your mouth. Call your doctor if these symptoms persist or become severe.

Make sure you know how you react to Tavist before you drive, use machines, or perform other activities that require alertness.

If you experience dry mouth, try using sugarless hard candy or gum, ice chips, or a saliva substitute. If your dry mouth lasts for more than 2 weeks, check with your doctor or dentist.

What you must know about alcohol and other drugs

Don't drink alcoholic beverages while taking this medication. Doing so could cause you to become oversedated.

Tell your doctor about other medications you're taking. Depressants (medications that slow down your central nervous system) may increase the sedative effect of Tavist. Don't use Tavist if you take a monoamine oxidase (MAO) inhibitor such as Marplan (isocarboxazid).

Also let your doctor know if you take large amounts of aspirin, such as for arthritis pain. Tavist may cover up warning signs of aspirin overdose.

Special directions

• Because this medication can aggravate certain conditions, tell your doctor if you have other medical problems, especially asthma, glaucoma, an enlarged prostate, bladder problems, or difficulty urinating. Also reveal if you have heart disease, an overactive thyroid, diabetes, or stomach ulcers.

• Inform the doctor that you're taking this medication before you have skin tests for allergies because Tavist may alter the test results.

Important reminders If you're pregnant or breast-feeding, don't use Tavist unless your doctor instructs you otherwise.

Children and older adults are especially sensitive to the effects of Tavist and therefore more likely to develop side effects.

Tegretol

This medication controls some types of seizures. It's also used to treat pain from trigeminal neuralgia. This drug's generic name is carbamazepine.

How to take Tegretol Tegretol comes in oral suspension, tablet, and chewable tablet forms. Carefully read your medication label. Follow the directions exactly. Take Tegretol with meals.

What to do if you miss a dose Take the missed dose as soon as you remember. However, if it's almost time for your next dose, skip the dose you missed and take the next dose at the scheduled time. Never take a double dose. If you miss more than one dose a day, check with your doctor.

What to do about side effects Consult the doctor *at once* if you have signs of infection (fever, chills, cough) or unusual bleeding (bruises or bloody urine or stools).

Common side effects include dizziness, drowsiness, clumsiness, nausea, vertigo (sensation that objects are spinning), mouth sores, and rashes. If these symptoms persist or worsen, notify your doctor.

Make sure you know how you react to Tegretol before driving or performing other activities requiring alertness.

Your sensitivity to sunlight may increase, especially at first. Protect yourself from the sun. If you have a severe reaction, notify your doctor.

What you must know about alcohol and other drugs Be sure to tell your doctor about other medications you're taking. Alcoholic beverages and central nervous system depressants (such as sleeping pills and cold remedies) may reduce alertness and coordination. Some drugs may decrease or increase Tegretol's effects and the effects of other drugs you take.

Special directions • As a pain reliever, Tegretol works only for certain kinds of pain. Don't take it for other discomfort.

• If you're taking Tegretol for seizures, don't stop using it without consulting your doctor, who may reduce the dosage gradually.

• Have regular checkups to monitor your progress and make dosage changes.

• Before medical tests, surgery, dental work, or emergency treatment, tell your doctor or dentist that you're taking Tegretol.

• Carry an identification card or bracelet that states you're taking Tegretol.

Important reminders If you have diabetes, Tegretol may affect your urine glucose levels.

If you're pregnant or breast-feeding, consult the doctor before taking Tegretol.

Children and older adults may be especially sensitive to this medication.

If you're an athlete, you should know that the U.S. Olympic Committee and the National Collegiate Athletic Association ban the use of carbamazepine.

Tenormin

Tenormin is used to treat high blood pressure, relieve chest pain caused by angina, and prevent another heart attack in recent heart attack victims. This drug's generic name is atenolol.

How to take Tenormin Swallow the tablet whole; don't crush, break, or chew it.

Your doctor may tell you to check your pulse rate before and after taking Tenormin. If it's much slower than usual, call the doctor before taking the next dose.

Try not to miss doses. Some conditions become worse when this medication isn't taken regularly.

What to do if you miss a dose

Take the missed dose as soon as possible. However, if it's within 8 hours of your next dose, skip the missed dose and resume your regular dosage schedule. Don't take a double dose.

What to do about side effects

Contact the doctor *immediately* if you have trouble breathing, swollen ankles, or a sudden weight gain of 3 pounds (1.4 kilograms) or more (signs that you're retaining water) or if your blood pressure rises.

You may feel light-headed and extremely tired and have a slow pulse rate. If these symptoms persist or become severe, contact your doctor.

Because Tenormin may make you drowsy, avoid driving, using machinery, or performing other activities that require alertness.

You may be especially sensitive to cold while taking Tenormin, especially if you have blood circulation problems.

What you must know about other drugs

Tell your doctor if you're taking other medications. If you're taking other medications to lower your blood pressure, Tenormin may lower your blood pressure too much. If you're taking Lanoxin (digoxin), your pulse rate may become dangerously slow. Indocin (indomethacin) may make Tenormin less effective.

If you're taking an antidiabetic medication or insulin, check your blood sugar level carefully because Tenormin can hide low blood sugar levels.

Special directions

• Tell your doctor if you have other medical problems, especially breathing problems, diabetes, kidney or liver disease, depression, or thyroid problems.

• If you have allergies to medications, foods, preservatives, or dyes, this medication may worsen allergic reactions and make them harder to treat.

• Don't suddenly stop taking this medication because your condition may worsen. Your doctor may reduce the amount you're taking gradually.

• Before surgery, emergency treatment, or medical tests, tell the doctor or dentist that you're taking Tenormin.

• Check with your doctor before taking any nonprescription medications.

Important reminders   Contact your doctor if you become pregnant while taking Tenormin.

Older adults are especially sensitive to this medication and likely to experience side effects.

If you're an athlete, you should know that the U.S. Olympic Committee and the National Collegiate Athletic Association ban the use of atenolol.

Tenuate

Your doctor has prescribed short-term use of this medication to treat your obesity. This drug's generic name is diethylpropion.

How to take Tenuate   Tenuate comes in the form of tablets and extended-release tablets. Follow the directions on your prescription bottle exactly as ordered. Take the last dose of the day about 4 to 6 hours before bedtime to help prevent insomnia. Don't break, crush, or chew the tablets — swallow them whole.

Don't stop taking this medication suddenly without first checking with your doctor. Your doctor may want to decrease your dose gradually to prevent withdrawal symptoms.

What to do if you miss a dose   Before you start taking Tenuate, ask your doctor for instructions on what to do if you miss a dose.

What to do about side effects   Check with your doctor if you become nervous or experience a rapid heartbeat or palpitations while taking this medication, especially if your symptoms persist or become severe.

Because this medication may make you dizzy or drowsy, make sure you know how you react to it before you drive or use machines that could be dangerous if you're not fully alert.

If you're taking Tenuate for a long time and think you may be dependent on it, check with your doctor. Some signs of dependence are a strong desire or need to continue taking this medication, a need to increase the dose to receive its effects, or withdrawal side effects when you stop taking it.

What you must know about other drugs

Tell your doctor if you're taking other medications. Monoamine oxidase (MAO) inhibitors such as Marplan (isocarboxazid), which are used to treat depression, may increase your blood pressure to a dangerous level when used with Tenuate.

Special directions

• Before you begin using Tenuate, tell your doctor if you have other medical problems.

• See your doctor at regular intervals to make sure this medication doesn't cause unwanted effects.

• Before having any kind of surgery, dental treatment, or emergency treatment, tell the doctor or dentist that you're taking Tenuate.

Important reminders

If you're pregnant or breast-feeding, don't take this medication without your doctor's approval.

If you have diabetes, Tenuate may affect your blood sugar levels. If you notice a change in the results of your urine or blood glucose test, call your doctor.

If you're an athlete, you should know that the U.S. Olympic Committee and the National Collegiate Athletic Association ban the use of diethylpropion.

Terazol

Your doctor has ordered Terazol to treat your vaginal fungal infection. This drug's generic name is terconazole.

How to use Terazol

Terazol is available as a cream and a suppository. Both forms come with an applicator. Use the applicator to insert the medication into your vagina at bedtime. If you're inserting a vaginal suppository, remain lying down for at least 30 minutes after each dose to allow your vagina time to absorb the Terazol.

Use the medication for the number of nights prescribed by your doctor. Don't stop before then, even if your symptoms subside. If you stop using the medication too soon, your symptoms may return.

What to do if you miss a dose

Take the missed dose as soon as possible. But if it's almost time for your next dose, skip the missed dose and take your next dose as scheduled.

What to do about side effects

If your vagina becomes irritated or burns after using this medication and it wasn't irritated and didn't burn before, call your doctor as soon as possible.

Some women develop a headache after using Terazol. If this occurs, take Tylenol (acetaminophen) or another mild pain reliever.

Special directions

• Tell your doctor if you've ever had an allergic reaction to any antifungal drug. Also tell your doctor if you're using a douche or another type of vaginal medication.

• Keep using the medication, even if your period starts. But don't use tampons so you won't remove any of the medication from your vagina,

• To keep the medication from soiling your clothes, wear a minipad or sanitary napkin.

• If your symptoms don't subside or if they worsen after using the medication for several days, call your doctor.

• To keep your infection from returning, you need to develop good health habits: Wear panties made only of cotton, instead of nylon or rayon. Or choose pantyhose or panties that have a cotton crotch.

• It's possible to spread your infection to your sexual partner during intercourse. Also, your partner could be carrying the fungus in his genital tract. To keep from spreading the infection or to keep from becoming reinfected, have your partner wear a condom during intercourse.

Theo-Dur

Your doctor has prescribed Theo-Dur to help treat and prevent the symptoms of your asthma. This drug's generic name is theophylline. Another brand name is Slo-Bid.

How to take Theo-Dur

Theo-Dur is available as a liquid, tablet, and capsule. Follow your doctor's instructions exactly. Don't take more or less, and don't take it more often or longer than directed. Take your medication at the same time every day.

In general, take Theo-Dur 30 minutes to 1 hour before meals or 2 hours after meals, unless your doctor directs you otherwise. Theo-Dur works best on an empty stomach.

If you're taking the *extended-release* form of the medication, don't crush or break the capsules or tablets.

What to do if you miss a dose

For the medication to work properly, you need to take every dose on time. If you do miss a dose, though, take the missed dose as soon as possible. If it's almost time for your next dose, skip the missed dose and take your next dose on schedule.

What to do about side effects

Call the doctor *immediately* if you develop diarrhea or have a seizure. Also let the doctor know if you feel nervous or dizzy, have difficulty sleeping, have a rapid heartbeat, become nauseated or vomit, or lose your appetite.

What you must know about other drugs

Theo-Dur can interfere with the way some other drugs work. At the same time, some drugs can interfere with Theo-Dur's actions. Tell your doctor if you're taking birth control pills; drugs for seizures, heart problems, tuberculosis, or a stomach ulcer; or nonprescription medications.

Also tell the doctor if you've smoked tobacco or marijuana within the previous 2 years. Smoking may affect how much Theo-Dur you need.

Special directions

• Tell the doctor if you've ever had an allergic reaction to any drug for asthma.

• Because Theo-Dur can make some medical problems worse, tell the doctor if you have heart or circulatory problems, diabetes, glaucoma, high blood pressure, an overactive thyroid, stomach ulcers, or indigestion.

• Because charcoal-broiled foods may interfere with how Theo-Dur works, don't eat these foods every day. Also, don't eat or drink a large amount of foods containing caffeine, such as chocolate, tea, coffee, and colas. The extra caffeine may increase the stimulant effects of Theo-Dur.

• Call your doctor right away if you develop a fever or feel like you have the flu. These conditions could increase your risk for side effects.

Important reminders If you're pregnant or breast-feeding, check with your doctor before taking Theo-Dur.

If you're an older adult, you may be especially prone to side effects from Theo-Dur.

Thorazine

This medication is used to treat persistent hiccups, mild withdrawal from alcohol, tetanus, and certain mental and emotional disorders. This drug's generic name is chlorpromazine.

How to take Thorazine Thorazine comes in tablet, sustained-release capsule, concentrate, syrup, and suppository forms. Follow the directions on the medication label exactly. You may take oral forms of this medication with food, milk, or water to minimize stomach upset.

If you're taking the *sustained-release capsule*, swallow it whole. Don't crush, chew, or break it.

If you're taking the *concentrate*, mix it in 2 to 4 ounces (50 to 125 milliliters) of water, soda, juice, milk, pudding, or applesauce.

If you're using a *suppository* and it's too soft to insert, chill it in the refrigerator for 30 minutes or run cold water over it before removing the foil wrapper. Then moisten it with water, lie down on your side, and use your finger to push the suppository well up into your rectum.

What to do if you miss a dose If you're taking one dose a day, take the missed dose as soon as you remember that day. If you don't remember until the next day, skip the dose you missed and take your next regular dose.

If you're taking more than one dose a day and you remember within 1 hour or so of the scheduled time, take the missed dose right away. If you don't remember until later, skip the missed dose and take your next dose at the regular time.

What to do about side effects

If you have a persistent fever, sore throat, joint pain, or unusual bruising or bleeding, stop taking this medication and call the doctor *at once*.

Other possible side effects of Thorazine include unusual movements, such as lip smacking or jumpy arms and legs, blurred vision, dry mouth, constipation, inability to urinate, and sensitivity to sunlight. If any of these symptoms persist or worsen, call your doctor.

Be sure of your response to Thorazine before performing activities requiring alertness and clear vision.

If you become extra sensitive to light, protect yourself from direct sunlight.

To relieve dry mouth, use ice chips or sugarless gum or hard candy.

What you must know about alcohol and other drugs

Avoid alcoholic beverages or other drugs that depress the central nervous system because Thorazine intensifies their effect.

Tell the doctor about other medications you're taking because Thorazine may change the effects of other drugs. For example, it decreases the effects of drugs that lower blood pressure and prevent blood clots.

Special directions

• Check with your doctor before taking new medications (prescription or nonprescription).

• Before surgery, dental work, or emergency treatment, tell the doctor or dentist that you're taking this drug.

Important reminders

If you're pregnant or breast-feeding, tell your doctor before using Thorazine.

Children and older adults are especially sensitive to side effects from Thorazine.

Tigan

Your doctor has prescribed Tigan to help treat your nausea and vomiting. This drug's generic name is trimethobenzamide.

How to take Tigan

Tigan comes in oral capsule, injection, and suppository forms. Follow your doctor's instructions exactly. Don't use more of this medication or take it more often than your doctor has ordered.

If you're using the *suppository*, remove the foil wrapper and moisten the suppository with cold water. Lie down on your side and use your finger to push the suppository well up into your rectum. If the suppository is too soft to insert, place it in the refrigerator for 30 minutes or run cold water over it before removing the wrapper. Wash your hands before and after inserting the suppository.

What to do if you miss a dose

Take the missed dose as soon as possible. But if it's almost time for your next dose, skip the missed dose and take your next dose as scheduled. Don't take a double dose.

What to do about side effects

Tigan commonly causes drowsiness.

Call your doctor *immediately* if you develop any of the following uncommon side effects: skin rash, shakiness or tremor, severe or continued vomiting, unusual tiredness, or yellow eyes or skin.

Because this medication may make you dizzy or lightheaded, don't drive or perform any activities that could be dangerous if you're dizzy or not alert.

Special directions

Tell your doctor if you've ever had an allergic reaction to benzocaine or a local anesthetic. Also mention whether you have other medical problems, particularly a high fever or an intestinal infection.

Important reminders

Don't give Tigan to a child unless the cause of vomiting is known and your doctor approves. When given to a child with a viral illness (a common cause of vomiting), this medication may lead to Reye's syndrome, which is a potentially fatal brain disorder.

If you're pregnant or breast-feeding, don't take Tigan without first talking with your doctor.

Timoptic

These eyedrops are prescribed to treat glaucoma. The drug's generic name is timolol.

How to instill Timoptic

To instill Timoptic eyedrops, follow these steps. First wash your hands. Then tilt your head back. Using your middle finger, apply pressure to the inside corner of your eye. Then, with the index finger of your same hand, pull the lower eyelid away from your eye to form a pouch. Instill the prescribed number of drops into the pouch without touching the applicator to your eye or the surrounding tissue. Gently close your eyes, but don't blink. With your eyes closed, keep your middle finger pressed against the inside corner for 1 minute. This will help the medication stay in your eye and keep your body from absorbing it. Wash your hands again.

What to do if you miss a dose

If you take one dose a day, take the missed dose as soon as possible. But if you don't remember until the next day, skip the missed dose and take your next dose as scheduled.

If you take more than one dose a day, take the missed dose as soon as possible. But if it's almost time for your next dose, skip the missed dose and take your next dose as scheduled.

What to do about side effects

Call your doctor *right away* if you develop any of these side effects: dizziness or feeling faint; irregular, slow, or pounding heartbeat; wheezing or trouble breathing; swelling of feet or lower legs; unusual tiredness or weakness; skin rash or itching; severe eye irritation; or vision disturbances.

What you must know about other drugs

Because Timoptic may affect how some other drugs work, tell your doctor if you're taking a beta blocker, such as Inderal (propranolol).

Because Timoptic may interact with some anesthetics, tell your doctor or dentist you're taking Timoptic before you undergo any kind of surgery or emergency treatment.

Special directions Because Timoptic may make some medical problems worse, tell your doctor if you have a history of asthma, diabetes, heart or blood vessel disease, myasthenia gravis, kidney or liver disease, or an overactive thyroid.

Important reminders If you have diabetes, Timoptic may affect your blood sugar levels. It may also cover up some signs of low blood sugar, such as trembling and increased heart rate and blood pressure. If you notice a change in your blood or urine glucose tests, call your doctor.

If you're an athlete, you should know that the National Collegiate Athletic Association bans timolol.

Tinactin

Your doctor has prescribed Tinactin to treat your fungal skin infection. This drug's generic name is tolnaftate.

How to use Tinactin Tinactin comes in cream, gel, powder, lotion, pump-spray liquid, and aerosol forms. It's available without a prescription.

To use Tinactin, first wash the affected area and dry it thoroughly. Then apply enough medication to cover the area. Usually, a ¼- to ½-inch ribbon of *cream* or *gel* or three drops of *lotion* will cover an area the size of your hand.

If you're using Tinactin *powder* on your feet, sprinkle it between your toes, on your feet, and in your socks and shoes.

If you're using a *pump-spray liquid,* hold the container 4 to 6 inches (10 to 15 centimeters) away from the area and spray.

If you're using the *aerosol liquid* or the *aerosol powder*, shake the can well. Then, holding the can 6 to 10 inches (15 to 25.5 centimeters) away, spray the affected area. Don't inhale the vapor or powder from the spray. Also, don't use it near heat, an open flame, or while you're smoking.

Keep using the medication for 2 weeks after burning, itching, or other symptoms have disappeared. This will help you clear up the infection completely.

What to do if you miss a dose Take the missed dose as soon as possible. Then return to your regular dosage schedule.

What to do about side effects Check with your doctor or pharmacist if skin irritation occurs that wasn't present before you used this medication. If you're using the spray solution form of Tinactin, you may experience a mild, temporary stinging sensation.

Special directions • If you have a fungal infection of your hair or nails, see your doctor. Tinactin alone won't cure these types of infections.

• If you're treating athlete's foot and your symptoms haven't subsided after using the medication for 10 days, call your doctor. If you're treating another type of fungal infection and you've used the medication for 4 weeks without improvement or if your symptoms have worsened, call your doctor.

• To help prevent reinfection after you've finished your treatment, use the powder or spray powder each day after bathing. Also sprinkle the powder or spray the aerosol inside your socks and shoes.

Important reminder Don't use Tinactin on a child younger than age 2, unless your doctor orders otherwise.

Tobrex

This medication is prescribed to treat eye infections. This drug's generic name is tobramycin.

How to use Tobrex Tobrex is available in eyedrop and ointment forms.

If you're using the *eyedrop* form of the drug, follow these steps. First, wash your hands. Then tilt your head back. With your middle finger, press on the inside corner of your eye. At the same time, use your index finger to pull your lower eyelid away from your eye, forming a pouch. Without touching your eye with the applicator, instill the prescribed amount of drops into the pouch. Gently close your eye and don't blink. Keep your eye closed and your finger pressed against the inside corner for 1 minute to give the medication time to saturate the area.

If your doctor has ordered another solution to be used with this one, wait at least 5 minutes before using the second medication. This will help keep the second medication from washing away the first.

If you're using the *eye ointment* form of the drug, follow these steps. Wash your hands. Then pull your lower eyelid away from your eye to form a pouch. Without touching your eye with the applicator tip, squeeze a thin strip of ointment, about 1 inch (2.5 centimeters) long, into the pouch. Gently close your eye. Keep your eye closed for 1 to 2 minutes. After you finish applying the medication, wash your hands again.

Use all of the medication as prescribed by your doctor, even if your symptoms improve after a few days.

What to do if you miss a dose

Take the missed dose as soon as possible. However, if it's almost time for your next dose, skip the missed dose and take the next dose on schedule.

What to do about side effects

Your eyes may sting or burn for a few minutes after you apply the drops or ointment. This is to be expected. Also expect your vision to blur briefly after applying eye ointment.

Call your doctor if your eyelids swell, itch, or burn constantly. This may signal that you're allergic to Tobrex.

What you must know about other drugs

Don't use Tobrex if you're using an eye medication containing tetracycline. The two drugs don't work well together.

Special directions

Tell your doctor if you have a history of kidney disease; ear problems, such as ringing or hearing loss; myasthenia gravis; Parkinson's disease; or low calcium levels.

Tofranil

Prescribed to treat depression and to relieve severe, chronic pain, Tofranil may also be prescribed to treat childhood bed-wetting. This drug's generic name is imipramine. Another brand name is Janimine.

How to take Tofranil   Unless your doctor instructs otherwise, take Tofranil with food (even at bedtime) to reduce stomach upset.

What to do if you miss a dose   If you take your medication once a day at bedtime, check with your doctor about how to handle a missed dose.

If you take more than one dose a day, take the missed dose as soon as possible. But if it's almost time for your next dose, skip the missed dose and resume your schedule. Don't take a double dose.

What to do about side effects   If you develop blurred vision, constipation, a fast heartbeat, or trouble urinating, call your doctor *immediately*.

If you think you've taken an overdose or experience symptoms of overdose, such as seizures, confusion, severe drowsiness, or fast, slow, or irregular heartbeat, stop taking Tofranil and get emergency care *immediately*.

Dizziness, drowsiness, dry mouth, headache, and increased sweating may occur but should go away as your body adjusts to the medication. If they persist, tell your doctor.

Call your doctor if you can't sleep or have uncontrolled lip, arm, or leg movements after you stop taking Tofranil.

What you must know about alcohol and other drugs   Don't drink alcoholic beverages while taking Tofranil. Check with your doctor if you're taking other prescription or nonprescription medications. They can interact with Tofranil and possibly cause problems.

Special directions   • Tell your doctor about other medical conditions you have. They may affect the use of Tofranil.

• Don't stop taking Tofranil without first consulting your doctor, who may decrease your dosage gradually to minimize withdrawal effects.

• Make sure you know how you react to Tofranil before you drive or perform other activities requiring alertness and the ability to see clearly.

If you feel dizzy or faint when arising from a sitting or lying position, get up slowly.

Because Tofranil may increase your skin's sensitivity to sunlight, limit your sun exposure. When outdoors, wear protective clothing and sunglasses and use a sunblock.

Unless your doctor instructs otherwise, drink plenty of liquids and eat a high-fiber diet to prevent constipation.

Relieve mouth dryness with sugarless hard candy or gum, ice chips, mouthwash, or a saliva substitute. If dryness continues for more than 2 weeks, tell your doctor or dentist because it puts you at risk for tooth or gum problems.

Important reminders If you're pregnant or breast-feeding, check with your doctor before starting this medication.

Children and older adults are at special risk for Tofranil's side effects.

If you have diabetes, Tofranil can affect your blood sugar levels. If it does, call your doctor.

Tolectin

This medication helps control both inflammation and pain. The drug's generic name is tolmetin.

How to take Tolectin Take your medication with milk, meals, or an antacid. This will help prevent stomach upset, which could occur if you take the drug on an empty stomach. If you use an antacid, choose one containing magnesium and aluminum hydroxides, such as Maalox.

Also drink a full glass (8 ounces) of water with each dose. Don't lie down for 15 to 30 minutes after taking the medication. This will help prevent irritation that could cause you to have difficulty swallowing.

What to do if you miss a dose If your doctor has prescribed Tolectin on a regular schedule and if you miss a dose, take the missed dose as soon as you remember. But if it's almost time for your next dose, skip the missed dose and take your next dose as scheduled. Don't take a double dose.

What to do about side effects

Notify your doctor immediately if you notice any of these side effects:
- stomach pain or burning
- bloody or black, tarry stools
- easy bruising and bleeding
- changes in vision
- swelling in your face, feet, or lower legs
- persistent nausea or vomiting
- loss of appetite or weight loss.

What you must know about other drugs

Because Tolectin may interact with other medications, tell your doctor and pharmacist about other medications you're taking. In particular, tell your doctor if you're taking aspirin, Dilantin (phenytoin), thyroid medication, another anti-inflammatory medication, or a blood thinner.

Special directions

- Tell your doctor if aspirin or another anti-inflammatory medication has ever caused you to experience asthma-like symptoms, a runny nose, or itching.
- Also tell the doctor if you have a history of gastrointestinal bleeding, liver or kidney disease, asthma, heart disease, or high blood pressure.
- Although Tolectin should begin working in 1 week, you may not feel its full effects for 2 to 4 weeks. But if your pain persists or worsens, let your doctor know.

Important reminder

Tolectin can hide the symptoms of an infection. Therefore, if you have diabetes, you need to be especially careful about caring for your feet and watching for any abnormality that might be caused by an infection.

Tolinase

This medication is prescribed to help control your diabetes. This drug's generic name is tolazamide.

How to take Tolinase

Take each dose with food. If your doctor prescribes one dose a day, take it with breakfast. If two doses a day are prescribed, take one dose with breakfast and the second dose with your evening meal.

Keep taking the medication, even if you feel well. Tolinase doesn't cure diabetes; it only relieves the symptoms.

What to do if you miss a dose

Take the missed dose as soon as you remember. But if it's almost time for your next dose, skip the missed dose and take your next dose as scheduled. Don't take two doses at once.

What to do about side effects

Taking too much Tolinase may cause a condition called low blood sugar (hypoglycemia), which can produce symptoms such as drowsiness, headache, nervousness, cold sweats, and confusion. If these symptoms occur, eat or drink something sweet, such as orange juice, and call your doctor.

Tolinase may increase your sensitivity to sunlight. Take precautions to protect your skin when outdoors.

What you must know about alcohol and other drugs

Avoid drinking alcoholic beverages while you're taking Tolinase. The combination could cause unpleasant side effects. Keep in mind that many foods and drugs contain alcohol.

Tell your doctor if you're taking other medications. Tolinase may interfere with the way some medications work, and other medications may interfere with the way Tolinase works. Especially tell your doctor if you're taking a blood thinner; diet pills; medication for asthma, colds, allergies, high blood pressure, or tuberculosis; sulfa medication; aspirin; steroids; or a thiazide diuretic (a type of water pill).

Special directions

• Tell your doctor if you've ever had an allergic reaction to an oral medication used for treating diabetes or to a diuretic.

• Because some medical conditions may prevent you from taking Tolinase, tell the doctor if you have a disorder that affects your liver, kidneys, adrenal glands, pituitary gland, or thyroid gland.

• Follow your doctor's instructions for testing your blood or urine for glucose. Also closely follow your instructions for diet and exercise.

• At all times, wear a medical identification bracelet stating that you have diabetes and listing your medication.

Important reminder   Tell your doctor if you're breast-feeding or pregnant. Your doctor may need to prescribe a different medication.

Tonocard

Your doctor has prescribed Tonocard to correct your irregular heartbeat. This drug's generic name is tocainide.

How to take   Take the exact amount of medication prescribed by your
Tonocard   doctor. Try to take your medication at the same time every day, and space your doses evenly throughout the day and night. If the medication upsets your stomach, take it with food or milk.

Continue to take the medication as directed, even if you feel well.

What to do if you   If you remember your missed dose within 4 hours, take
miss a dose   it as soon as possible. But if you don't remember until later, skip the missed dose and take your next dose as scheduled. Don't take a double dose.

What to do about   Call your doctor *right away* if you develop any of the fol-
side effects   lowing side effects: trembling or shaking, coughing or shortness of breath, fever or chills, unusual bleeding or bruising, or unusual tiredness.

Also let your doctor know if you experience nausea, vomiting, stomach pain, dizziness, or light-headedness.

Make sure you know how you react to Tonocard before driving or performing other activities requiring alertness.

What you must   Tonocard may interfere with how some other medica-
know about other   tions work. For this reason, tell your doctor if you're tak-
drugs   ing a beta blocker, such as Inderal (propranolol) or Lopressor (metoprolol). Also, before beginning any new medications, talk with your doctor or pharmacist.

Tell your doctor or dentist you're taking Tonocard before having any kind of surgery or emergency treatment.

Special directions
• Tonocard may make some medical conditions worse. Tell your doctor if you have a history of kidney or liver disease, a bone marrow disorder, congestive heart failure, or some other heart problem.
• Also tell your doctor if you've ever had an allergic reaction to an anesthetic.

Important reminders
If you're pregnant or breast-feeding, talk with your doctor before taking Tonocard.

If you're an older adult, be careful when walking or first getting up out of a chair. You may be especially prone to the side effect of dizziness, which could place you at risk for a fall.

Totacillin

This medication is prescribed to treat bacterial infections. Its generic name is ampicillin. Another brand name is Omnipen.

How to take Totacillin
Totacillin comes in liquid and capsule forms. Take it at evenly spaced times day and night.

Take it with a full glass (8 ounces) of water on an empty stomach either 1 hour before or 2 hours after a meal unless otherwise directed.

If you're taking the *liquid*, use a specially marked measuring spoon, not a household teaspoon, to measure the correct dose.

If you're taking the *capsules*, don't break, chew, or crush them. Swallow them whole.

Take all the prescribed medication, even if you feel better. If you stop it too soon, your symptoms may return. Try not to miss a dose because Totacillin works best when you have a constant amount in your blood.

What to do if you miss a dose
Take the missed dose as soon as possible. But if it's almost time for your next dose and you normally take two doses daily, space the missed dose and the next dose 5 to 6 hours apart. If you take three or more doses a day, space the missed dose and the next dose 2 to 4 hours apart. Then go back to your regular schedule.

What to do about side effects

Contact your doctor *immediately* and stop taking the medication if you have difficulty breathing, a rash, hives, itching, or wheezing. These effects may mean that you're allergic to Totacillin.

You may also have nausea and diarrhea. If these symptoms persist or become severe, notify your doctor.

What you must know about other drugs

Tell your doctor about other medications you're taking. Zyloprim (allopurinol) taken with Totacillin may increase your risk of developing a rash. Probalan (probenecid) increases blood levels of Totacillin — a beneficial side effect.

• If your symptoms don't improve within a few days or if they become worse, check with your doctor.

• Tell your doctor if you're allergic to other penicillins or cephalosporins, Fulvicin (griseofulvin), or Cuprimine (penicillamine). If you're allergic to Totacillin, carry medical identification that describes your allergy.

• Totacillin may interfere with the effectiveness of oral contraceptives (birth control pills) containing estrogen. Use a different or additional birth control method while you're taking Totacillin.

• If you develop severe diarrhea, don't take any diarrhea medication without checking first with your doctor. Diarrhea medications may make your diarrhea worse or last longer.

Important reminders

If you have diabetes, Totacillin may cause false test results with some urine glucose tests. Check with your doctor before changing your diet or the dosage of your diabetes medication.

If you're breast-feeding, tell your doctor before taking Totacillin.

Trandate

One of a group of medications commonly called beta blockers, Trandate is prescribed to control your blood pressure. This drug's generic name is labetalol. Another brand name is Normodyne.

How to take Trandate

Take your medication exactly as prescribed, either with food or on an empty stomach, as you prefer. Swallow the tablets whole; don't break, crush, or chew them.

What to do if you miss a dose

Take the missed dose as soon as you remember unless it's within 8 hours of your next dose. If so, skip the missed dose and take the next one at the scheduled time. Never take a double dose.

What to do about side effects

Trandate may cause dizziness and a sudden blood pressure drop when you stand up quickly. To minimize dizziness, get up slowly from a sitting or lying position. If these side effects become bothersome, tell your doctor.

What you must know about alcohol and other drugs

Avoid alcoholic beverages, which in combination with Trandate may cause an excessive drop in blood pressure. Check with your doctor before taking Tagamet (cimetidine), insulin, or oral diabetes drugs with Trandate.

Because Trandate may make you dizzy, don't drive or perform other activities requiring alertness until you know how you respond to this medication.

Special directions

• Tell your doctor about other medical problems you have. They may affect the use of this medication.
• Keep in mind that Trandate controls high blood pressure but doesn't cure it. For this reason, keep taking it as prescribed, even if you think you don't need it anymore.
• Make sure you always have enough Trandate on hand, especially when you're away from home, so you don't have to interrupt your dosing schedule because you run out.
• Carry medical identification stating that you're taking Trandate.
• Reduce your intake of salt if your doctor has instructed you to do so.

Important reminders

If you're pregnant or breast-feeding, check with your doctor before taking Trandate.

If you're an older adult, you may be especially sensitive to Trandate's side effects.

If you have diabetes, be aware that Trandate may cause your blood sugar level to drop and also may mask signs of low blood sugar such as an altered pulse rate.

If you're an athlete, be aware that the U.S. Olympic Committee and the National Collegiate Athletic Association ban beta blockers.

Transderm-Scop

This skin patch is prescribed to prevent nausea and vomiting caused by motion sickness. The drug's generic name is scopolamine.

How to apply Transderm-Scop

This medication comes in the form of a small patch a transdermal disk that you wear behind your ear. First, carefully read the patient directions that come with the transdermal disk. Wash and dry your hands well before and after handling the disk. Apply the disk to a hairless skin area behind the ear.

Apply the disk the night before or several hours before your trip. Don't place it over any cuts or irritations on your skin.

If the disk loosens, remove it and replace it with a new disk on another clean area of skin behind the ear.

When you no longer need the medication, remove and discard the patch. Wash your hands and the skin that was beneath the disk. The disks are designed to deliver medication for up to 3 days.

What to do about side effects

Check with your doctor if Transderm-Scop makes you drowsy or dries your mouth, especially if these symptoms continue or bother you.

Also, while using the disk or even after removing it, your eyes may be more sensitive than usual to light. You may also notice the pupil in one eye is larger than the pupil in the other eye. Call your doctor if this side effect persists or troubles you.

Because Transderm-Scop may make you drowsy, make sure you know how you react to it before you drive or perform other activities that might be dangerous if you're not fully alert.

If Transderm-Scop makes your mouth feel dry, use sugarless gum or hard candy, ice chips, or a saliva substitute. If your mouth still feels dry after 2 weeks, see your dentist.

Special directions

• Tell your doctor if you have other medical problems, especially glaucoma, asthma, lung disease, myasthenia gravis, or intestinal disease. Other medical problems may affect the use of this medication.

• This product comes with a patient brochure containing helpful information. You may want to request it from your pharmacist.

Important reminders

If you're breast-feeding, check with your doctor before using Transderm-Scop.

Don't use the transdermal disk on children.

If you're an athlete, you should know that the U.S. Olympic Committee bans and sometimes tests for scopolamine in biathlon and modern pentathlon events.

Tranxene

This medication is used to prevent seizures in people with seizure disorders and to relieve extreme feelings of nervousness or tension. The drug's generic name is clorazepate.

How to take Tranxene

Tranxene comes in tablet or capsule form.

Follow your doctor's instructions exactly. Because this medication can be habit-forming, don't take more, and don't take it more often or longer than the label directs.

If you're taking Tranxene for a seizure disorder, take it every day in regularly spaced doses as ordered.

What to do if you miss a dose

Take the missed dose as soon as possible. But if it's almost time for your next dose, skip the missed dose and take your next dose on schedule. Don't take a double dose.

What to do about side effects

Get emergency help *at once* if you have these symptoms of an overdose: slurred speech, confusion, severe drowsiness, and staggering. Check with your doctor if this medication makes you feel drowsy, sluggish, or like you have a hangover.

Because this medication can make you drowsy, make sure you know how you react to it before you drive, use machines, or perform other potentially hazardous activities that require alertness.

What you must know about alcohol and other drugs

Tell your doctor about other medications you're taking. Avoid alcoholic beverages and other medications that slow down your central nervous system (such as antihistamines or medications for hay fever, other allergies, or colds) while taking Tranxene because this combination may cause oversedation. Tagamet (cimetidine), an ulcer medication, may also cause increased drowsiness when used with Tranxene.

Special directions

• Tell your doctor if you have other medical problems, especially glaucoma, myasthenia gravis, Parkinson's disease, or kidney or liver disease. Also reveal if you have a history of mental illness or drug abuse.
• If you've been taking this medication for a long time, don't stop taking it without first checking with your doctor.
• If you're taking Tranxene for a seizure disorder, your doctor may want you to carry medical identification stating that you're taking it.
• Before you have medical tests, tell the doctor that you're taking Tranxene because this drug may alter the test results.

Important reminders

If you're pregnant or breast-feeding, check with your doctor before taking this medication.

If you're an older adult, be aware that you may be especially prone to side effects.

If you're an athlete, you should know that the U.S. Olympic Committee and the National Collegiate Athletic Association ban the use of clorazepate.

Trental

By relieving leg pain and cramps caused by poor circulation, Trental can improve your blood circulation. Trental's generic name is pentoxifylline.

How to take Trental

Trental comes in extended-release tablets. Take your medication with meals to lessen the chance of stomach upset. You may also take the tablets with an antacid unless your doctor tells you otherwise.

Swallow the tablet whole — don't chew, crush, or break it.

Don't stop taking this medication suddenly without first checking with your doctor. Also, realize that it may take several weeks before you feel that Trental is working.

What to do if you miss a dose

Take the missed dose as soon as possible. But if it's almost time for your next dose, skip the missed dose and take your next dose on schedule. Don't take a double dose.

What to do about side effects

Trental can cause headache, dizziness, heartburn, nausea, or vomiting. Check with your doctor if these symptoms continue or bother you.

Rarely, this medication causes chest pain or an irregular heartbeat. If you have these symptoms, call your doctor *as soon as possible*.

What you must know about other drugs

Tell your doctor about other medications you're taking. Taking Trental with blood thinners may increase your risk of bleeding. If you take medications for high blood pressure, your doctor may need to adjust your dosage of these medications because Trental can increase their effect.

Special directions

• Tell your doctor if you have other medical problems, especially stomach ulcers and kidney or liver disease. Also mention if you've ever had an unusual or allergic reaction to caffeine or any foods or medications.
• Because nicotine can narrow your blood vessels, cigarette smoking may worsen your condition. Therefore, if

you smoke, make an effort to quit such as by joining a stop-smoking program.

Important reminders

If you're pregnant or breast-feeding, check with your doctor before you take Trental.

If you're an older adult, you may be especially prone to side effects from Trental.

Triavil

This medication is used to treat certain mental and emotional disorders. This drug's generic name is amitriptyline with perphenazine.

How to take Triavil

Take Triavil with food or right after meals, unless otherwise directed. Don't increase the dose or take it more often than prescribed.

What to do if you miss a dose

Take the missed dose as soon as you remember. However, if you remember within 2 hours of your next dose, skip the missed dose and go back to your regular schedule. Don't take a double dose.

What to do about side effects

Call the doctor *immediately* if you develop a fever, bleeding gums, or mouth sores or if you feel extremely tired.

You may also experience dizziness, drowsiness, uncontrolled movements of the arms or legs, light-headedness when changing position, increased pulse rate, constipation, dry mouth, blurred vision, sensitivity to sunlight, and sweating. Contact the doctor if these effects persist or become severe.

Triavil can cause drowsiness, so make sure you know how it affects you before you drive a car or perform other activities that require alertness.

Get up slowly from a lying or sitting position to prevent dizziness.

Avoid direct sunlight as much as possible. Wear protective clothing, including sunglasses and a hat, and use a sunblock with a skin protection factor (SPF) of 15 or higher.

What you must know about alcohol and other drugs Avoid alcoholic beverages or other medications that make you sleepy or relaxed, such as allergy, hay fever, and cold medications; prescription pain and seizure medications; and anesthetics.

Don't take Triavil within 2 hours of taking antacids or medication to treat diarrhea. Taking these medications too close together may lessen the effectiveness of Triavil.

Special directions • Be sure to tell your doctor if you have other medical problems. They may affect the use of Triavil.

• Tell your doctor about previous allergic or unusual reactions to other antipsychotics or to Elavil or other antidepressants.

• Before you have surgery, dental work, or emergency treatment, tell the doctor or dentist that you're taking Triavil.

Important reminders If you're breast-feeding or you become pregnant while taking Triavil, notify your doctor as soon as possible.

Teenagers and older adults may be especially sensitive to the effects of Triavil.

If you're an athlete, you should know that the U.S. Olympic Committee and the National Collegiate Athletic Association ban the use of perphenazine.

Trilafon

This medication is used to treat psychological disorders and to relieve severe nausea, vomiting, or hiccups. This drug's generic name is perphenazine.

How to take Trilafon Trilafon comes in tablets and a concentrated oral solution. Take your medication exactly as your doctor directs. Take your dose with food, water, or milk to prevent stomach irritation.

To use the concentrated oral solution, dilute your dose in fruit juice, ginger ale, or semisolid food such as applesauce. Don't mix your medication with colas, black coffee, grape or apple juice, or tea.

Don't stop taking Trilafon without first checking with your doctor.

What to do if you miss a dose

If you take one dose daily, take the missed dose as soon as possible. If you don't remember until the next day, skip it and go back to your regular schedule.

If you take more than one dose a day, take the missed dose within 1 hour of the scheduled time if you remember it. If not, skip the missed dose and go back to your regular dosage schedule. Don't take a double dose.

What to do about side effects

Call your doctor *right away* if you develop a fever, a fast heartbeat, difficulty breathing, and increased sweating. Also call *immediately* if you start to feel extremely tired or unwell.

Tell your doctor if this medication causes uncontrolled movements of your mouth, tongue, or other body parts or if you have blurred vision, a dry mouth, difficulty urinating, or constipation. Let your doctor know if Trilafon makes you feel dizzy or faint, especially when you get up from a sitting or lying position.

Because Trilafon may make you dizzy, make sure you know how you react to it before you drive or perform other activities that require alertness.

Don't drink alcoholic beverages while taking this medication because it could cause oversedation. For the same reason, avoid other medications that depress the central nervous system, including tranquilizers and sleeping pills.

What you must know about alcohol and other drugs

To avoid harmful drug interactions, check with your doctor before you use other medications. If you take antacids, take them at least 2 hours before or after taking Trilafon.

Special directions

• Tell your doctor if you have other medical problems because Trilafon can aggravate many medical conditions.

• Before you have medical tests, tell the doctor that you're taking Trilafon because it may affect the test results.

Important reminders

If you're pregnant or breast-feeding, check with your doctor before taking Trilafon.

Children and older adults are especially prone to Trilafon's side effects.

If you're an athlete, be aware that the U.S. Olympic Committee and the National Collegiate Athletic Association ban and sometimes test for perphenazine in shooting events.

Tylenol

Tylenol relieves mild pain and fever. This drug's generic name is acetaminophen.

How to take Tylenol

Tylenol comes in many forms: capsule, oral liquid, tablet, chewable tablet, wafer, and suppository.

Carefully follow the precautions listed on the package label. If you're an adult, you can take a dose of Tylenol every 4 hours as needed, but don't exceed eight tablets a day. For a child, you can repeat the dose every 4 hours, but don't exceed five doses a day.

If you're using a *suppository* and it's too soft to insert, run cold water over it or refrigerate it for a few minutes before removing the wrapper.

What to do if you miss a dose

Take the missed dose as soon as you remember. But if it's almost time for your next dose, skip the missed dose and resume your regular dosage schedule. Don't take a double dose.

What to do about side effects

Keep in mind that large doses of Tylenol may cause liver damage. Call the doctor if you develop a rash or hives or if your skin turns yellowish.

What you must know about alcohol and other drugs

Don't drink alcoholic beverages when taking Tylenol because this combination may cause liver damage, especially if you take Tylenol regularly for a long time.

Check with the doctor or pharmacist before taking any nonprescription drugs. Many contain acetaminophen that must count toward your total daily dosage.

Tell your doctor if you're taking Dolobid (diflunisal), which may increase Tylenol's effects, or Coumadin (warfarin), which may cause bleeding with long-term Tylenol use.

Special directions

• Tell the doctor if you have medical problems, particularly if you have diabetes, kidney or liver disease, or blood disorders.

• If Tylenol doesn't relieve pain after 10 days (for adults, or 5 days for children), notify the doctor. If you have new symptoms, if the pain gets worse, or if the pain site appears red and swollen, also contact the doctor.

• If Tylenol doesn't make a fever go away within 3 days, call the doctor. Also call if the fever returns or rises or if new symptoms, redness, or swelling occur.

Important reminders

Give this medication to a child under age 2 only as prescribed by a doctor.

If you have diabetes, check your blood sugar level carefully. Tylenol can affect test results, so contact your doctor about unusual changes.

Tylenol with Codeine

This medication relieves moderately severe pain. A compound drug, it combines the generic products acetaminophen and codeine.

How to take Tylenol with Codeine

Tylenol with Codeine is available as a tablet, capsule, or liquid. Follow the directions on your medication label exactly. Usually, you may take this medication every 4 to 6 hours. To minimize stomach upset, you may take it with milk or meals.

If you don't begin to feel better, call the doctor. Don't increase the dose on your own.

What to do if you miss a dose

Take the missed dose as soon as you remember. But if it's almost time for your next dose, skip the missed dose and resume your regular dosage schedule. Don't take a double dose.

What to do about side effects

If you develop a rash, have difficulty breathing or swallowing, or show other signs of an allergic reaction, stop taking this medication and get medical help *right away*.

Tylenol with Codeine may cause confusion, dizziness, drowsiness, light-headedness, stomach pain, nausea, vomiting, and constipation. If any of these symptoms persists, call the doctor.

Avoid driving and other activities that require mental alertness until you know how this medication affects you.

To avoid possible constipation, include plenty of fluids and fiber in your diet.

What you must know about alcohol and other drugs

While you're taking Tylenol with Codeine, don't drink alcoholic beverages or take sedatives, antihistamines, or other drugs that decrease your activity.

Check with the doctor or pharmacist before taking nonprescription medications. Many contain acetaminophen and should be counted toward your total daily dosage. In normal amounts, Tylenol with Codeine is safe; in high doses, it can damage the liver.

Tell your doctor if you're taking Dolobid (diflunisal) because it may increase the effects of Tylenol with Codeine.

Special directions

• Tell the doctor about your medical history, particularly head injury, severe headaches, diabetes, kidney or liver disease, or blood disorders.
• Tylenol with Codeine can be habit-forming. Take just the prescribed amount for only as long as directed.
• Don't take this medication if you're allergic to morphine or other opiates.

Important reminders

If you're breast-feeding or pregnant, talk to your doctor before taking Tylenol with Codeine.

Sharing this medication is against federal law.

If you're an athlete, you should know that the U.S. Olympic Committee and the National Collegiate Athletic Association ban the use of this medication.

U

Urecholine

This medication is used to treat certain bladder or urinary tract disorders. Its generic name is bethanechol.

How to take Urecholine

Urecholine comes in tablet form. Carefully follow the dosage directions on the prescription label.

Unless your doctor directs otherwise, take Urecholine on an empty stomach (either 1 hour before or 2 hours after meals) to minimize possible nausea and vomiting.

What to do if you miss a dose

If you remember within an hour or so of the scheduled dosing time, take your medication right away. But if you don't remember until 2 or more hours after your scheduled dosing time, skip the dose you missed and resume your normal dosing schedule. Don't take a double dose.

What to do about side effects

Common side effects with Urecholine include abdominal cramps and diarrhea. If these symptoms persist or become severe, contact your doctor.

Less common side effects include tearing, headache, flushing, sweating and, rarely, shortness of breath or wheezing. If you experience a breathing problem, contact your doctor right away.

You may feel dizzy, light-headed, or faint, especially when arising from a lying or sitting position. To minimize this problem, try getting up slowly.

What you must know about other drugs

You should tell your doctor about any other medications that you're taking. For example, anticholinergic agents — such as Atropisol (atropine) or Pro-Banthine (propantheline), Pronestyl (procainamide), and Cardioquin (quinidine) — may decrease Urecholine's effectiveness.

Special directions Inform your doctor if you have other medical problems because Urecholine may aggravate some disorders.

Important reminder Contact your doctor if you become pregnant while taking Urecholine.

V W

Because Valium causes relaxation, it's helpful for treating severe tension or anxiety as well as muscle spasms. It's also used to prevent seizures. This drug's generic name is diazepam.

How to take Valium

Valium comes in extended-release capsules, an oral solution, and tablets. Follow the directions exactly as ordered on your prescription label. Don't increase your dose.

If you're taking the *extended-release capsules,* don't crush, break, or chew them; swallow them whole.

If you're taking Valium regularly, don't suddenly stop taking your medication without first checking with your doctor.

What to do if you miss a dose

Take the missed dose right away if you remember within 1 hour or so of the missed dose. However, if you don't remember until later, skip the missed dose and take your next dose on schedule. Don't take a double dose.

What to do about side effects

Get emergency help *at once* if you suddenly start to feel very ill and experience difficulty breathing, faintness, or a dramatic change in your heart or pulse rate.

Check with your doctor if this medication makes you feel drowsy, lethargic, or like you have a hangover. Also call if you start to stagger when you walk.

Make sure you know how you react to Valium before you drive, use machines, or perform other activities that requires alertness.

What you must know about alcohol and other drugs

Don't drink alcoholic beverages while taking Valium because the combination may cause oversedation. For the same reason, avoid other central nervous system depressants (medications that slow down your central nervous system), such as sleeping pills, tranquilizers, and many cold and flu medications. Taking Valium with the ulcer drug Tagamet (cimetidine) may also lead to increased drowsiness.

Special directions
• Tell your doctor if you have other medical problems, such as glaucoma, myasthenia gravis, Parkinson's disease, and liver or kidney problems. Also mention if you have a history of drug addiction or psychological problems.
• See your doctor regularly to determine if you need to continue taking this medication because, if too much is taken, it may become habit-forming.
• Before you have medical tests, tell the doctor that you're taking Valium because it may alter the test results.

Important reminders
If you're pregnant or breast-feeding, check with your doctor before taking this medication.

If you're an older adult, realize that you may be especially prone to Valium's side effects.

If you're an athlete, you should know that the National Collegiate Athletic Association and the U.S. Olympic Committee ban the use of diazepam.

Vancocin

Your doctor has prescribed Vancocin to treat your bacterial infection. This drug's generic name is vancomycin.

How to take Vancocin
Vancocin comes in the form of an oral liquid and capsules. Take it only as your doctor directs.

If you're taking the *oral liquid* form of the medication, use a specially marked measuring spoon — not a household teaspoon — to accurately measure each dose.

Keep taking this medication even after you begin to feel better. Stopping too soon allows your infection to return.

What to do if you miss a dose
Take the missed dose as soon as possible. However, if it's almost time for your next dose, skip the missed dose and take your next dose as scheduled. Don't take a double dose.

What to do about side effects

Call your doctor *right away* if you develop any of the following side effects: ringing or buzzing in your ears, a feeling of fullness in your ears, a rash or itching, or difficulty breathing.

Also check with your doctor if you experience nausea and vomiting after taking the medication.

What you must know about other drugs

Taking certain medications at the same time you're taking Vancocin may increase your risk for side effects. So be sure to tell your doctor if you're taking any of these medications: antibiotics called aminoglycosides, such as Amikin (amikacin); Fungizone (amphotericin B); Platinol (cisplatin); or NebuPent (pentamidine).

Tell your doctor if you're taking Questran (cholestyramine) or Colestid (colestipol). Both of these medications may prevent Vancocin from working properly.

Special directions

• Because certain medical conditions may prevent your using this drug, tell your doctor if you have a history of kidney disease, hearing loss, or an inflammatory bowel disorder.

• Before using new medication, or if you develop a new medical problem while you're taking Vancocin, check with your doctor or pharmacist.

Important reminder

If you're pregnant or breast-feeding, check with your doctor before taking Vancocin.

Vaseretic

Your doctor has prescribed this combination medication to lower your high blood pressure. This drug's generic name is enalapril with hydrochlorothiazide.

How to take Vaseretic

Vaseretic comes in tablet form. Carefully check the your prescription label to determine your dosage.

This medication usually increases urination. If you take one dose per day, take it in the morning after breakfast. If you take two or more doses per day, take the last dose no later than 6 p.m. to prevent you from awakening during the night to urinate.

What to do if you miss a dose

Take the missed dose as soon as possible. But if it's almost time for your next dose, skip the missed dose and take your next dose on schedule. Don't take a double dose.

What to do about side effects

Call your doctor *right away* and stop taking this medication if you have any of these symptoms: a fever that persists, a sore throat, joint pain, easy bleeding or bruising, or swelling of your face, mouth, hands, ankles, or feet.

Check with your doctor if you feel dizzy or very tired or if you have a headache, muscle cramps, or low blood pressure, especially if these symptoms continue or bother you.

Make sure you know how you react to Vaseretic before you drive, use machinery, or perform other activities that require alertness.

What you must know about other drugs

Don't take this medication with Eskalith (lithium) because lithium toxicity may occur. You may also be instructed to avoid certain pain relievers called nonsteroidal anti-inflammatory drugs, such as Advil (ibuprofen), because these medications can prevent Vaseretic from working well.

Potassium supplements used with this medication may lead to dangerously high potassium levels. Also, avoid using Questran (cholestyramine) or Colestid (colestipol) — cholesterol-lowering drugs — because they reduce the absorption of this medication. Taking Proglycem (diazoxide) with this medication may cause high blood sugar levels and other problems.

Special directions

• Tell your doctor if you have other medical problems, especially diabetes, immune diseases, pancreatitis, and kidney or liver disease.

• Your doctor may instruct you to eat a diet that is low in salt because too much dietary salt can increase blood pressure.

• If you become sick and have persistent diarrhea or vomiting, call your doctor *right away.* These problems can make you lose too much water, leading to low blood pressure.

Important reminders If you're pregnant, check with your doctor before taking this medication.

If you're an older adult, be aware that you may be especially prone to Vaseretic's side effects.

Vasotec

Your doctor has prescribed Vasotec to treat your condition. This medication is used to lower high blood pressure. It's also prescribed to treat heart problems, when used along with other medications. This drug's generic name is enalapril.

How to take Vasotec Vasotec comes in tablet form. Follow the directions on your prescription label exactly, unless your doctor changes your dosage. Don't suddenly stop taking this medication without checking first with your doctor.

What to do if you miss a dose Take the missed dose as soon as possible. But if it's almost time for your next dose, skip the missed dose and take your next dose on schedule. Don't take a double dose.

What to do about side effects Get emergency help *at once* and stop taking your medication if you have any of the following symptoms: difficulty swallowing, difficulty breathing, or swelling of your face, eyes, lips, hands, feet, or tongue.

Check with your doctor as soon as possible if you feel dizzy or light-headed. Headaches and unusual tiredness also may occur, but these symptoms usually go away as your body adjusts to Vasotec. However, if these symptoms persist or bother you, check with your doctor.

Make sure you know how you react to Vasotec before driving, using machines, or performing other activities that require alertness.

A blood problem that can cause severe infections is a rare but serious complication. Report fever, chills, weakness, or a sore throat to your doctor *right away*.

What you must know about other drugs

Don't use salt substitutes or low-salt milk unless your doctor directs you to do so. It may alter your heart rhythm or cause other problems due to a buildup of potassium in your body.

Check with your doctor before taking any nonprescription medications, and be sure your doctor is aware of all prescription medications you're taking. If you're taking Eskalith (lithium), your doctor will closely watch your lithium level and may adjust your lithium dosage. The doctor may tell you to use certain painkillers cautiously because they can prevent Vasotec from working well.

Special directions

• Tell your doctor about any medical conditions you have, especially kidney, liver, or immune disease; if you have diabetes or heart or blood vessel disease; or if you've recently had a heart attack or stroke.

• Your doctor may prescribe a low-salt diet for you. If so, you need to limit canned soups, pickles, and other salty foods. Check with your doctor first because too little salt in your body can also cause problems.

Important reminder

If you're pregnant or think you may be, check with your doctor before taking this medication.

Vermox

Vermox is usually prescribed to treat worm infections, such as pinworm, roundworm, whipworm, and hookworm. This drug's generic name is mebendazole.

How to take Vermox

This medication is available in tablets and an oral suspension. Carefully check the prescription label. Take only the prescribed amount.

If you're taking the tablets, you may chew them, swallow them whole, or crush them and mix them with food.

If the doctor has prescribed high doses of this medication, take the doses with meals. Fatty foods, such as ice cream and whole milk, help the medication work better. However, if you're on a low-fat diet, check with your doctor before taking the drug with fatty foods.

What to do if you miss a dose
Take the missed dose as soon as possible. However, if it's almost time for your next scheduled dose and the doctor has prescribed two doses a day, space the missed dose and the next dose 4 to 5 hours apart. If the doctor has prescribed eight doses a day, space the missed dose and the next dose 1½ hours apart. Then resume your normal dosage schedule.

What to do about side effects
Contact your doctor *immediately* if you have a fever, itching, a rash, a sore throat, or unusual weakness or fatigue.

Special directions
• Wash your hands often and thoroughly to avoid spreading the infection. Be sure to wash your hands and clean your fingernails before meals and after bowel movements.

• Don't prepare food as long as your infection lasts.

• If your symptoms don't improve within a few days or if they get worse, notify your doctor.

• If you have anemia caused by whipworm or hookworm, the doctor may prescribe an iron supplement in addition to Vermox. Be sure to take the supplement every day and to take all prescribed doses of it. You may need to take the iron supplement for several months after you've finished Vermox treatment.

• To prevent reinfection, the doctor may want members of your household to take Vermox while you're being treated with it. To eliminate the infection completely, a second treatment 2 to 3 weeks after the first treatment may be required .

• If you're being treated for pinworm but the infection returns after Vermox treatment, wash all bedding and pajamas to help prevent a recurrence after a second treatment.

• See your doctor regularly to make sure the infection has gone away and to check for any side effects of this medication.

Important reminder
If you're pregnant, check with your doctor before taking this medication.

Vibramycin

Your doctor has prescribed this antibiotic medication to treat your bacterial infection. This drug's generic name is doxycycline. Another brand name is Vibra-Tabs.

How to take Vibramycin

Vibramycin comes in capsule, delayed-release capsule, oral suspension, and tablet forms. Take your dose with food, milk, or a full glass (8 ounces) of water to prevent irritation of your esophagus (food tube) or stomach.

If you're taking the *oral suspension,* use a specially marked spoon — not a household teaspoon — to measure each dose accurately.

Try to take your doses at evenly spaced times day and night.

Continue to take your medication, even if you start to feel better after a few days. Stopping too soon may allow your infection to return.

Store your medication away from heat and direct light. Don't keep it in the bathroom, near the kitchen sink, or in other damp places. Heat or moisture may cause the medication to break down. Keep the oral liquid forms of the medication from freezing.

What to do if you miss a dose

Take the missed dose as soon as possible. But if it's almost time for your next dose, adjust your dosage schedule as follows.

If you take one dose a day, space the missed dose and the next dose 10 to 12 hours apart.

If you take two doses a day, space the missed dose and the next dose 5 to 6 hours apart.

If you take three or more doses a day, space the missed dose and the next dose 2 to 4 hours apart. Then resume your regular dosage schedule.

What to do about side effects

Call your doctor *right away* if you develop any of the following symptoms of an allergic reaction to Vibramycin: severe headache, vision changes, difficulty breathing, wheezing, hives, or itching.

Also check with your doctor if you experience heartburn, nausea, diarrhea, rashes, or increased light sensitivity, especially if these symptoms persist or become severe.

Because this medication may make your skin more sensitive to sunlight, limit your exposure to the sun.

What you must know about alcohol and other drugs

Avoid drinking alcoholic beverages because it may prevent Vibramycin from working well. Other medications that may reduce the effectiveness of Vibramycin are antacids, iron preparations (such as iron-containing vitamins), and some seizure medications.

If you use birth control pills, Vibramycin may keep them from working effectively. Use another form of birth control.

Special directions

• Tell your doctor if you have other medical problems, especially kidney disease, or if you're allergic to a tetracycline antibiotic.

• If your medication has changed color, tastes or looks different, has become outdated, or has been stored incorrectly (in a place too warm or too damp), don't use it; it could cause serious side effects. Discard the bottle and obtain a fresh supply.

Important reminder

If you're pregnant or breast-feeding, don't take Vibramycin. It could stain your developing baby's teeth.

Voltaren

Your doctor has prescribed Voltaren to relieve joint pain, swelling, and stiffness caused by arthritis. This drug's generic name is diclofenac.

How to take Voltaren

Take this medication with milk, meals, or a full glass (8 ounces) of water. Also, avoid lying down for about 15 to 30 minutes after taking this medication. This helps prevent irritation of your esophagus. Swallow the tablets whole — don't chew or break them.

What to do if you miss a dose

Take the missed dose as soon as possible. However, if it's almost time for your next dose, skip the missed dose and take your next dose on schedule. Don't take a double dose.

What to do about side effects

Get emergency help *at once* if you have symptoms of an allergic reaction, such as wheezing, difficulty breathing, hives, itching, or a rash. Also call your doctor *right away* if you hear ringing or buzzing in your ears.

Be aware that Voltaren can cause serious bleeding from the digestive tract, including ulcers. Stop taking this medication and check with your doctor *at once* if you have any of these warning signs: severe abdominal or stomach pain; black, tarry stools; severe, continuing nausea or heartburn; or vomiting of blood or material that looks like coffee grounds.

Check with your doctor if you feel drowsy or have a headache, abdominal discomfort, or diarrhea.

Make sure you know how you react to Voltaren before you drive, use machines, or perform other activities that could be dangerous if you're not fully alert.

What you must know about alcohol and other drugs

Avoid alcoholic beverages while taking Voltaren because stomach problems are more likely to occur.

Tell your doctor about other medications you're taking. If you take blood thinners, taking Voltaren may increase your risk of bleeding. Also, don't take aspirin or Tylenol (acetaminophen) for more than a few days while taking Voltaren, unless your doctor tells you otherwise.

Voltaren may increase the toxicity of certain drugs, including Sandimmune (cyclosporine), an antibiotic; Lanoxin (digoxin), a heart medication; Eskalith (lithium), a drug for manic-depressive disorder; and Rheumatrex (methotrexate).

Voltaren may also interfere with the effects of water pills (diuretics).

If you have diabetes, your doctor may need to adjust your medications for this disease while you're taking Voltaren.

Special directions

• Tell your doctor if you have other medical problems, especially ulcers, porphyria, or liver or kidney disease.
• Also tell the doctor if you're allergic to aspirin or any other medications.

Important reminders   If you're pregnant or breast-feeding, don't take Voltaren without your doctor's consent.

    If you're an older adult, realize that you may be especially prone to side effects from Voltaren.

X Y

Xanax

This medication is used to relieve anxiety or tension caused by unusual stress. This drug's generic name is alprazolam.

How to take Xanax

This medication is available as a tablet. Follow the directions on your medication label exactly.

What to do if you miss a dose

If you're using this medication regularly and you miss a dose, take the missed dose right away if it's within 1 hour or so of the scheduled time. If more than 1 hour has passed, skip the missed dose and take the next dose at the regular time. Don't take a double dose.

What to do about side effects

If you think you may have taken an overdose, get emergency help *immediately*. Overdose signs include continuing slurred speech or confusion, severe drowsiness, and staggering.

Xanax may make you feel drowsy, dizzy, light-headed, clumsy, unsteady, or less alert than usual. Even if you take this medication at bedtime, you may feel drowsy or sluggish when you wake up. If these feelings persist or become severe, contact your doctor.

Make sure you know how this medication affects you before you drive or perform other activities requiring alertness.

What you must know about alcohol and other drugs

Avoid alcoholic beverages and other central nervous system depressants (including hay fever, allergy, or cold remedies), which may cause excessive drowsiness. When taken with Xanax, the ulcer drug Tagamet (cimetidine) may also increase drowsiness.

Tell your doctor about other medications you're taking. Their dosages may need to be adjusted because of combined effects with Xanax.

Special directions
- See your doctor regularly (at least every 4 months) to evaluate whether you need to continue this medication.
- Let your doctor know that you're taking Xanax because it may change certain medical test results.
- If you're having dental work that will require an anesthetic, tell your dentist that you're taking Xanax.
- Don't abruptly stop taking this medication without consulting your doctor. To prevent withdrawal effects, your doctor may reduce your dosage gradually.

Important reminders

If you're breast-feeding or pregnant, be sure to tell your doctor before taking this medication.

Children and older adults are more likely to experience side effects with Xanax.

If you're an athlete, you should know that alprazolam use is banned in most athletic events sponsored by the National Collegiate Athletic Association and the U.S. Olympic Committee.

Z

Zantac

This medication is prescribed to treat duodenal and gastric ulcers and to prevent their return. It's also used to treat some conditions in which the stomach makes too much acid. This drug's generic name is ranitidine.

How to take Zantac

Zantac comes in syrup and tablet forms. Follow your doctor's directions for taking this medication exactly. If you're taking one dose daily, take it at bedtime, unless otherwise directed. If you're taking two doses daily, take one in the morning and one at bedtime. If you're taking several doses a day, take them with meals and at bedtime for best results.

Take this medication for the full time of treatment, even after you start to feel better.

What to do if you miss a dose

Take the missed dose as soon as possible. However, if it's almost time for your next dose, skip the missed dose and take your next dose on schedule. Don't take a double dose.

What to do about side effects

Check with your doctor if this medication makes you feel dizzy, confused, nauseous, or constipated. Also let your doctor know if you get a rash or headache or if your heart starts to beat very slowly.

Make sure you know how you react to Zantac before you drive or perform other activities that might be dangerous if you're not fully alert.

What you must know about other drugs

Tell your doctor if you're taking other medications. Also check before you take new medications. If you're using antacids to relieve stomach pain, wait 30 minutes to 1 hour between taking the antacid and Zantac.

To prevent harmful drug interactions, your doctor also needs to know if you use blood thinners, muscle relaxants, or medications for diabetes or an irregular heartbeat.

Special directions
- Tell your doctor if you have other medical problems, especially kidney or liver disease. Other medical problems may affect the use of this medication.
- Before you have skin tests or tests to determine how much acid your stomach produces, tell the doctor you're taking Zantac. This medication may affect the test results.
- Don't smoke while taking Zantac because cigarette smoking reduces the drug's effectiveness.
- Stay away from foods and other substances that can irritate your stomach, such as aspirin, citrus products, and carbonated drinks.

Important reminders
If you're pregnant, check with your doctor before using Zantac. If you're breast-feeding, don't use this medication unless instructed to do so by your doctor.

Older adults may be especially prone to Zantac's side effects, particularly confusion and dizziness.

Zaroxolyn

This medication is usually prescribed to treat high blood pressure. It may also be used to treat heart failure or kidney disease. This drug's generic name is metolazone.

How to take Zaroxolyn
This medication is available in tablets. Carefully check the prescription label. Take only the prescribed amount.

What to do if you miss a dose
Take the missed dose right away. However, if it's almost time for your next regular dose, skip the missed dose and resume your regular dosage schedule. Don't take a double dose.

What to do about side effects
Call your doctor *right away* if you have fever; chills; lower back, side, or joint pain; severe stomach pain; a rash; hives; red spots on the skin; unusual bleeding or bruising; yellow skin or eyes; bloody urine or stools; or black, tarry stools.

Also call your doctor if you experience increased thirst, irregular heartbeat, muscle pain or cramps, nausea or vomiting, unusual fatigue or weakness, or mood or mental changes.

You may notice appetite loss, diarrhea, decreased sexual performance, stomach upset, and increased sensitivity to sunlight. Also, you may feel dizzy or light-headed when getting up from a sitting or lying position. Check with your doctor if these side effects persist or become bothersome.

What you must know about other drugs

Check with your doctor or pharmacist before taking another drug, especially nonprescription medications for colds, cough, hay fever, asthma, or appetite control.

Questran (cholestyramine) and Colestid (colestipol), medications used to lower cholesterol levels, may prevent Zaroxolyn from working properly. Zaroxolyn may increase the chance for side effects from digitalis glycosides (heart medications) when used with them. Nonsteroidal anti-inflammatory drugs — such as Advil (ibuprofen), Indocin (indomethacin), and Anaprox (naproxen) — may decrease the effects of Zaroxolyn.

Special directions

• Tell your doctor about other medical problems you have, especially diabetes, gout, lupus, inflammation of the pancreas, or heart, blood vessel, liver, or kidney disease.

• Follow any special diet the doctor has prescribed, such as a low-salt, high-potassium diet.

• Keep taking this medication exactly as directed, even if you feel well.

Important reminders

If you're breast-feeding or you become pregnant while taking this medication, check with your doctor.

If you're an older adult, you may be especially likely to feel dizzy and light-headed and to lose too much potassium when taking this medication.

If you have diabetes, this medication may increase your blood sugar level. Be sure to test your blood or urine for glucose regularly.

If you're an athlete, you should know that the U.S. Olympic Committee and the National Collegiate Athletic Association ban the use of metolazone.

Zovirax

This medication treats infections caused by the herpes virus, such as genital herpes and shingles. It's also given for chickenpox. Although this medication won't cure you, it will make you feel more comfortable and shorten your illness. This drug's generic name is acyclovir.

How to take Zovirax Zovirax is available in capsule, tablet, liquid, and ointment forms. Follow the directions on your medication exactly.

Take Zovirax until your prescription is finished, even if your symptoms subside and you begin to feel better. Try not to miss any doses, but don't take the drug more often or longer than directed.

Take the *capsule, tablet,* or *liquid* form of Zovirax with meals to minimize possible stomach upset. If you're taking *liquid* Zovirax, measure each dose accurately by using a measuring spoon. Don't use a household teaspoon.

If you're using Zovirax *ointment,* wear a disposable glove to apply the medication. Doing this helps prevent spreading the infection to other body areas. Apply enough ointment to cover each herpes blister. A 1-inch (2.5-centimeter) strip of ointment will cover about 2 square inches.

What to do if you miss a dose Take the missed dose as soon as you remember. But if it's almost time for your next dose, skip the missed one and take the next one at your regularly scheduled time. Don't take two doses together.

What to do about side effects Zovirax may cause nausea and vomiting. If these symptoms persist or become worse, contact your doctor.

What you must know about other drugs Be sure to tell the doctor what other medications you're taking especially Probalan (probenecid), which may make Zovirax's effects stronger. Also tell the doctor if you're taking Retrovir (zidovudine) because this combination may cause drowsiness.

Special directions • Avoid sexual activity if either you or your partner has herpes symptoms. Zovirax will not prevent the spread of herpes between partners. Using a latex condom may help prevent the spread of herpes, but using a spermicidal jelly or a diaphragm probably won't.

• Keep the areas affected by herpes clean and dry. Also, wear loose-fitting clothing to avoid irritating the sores.

• Never apply the ointment form of Zovirax to your eyes.

Important reminder If you're a woman and have genital herpes, be sure to have a Pap test at least once a year.

Zyloprim

This medication is prescribed to treat chronic gout (gouty arthritis). The drug's generic name is allopurinol.

How to take Zyloprim This medication is available as a tablet. Follow the directions on your medication label exactly. To work effectively, Zyloprim must be taken regularly as directed by your doctor.

Take Zyloprim after a meal if you find that it upsets your stomach. Drink 10 to 12 glasses (8 ounces each) of liquid each day unless your doctor directs otherwise. And continue to take Zyloprim, even if you take another medication for gout attacks.

What to do if you miss a dose Take the missed dose as soon as you remember. But if it's almost time for your next dose, skip the missed dose and take the next dose at the regular time. Don't take a double dose.

What to do about side effects Contact your doctor *immediately* if you have a rash, skin ulcers, hives, itching, blood in your urine, trouble breathing, chest tightness, or unusual bruising, bleeding, or weakness.

Common side effects include drowsiness, diarrhea, nausea, and vomiting. If any of these symptoms persist or become worse, call your doctor.

Until you know how Zyloprim affects you, avoid driving and other activities that require alertness.

What you must know about alcohol and other drugs

Avoid alcoholic beverages or limit the amount you drink. Too much alcohol may increase the uric acid in your blood and decrease the benefit of Zyloprim.

Inform your doctor about other medications that you're taking. Combining oral anticoagulants (blood thinners) and Zyloprim may increase your risk for abnormal bleeding. Taken with Zyloprim, drugs such as Imuran (azathioprine) or Purinethol (mercaptopurine) may increase the chance of serious side effects.

Also consult your doctor before taking nonprescription preparations. Taking too much vitamin C, for instance, may increase your risk for kidney stones.

Special directions

• Tell the doctor about any other medical problems you may have, particularly diabetes, high blood pressure, or kidney disease, because your dosage of Zyloprim may need to be adjusted.

• Have regular checkups so your doctor can monitor your progress and the effects of Zyloprim.

Index